The

Good Housekeeping

Illustrated Book of

Pregnancy
&Baby Care

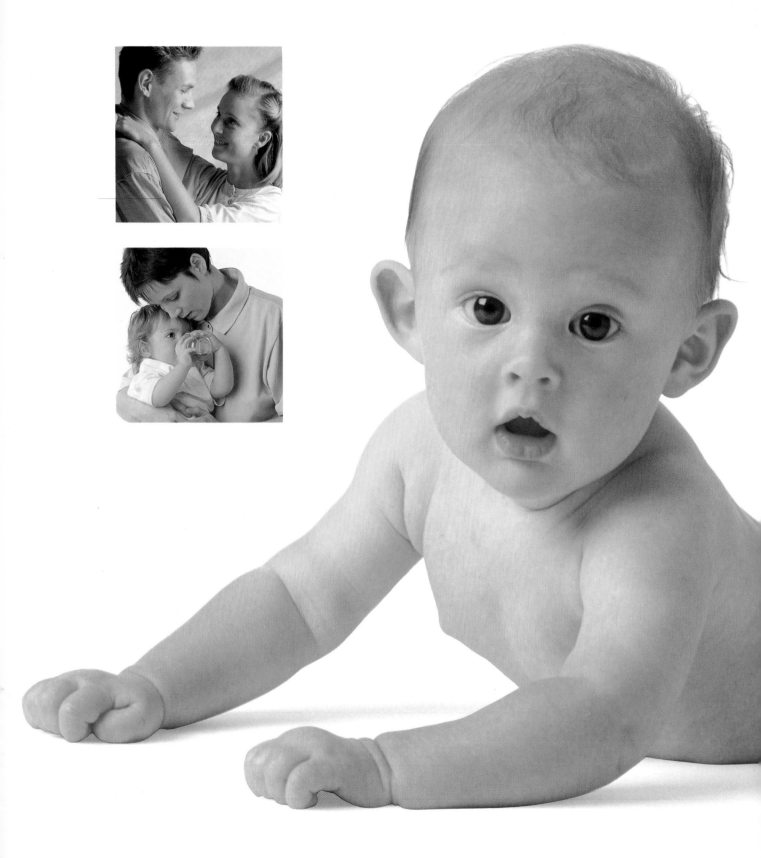

The 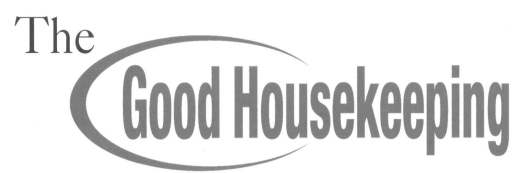 Good Housekeeping
Illustrated Book of
Pregnancy
& Baby Care

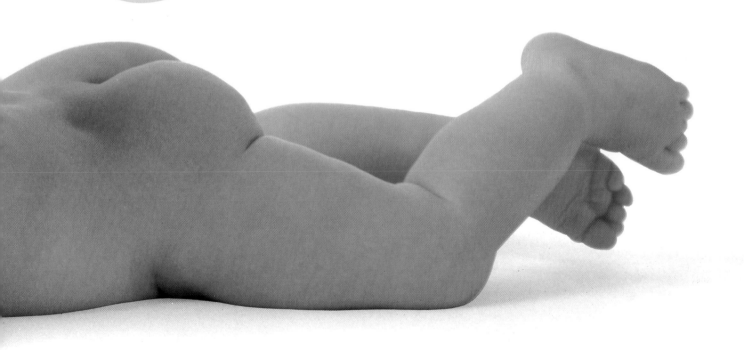

Hearst Books
A Division of Sterling Publishing Co., Inc.
New York

For Good Housekeeping
Editor in Chief: Ellen Levine

Medical Editors:
Mert Ozan Bahtiyar, M.D.
Clinic Instructor, Division of Maternal and Fetal Medicine,
Dept. of Obstetrics and Gynecology
Yale University School of Medicine

Svena D. Julien, M.D.
Clinic Instructor, Division of Maternal and Fetal Medicine,
Dept. of Obstetrics and Gynecology
Yale University School of Medicine

Marlene R. Miller, M.D., M.Sc.
Director of Quality and Safety Initiatives,
Johns Hopkins Children's Center

Medical Writer/Project Editor:
Joseph Gonzalez

Produced by Dorling Kindersley

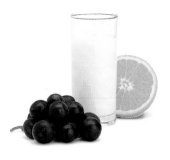

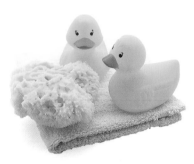

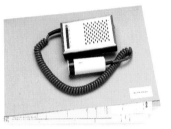

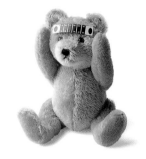

Publisher's note
Throughout this book, the pronouns "he" and
"she" refer to both sexes, except where a topic
applies specifically to a boy or a girl.

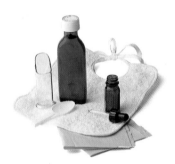

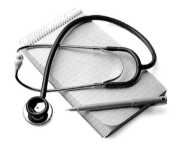

The Library of Congress has cataloged the
second hardcover edition as follows:
The Good Housekeeping illustrated book of
pregnancy and baby care.
p. cm.
"Completely revised and updated."
Includes index.
ISBN 0-688-16558-3
1. Pregnancy. 2. Childbirth. 3. Infants—Care. 4. Child care.
I. Good housekeeping (New York, NY)
RG525.G53 1999
618.2'4—dc21   98-23749
                                                      CIP

Third Edition
10 9 8 7 6 5 4

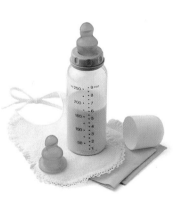

First Paperback Edition 2004
Published by Hearst Books
A Division of Sterling Publishing Co., Inc.
387 Park Avenue South, New York, NY 10016

Good Housekeeping and Hearst Books are trademarks owned
by Hearst Communications, Inc.

www.goodhousekeeping.com

Distributed in Canada by Sterling Publishing
c/o Canadian Manda Group, 165 Dufferin Street
Toronto, Ontario, Canada M6K 3H6

Distributed in Australia by Capricorn Link (Australia) Pty. Ltd.
P.O. Box 704, Windsor, NSW 2756 Australia

Printed in China

Sterling ISBN-13: 978-1-58816-376-9
ISBN-10: 1-58816-376-8

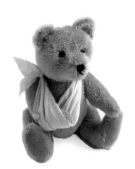

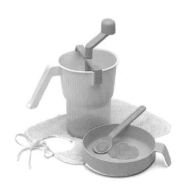

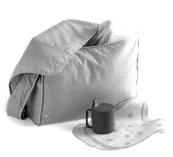

FOREWORD

We hope this book will show you in a very practical way how to care for your child. Having a baby opens up a whole new and exciting world—but it can be a terribly unfamiliar one, too. Most of us know very little about pregnancy and baby care at first, and we quickly find that there's seldom a "right" or a "wrong" way of doing things. But there's often an easy way. So what we have tried to do is show you what other mothers have found worked best, and what makes life easiest.

Every pregnancy is special. Even though it's an experience that has happened countless times, to countless couples, it will still be momentous for you. This book guides you through your pregnancy stage by stage, showing you how to make it a happy, healthy time for yourself and how to give your baby the best possible start in life.

Every baby is special too, a personality in his or her own right from the moment of birth. By showing you all the basics of baby care, by offering practical solutions to common problems and plenty of reassuring advice, this book will help you care for your baby, and find out all there is to know about his or her own particular character.

We hope you will quickly discover that parenthood, for all its responsibilities, can be fun. You don't have to aim to be the "perfect parents"; if you and your baby can learn to love each other and get along together, then you can be assured that you are the perfect parents for your child.

CONTENTS

1 PREGNANCY
AND BIRTH
8-73

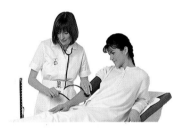

2 BABY CARE
74-171

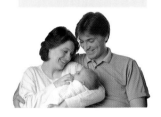

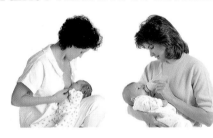

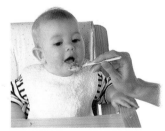

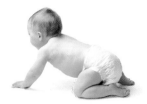
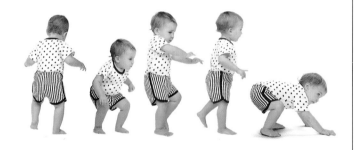

3
HEALTH CARE
172-245

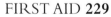
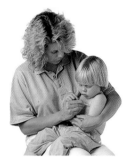

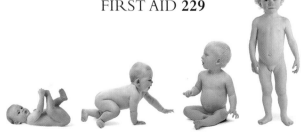

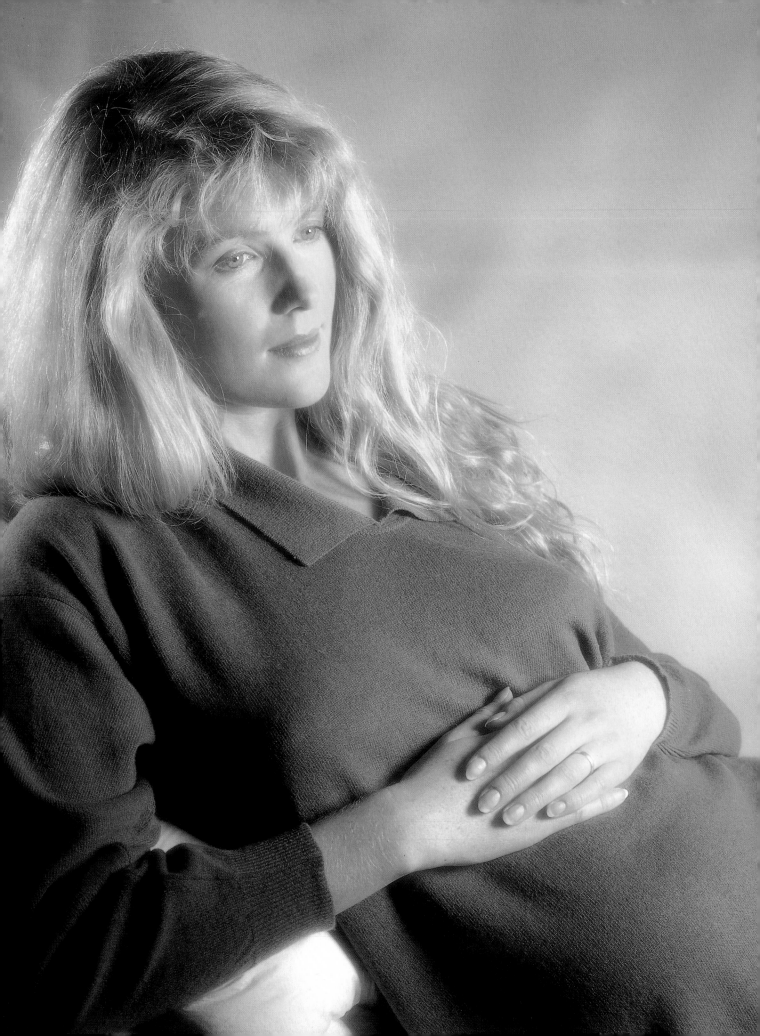

1

PREGNANCY
AND
BIRTH

∎ ∎ ∎ ∎ ∎ ∎

*An illustrated guide to a healthy and happy
pregnancy, incorporating practical
self-help advice for labor and birth.*

THINKING ABOUT PREGNANCY

To give any pregnancy the best possible start, try to plan ahead. There are a number of steps you can take to help ensure a normal healthy baby. Many obstetricians prescribe vitamins and folic acid if you are trying to conceive. Ideally, you and your partner should talk about pregnancy at least three months before you conceive. It is in the first few weeks, when you may not even know you are pregnant, that a baby's development

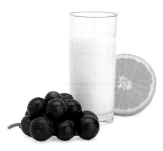

can be most easily affected. So keeping fit and eating healthy will ensure that you have done your best to nourish and protect a baby in your womb. Check whether there are hazards at work that could affect the fetus's health, and whether you had or were vaccinated against rubella as a child. Planning for pregnancy gives you time to consider any risks and, if necessary, to do something to reduce them.

CHECKLIST FOR PREGNANCY

USE THESE QUESTIONS as a checklist if you want to have a baby or have just discovered that you are pregnant. A few may not apply to you, but it is important to ask yourself all of them. Talk to your partner too, because some of the questions relate directly to him. If any frighten you, see your doctor.

Are you immune to rubella?
Rubella, or German measles, can cause serious defects in the baby if you develop it in pregnancy, especially early pregnancy, when the baby's internal organs are forming. So before you become pregnant, ask your doctor for a blood test to make sure that you are immune to the disease. If you are not, your doctor can vaccinate you. Arrange for the test right away because you shouldn't try to become pregnant for at least three months after a vaccination.

Do you or your partner have a family history of inherited disease?
Some medical conditions, such as hemophilia and cystic fibrosis, are inherited. If either you or your partner has a close relative with an inherited disease, there is a chance that it might be passed on to your baby. See your doctor before trying to become pregnant, and if recommended, see a genetic counselor, who can assess the level of risk that you will be taking. In most cases it takes both partners carrying the gene to cause substantial risk of passing the disease to a child.

Do you have a long-standing medical condition?
If you have a medical disorder, such as diabetes or epilepsy, you should talk to your doctor before trying to become pregnant. Your doctor may want to change your drug treatment, either because the drugs you are taking might affect the baby or because they might make it more difficult for you to conceive.

QUESTION & ANSWER

"How important is folic acid in pregnancy?"
Folic acid is a vitamin that has been shown to be *very* important in the formation of the fetus's spine and spinal cord. This formation takes place in the first four weeks of pregnancy, so it is strongly recommended that all women of childbearing potential ensure adequate folic acid in their diets. It is very important to do this before becoming pregnant and to continue until you have completed the first three months of pregnancy. The standard dose is 0.4mg each day.

If you're on the pill, when should you stop taking it?
It is best to stop taking the pill several months before you plan to conceive, to allow your body to return to its normal cycle. Wait until you have had three menstrual periods before trying to become pregnant. (Find alternative means of birth control, such as a condom or diaphragm, during this time.)

Does your work bring you into contact with any risks?
If you or your partner has a job that involves working with chemicals, lead, anesthesia, or X rays, this may affect your chances of conceiving, or involve a risk to the baby, so talk to your doctor. If possible, consider changing to a safer job, or at least avoid the risk as much as possible. Your doctor may also advise you to change jobs if yours involves heavy lifting. Standing for long periods of time in occupations such as bank teller, hairdresser, or supermarket cashier is not the best thing for a pregnancy. If you work at a daycare center, you may want to reconsider your position, since certain viruses that are known to harm the fetus are common in such centers.

How much do you weigh?

Ideally, your weight should be normal for your height for at least six months before conceiving, so if you are seriously over- or under-weight, see your doctor for advice on attaining the right weight. Obese women have an increased risk of having a child with a spinal defect—regardless of their folic acid intake. They are also at higher risk for pregnancy-induced hypertension and gestational diabetes.

Are you eating a balanced diet?

You will increase your chances of having a healthy baby if you eat a properly balanced diet, with plenty of fresh foods.

Do you smoke or drink?

Both you and your partner should stop smoking and drinking alcohol as soon as you decide to become pregnant. Smoking and drinking can harm the growing baby (see page 13).

Are you exercising regularly?

To keep fit, aim for at least 20 minutes of exercise each day. Walking and swimming are great before and during pregnancy.

Do you have insurance?

You should contact your insurance carrier or health maintenance organization (HMO) and obtain a list of participating hospitals, physicians, and prenatal services.

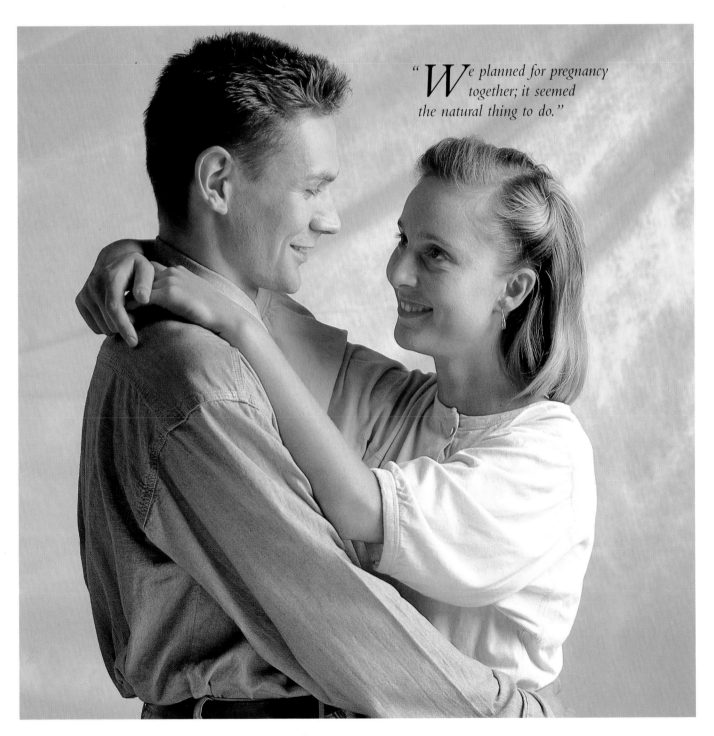

"We planned for pregnancy together; it seemed the natural thing to do."

A PREGNANCY CALENDAR

This month-by-month calendar charts the progress of one pregnancy. If you are pregnant, it will show the changes in your body and emotions as it follows the baby's development from conception to the last days in the womb. There is advice on what to do at each stage, as well as reassuring answers to questions and worries you might have. The text for each month explains at least one additional relevant aspect of pregnancy, such as options for prenatal classes or measuring yourself for a nursing bra. Every pregnancy varies, so don't be surprised if some of the changes don't happen to you exactly as they are described here. Your weight gain, for example, may differ from the one shown. The calendar counts day one of pregnancy as the first day of your last menstrual period, so two weeks after conception (according to the calendar), you are four weeks pregnant.

BECOMING PREGNANT

IF YOU ARE THINKING of becoming pregnant, make sure your lifestyle involves nothing that might harm the baby. All the major organs of his body are formed during the first three months, and it is then that his development can be harmed most easily. Once you have conceived, you will probably know or suspect that you are pregnant because of a number of different signs, such as heavy breasts or a feeling of nausea. Most of these changes are set off by the increase in certain hormone levels during the early weeks. The discomforts often lessen or even disappear completely around week 12.

EARLY SIGNS OF PREGNANCY

One or more of these changes can indicate that you are pregnant. You may not notice any of them at first, but still instinctively know you are pregnant because you "feel" different.

■ A missed period—but if your periods are normally irregular, or you are anxious, busy, or ill, this may not be a reliable guide. However, a missed period should be considered a sign of pregnancy unless proved otherwise. After you have become pregnant, it is possible to have slight bleeding around the time you would normally expect your period.

■ Enlarged, tender breasts, which may tingle a little.

■ A strange metallic taste in your mouth.

■ Tiredness, not just in the evening, but during the day.

■ Feeling faint, and perhaps dizzy.

■ An increase in normal vaginal discharge.

■ Nausea and perhaps vomiting; this may happen at any time of day.

■ A strong dislike of some things, such as alcohol, coffee, and cigarette smoke, and a craving for others.

■ Feeling unusually emotional.

■ A frequent need to urinate.

CONFIRMING THE PREGNANCY

Have the pregnancy confirmed as soon as possible. Your doctor or a family planning clinic can test a urine sample. About two weeks after conception, a hormone will appear in your urine, and this confirms the pregnancy.

Alternatively, buy a home pregnancy testing kit from a drugstore and do the test yourself. All kits contain a chemical solution that you mix with a few drops of urine. Various indicators, such as a color change, will suggest whether or not you are pregnant. These tests are fairly accurate if you follow the instructions carefully. However, be sure to see your doctor to confirm the pregnancy and to be sure it is in the uterus, not in the fallopian tube (an ectopic pregnancy). The doctor will probably give you a blood test, the most accurate indicator of pregnancy, and will examine you internally.

CALCULATING YOUR DELIVERY DATE

Pregnancy lasts about 266 days from conception to birth. The most likely time of conception is when you ovulate. In a normal 28-day cycle, this happens about 14 days before the next period is due, so to calculate your approximate delivery date, count 280 days (266 plus 14) from the first day of your last period. Remember, this is only a guide. A normal pregnancy can be anywhere from 38 to 42 weeks long. Therefore, you should calculate a "due month," rather than a "due day."

WHAT TO AVOID

Throughout pregnancy, avoid smoking, alcohol, and any form of medication, including over-the-counter medications such as aspirin or cough medicine, unless confirmed as safe by your doctor. This is especially important during the first three months, when the baby's organs are forming.

Smoking

Smoking deprives the baby of oxygen. Babies of mothers who smoke are more likely to be premature and have a low birthweight. Smoking also increases the chances of having a miscarriage, a stillbirth, a baby with restricted growth, or a baby who dies directly after birth. The more you smoke, the greater the risk. If you really can't give it up entirely, switch to a low-tar brand, ration the number of cigarettes you smoke, don't inhale, and stub out your cigarette when you've smoked half of it. Doctors now believe that the smoke you breathe in from other people's cigarettes (secondary smoke) is as harmful to your unborn child as if you smoked yourself. It could be a factor in crib death (Sudden Infant Death Syndrome, or SIDS).

Alcohol

Drinking during pregnancy can seriously affect the developing baby. No one knows what a "safe" level of drinking is, so it's best not to drink alcohol at all while pregnant. This includes beer, wine, and cough medicines that contain alcohol.

Medication

Many drugs can have harmful or unknown effects on the baby, so avoid taking any medication during pregnancy, unless it is prescribed by a doctor who knows you are pregnant. If you need medication to control a condition such as diabetes, your doctor may have to alter your dose.

Other risks

The feces of cats and some other mammals as well as raw meat and unpasturized goat milk may contain a parasite called toxoplasma, which can seriously harm the unborn baby. Avoid emptying cat-litter boxes. If you really have to, wear gloves and wash your hands well afterward. Wear gloves for gardening. Wash your hands well after handling raw meat.

THE START OF LIFE

DURING THE FIRST EIGHT WEEKS of pregnancy, the baby develops from a single cell at conception to a fetus that is starting to look like a human.

CONCEPTION TO WEEK FOUR

1 Ovulation

Around day 14 of your menstrual cycle, a ripe egg is released from one of your ovaries, and fertilization becomes possible. The egg is caught by the fingerlike ends of the fallopian tube and drawn into it. The egg can survive for up to 24 hours. If it isn't fertilized, it passes out of the vagina with the lining of the womb in your next monthly period.

The swim of the sperm

During orgasm, a man may ejaculate between 200 and 400 million sperm into a woman's vagina. Many spill out again, or are lost along the way, but some swim through the mucus secreted by the cervix (the neck of the womb), which becomes thin and soft around ovulation, and cross the womb into the fallopian tube. If an egg hasn't been released, the sperm can survive in the tube for up to 48 hours.

5 Implantation

The fertilized egg begins to implant itself in the soft, thick lining of the womb at about the end of week three of your cycle. Light bleeding may occur during implantation. When the egg is securely attached to the lining of the womb, conception is complete.

Sponge-like fingers from the embryo's outer cells burrow into the lining to link up with the mother's blood vessels. These later form the placenta. Some of the outer cells also develop into the umbilical cord and the membranes that protect the developing baby. Inner cells divide into three layers, which develop into different parts of the baby's body.

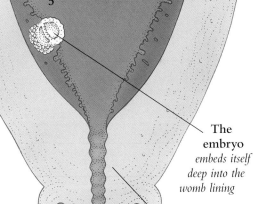

Position of the womb

Womb

Fallopian tube

The corpus luteum
produces hormones that prepare your body for pregnancy

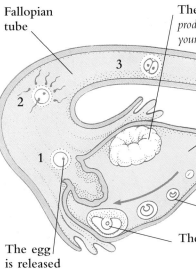

Ovary

3

2

1

The growing egg

The egg reaching maturity

The egg is released

4

5

2 Fertilization

Sperm carry a substance that can dissolve the outer covering of the egg, so that one of them can penetrate it. As soon as the successful sperm enters the egg, no other sperm can get through. The sperm loses its tail and its head and begins to swell. It fuses with the egg, forming a single cell.

3 The cell divides

Almost at once, the cell starts to divide. It continues to divide into more and more cells as it travels down the fallopian tube.

4 Reaching the womb

On about the fourth day after fertilization, the egg reaches the cavity of the womb. It has developed into a ball of about 100 cells with a hollow, fluid-filled center, but it is still too small to be seen by the naked eye. For the next few days, it floats around in the womb cavity.

The embryo
embeds itself deep into the womb lining

The cervix
becomes thin and soft around ovulation, so that sperm can pass through it more easily

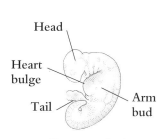

Head
Heart bulge
Tail
Arm bud

About week six

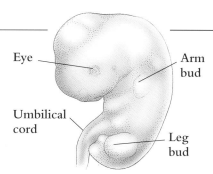

Eye
Arm bud
Umbilical cord
Leg bud

About week seven

Brain
Ear
Eye
Mouth
Hand
Arm
Elbow
Umbilical cord
Leg

About week eight

WEEKS FIVE TO SIX

■ The embryo is floating in a fluid-filled sac.
■ It has a simple brain, spine, and central nervous system.
■ Four shallow pits have appeared on the head; these will later become the baby's eyes and ears.
■ The embryo has the beginnings of a digestive system, a mouth, and a jaw.
■ The stomach and chest are developing. The heart can be seen as a large bulge at the front of the chest; by the end of the week it will start beating.
■ A system of blood vessels is forming.
■ Four tiny limb buds have developed.

Length: The embryo is now $\frac{1}{4}$ in (6mm), about the size of an apple seed.

WEEK SEVEN

■ The head looks large and is bent onto the chest. A face is forming, though the eyes are on the sides of the head and still sealed. Black pigment can be seen under the skin overlying the eyes.
■ The arms and legs are clearly visible, with clefts at the end, which will become fingers and toes.
■ The heart starts to circulate blood around the embryo's body.
■ The outline of the baby's nervous system is already nearly complete.
■ Bone cells are beginning to develop.
■ The embryo has lungs, an intestine, a liver, kidneys, and internal sex organs, but all are not yet fully formed.

Length: The embryo is now $\frac{1}{2}$ in (1.3cm), about the size of a small grape.

WEEK EIGHT

■ The embryo can now be called a fetus, which means "young one."
■ All the major internal organs have developed, although they are still in a simple form and may not be in their final position.
■ A face is recognizable: the nose seems to have a tip, the nostrils have formed, and the two sides of the jaw have joined to make a mouth. A tongue has already formed.
■ The inner parts of the ears, responsible for balance and hearing, are forming.
■ The fingers and toes are becoming more distinct, though they are joined by webs of skin.
■ The arms and legs have grown longer, and shoulders, elbows, hips, and knees are detectable.
■ The baby moves around a lot, although you can't feel him yet.

Length: The fetus is now 1in (2.5cm), about the size of a strawberry.

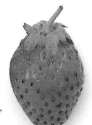

TWINS

About one in 80 pregnancies results in twins. If twins run in your family, your chances of having them are greater.
Fraternal twins occur when two separate eggs are fertilized by two separate sperm. They are three times as common as identical twins. Fraternal twins each have their own placenta, may or may not be the same sex, and are no more alike than any other brothers or sisters.
Identical twins are produced when the egg that is fertilized divides into two separate halves, each of which develops into an identical baby. The twins share a placenta, are always of the same sex, and have the same physical characteristics and genetic makeup.

QUESTION & ANSWER

"Can I do anything to influence the baby's sex?"
The baby's sex is determined by the man's sperm. Research suggests that male sperm swim faster but don't survive as long as female sperm, so your chances of having a boy may be *slightly* increased if you make love when you are most fertile (about 14 days before your period is due); and your chances of having a girl may be *slightly* greater if you have intercourse up to three days before you next expect to be fertile.

WEEK 12

THE BABY LOOKS much more human, although his head is still large in proportion to his body, and his limbs, although fully formed, are small. The discomforts of early pregnancy may begin to wear off. Make sure you have scheduled an appointment with an obstetrician or midwife by now.

Position of the womb

SEE ALSO:
Prenatal checkups
pages 34–36
Extra tests
page 37
Prenatal exercises
pages 45–47
Healthy eating
pages 50–53
Frequent urination
page 41
Morning sickness
pages 41
Pregnancy bra
page 23
Protecting your back
page 44

Your breasts *will feel heavier and may be tender*

Your shape *is probably still much the same as usual*

The top *of the womb can be felt just above your pubic bone*

■ CHANGES IN YOU ■

■ If you've been feeling nauseated because of morning sickness, this should start to ease.
■ You will probably feel that you don't need to urinate as often as you did in the early weeks of pregnancy.
■ You may still be emotional and easily upset by little things, because of hormone changes.
■ Constipation may be a problem, because bowel movements tend to slow down in pregnancy.
■ The volume of blood circulating in your body is increasing, so your lungs, kidneys, and heart have to work harder.

YOUR WEIGHT GAIN
The first three months
If vomiting has not been a problem for you, you may have gained 2lb (1kg), about 10% of total pregnancy weight gain. Model's total weight gain at week 12: 4½lb (2kg)   **10%**

YOUR BABY
Length 1–3in (2½–7½ cm)
Weight ⅝oz (18g)

The external ears *will be developed*

Tiny fingers *and toes have formed*

WHAT TO DO

- Buy a bra that will support your breasts well.
- Make sure you are eating a varied diet of fresh foods.
- Continue taking your prenatal vitamins.
- Guard against constipation by drinking plenty of water and eating high-fiber foods.
- Make an appointment with your dentist for a checkup.
- Tell your employer that you are pregnant so that you can adjust your work schedule.
- Find an obstetrician or midwife and arrange for your first checkup.
- Practice prenatal exercises. Go swimming or walking.
- Enroll in prenatal exercise classes.
- Find out about other prenatal classes in your area, such as prenatal yoga classes.

YOUR GROWING BABY

- All of the internal organs are formed and most are working.
- The eyelids have developed and are closed over the eyes.
- The baby has earlobes and limbs with fingers and toes.
- Miniature fingernails and toenails are growing.
- Muscles are developing, so the baby moves around much more. He can curl and fan his toes. He can make a fist.
- He can move the muscles of his mouth to open and close it, to frown, and to purse his lips.
- He can suck, and he swallows the fluid that surrounds him. He can urinate.
- The heartbeat can be heard using a special listening device (fetal Doppler).

PRENATAL CLASSES

START THINKING about the type of class that will best suit you and your partner. You might find an introductory class now—on ways to stay healthy in pregnancy, for example—but prepared childbirth classes usually start ten or more weeks before the baby is due. Prenatal exercise classes may continue throughout your pregnancy.

CHOOSING A CLASS

Prepared childbirth classes are run by hospitals and individual instructors, as well as by various organizations and local groups such as the YWCA. To find one, start by checking the professional section of a newspaper geared for your neighborhood, or any community bulletin boards you see regularly. Ask your doctor, midwife, or friends for recommendations. Make sure that you reserve a spot early in your second trimester, even if classes won't begin until you are 28 to 32 weeks pregnant. Most feature a weekly two-hour session, scheduled over a six- to eight-week period. To find the one that suits your feelings about pregnancy, labor, and delivery best, you might want to observe a session before you sign up.

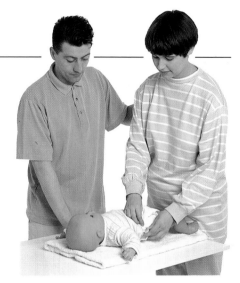

Basics of babycare
It's fun and helpful to learn how to take care of your baby in a class.

What will you learn?

Though the course content may vary, all childbirth classes teach couples basic information about pregnancy, labor and delivery, stress relaxation techniques, physical exercises, medication and anesthesia, and everything you might need to know about different hospital procedures and policies. In fact, a tour of the hospital is often part of the curriculum. Childbirth classes can be invaluable for first-time mothers and fathers, and even in a second or third pregnancy, the review is almost always worthwhile. Most emphasize the close working relationship the woman will want to have with the person she chooses to have by her side during the birth, her labor partner. Some classes cover the postnatal period and will include tips on caring for a newborn, breast-feeding, postpartum depression, and exercises for getting back into shape. If the class does not include information on infant cardiopulmonary resuscitation (CPR), you may want to take such a course separately.

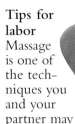

Tips for labor
Massage is one of the techniques you and your partner may be taught to help you cope with labor.

WEEK 16

NOW INTO THE second three months of pregnancy, you should be feeling healthier and more energetic than in your first trimester. You will begin to look pregnant, and you will need looser clothes. Your baby is fully formed and has been nourished by the placenta since week 12. Over the remaining weeks, he will grow and mature so that he is capable of an independent life at birth.

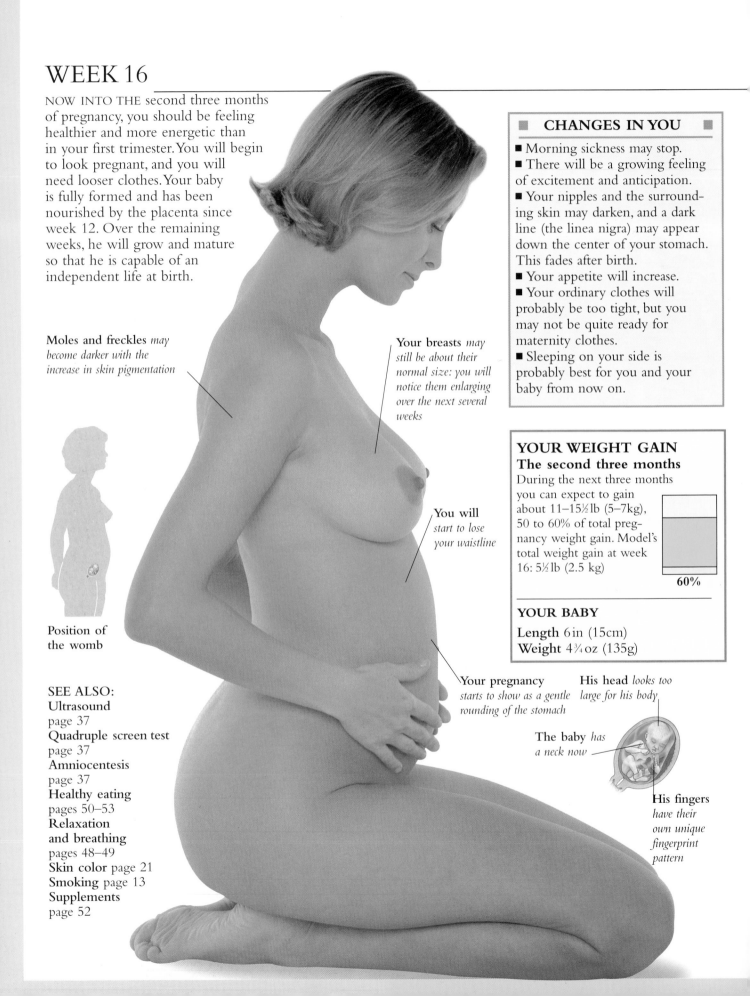

Moles and freckles *may become darker with the increase in skin pigmentation*

Position of the womb

SEE ALSO:
Ultrasound
page 37
Quadruple screen test
page 37
Amniocentesis
page 37
Healthy eating
pages 50–53
Relaxation and breathing
pages 48–49
Skin color page 21
Smoking page 13
Supplements
page 52

Your breasts *may still be about their normal size: you will notice them enlarging over the next several weeks*

You will *start to lose your waistline*

Your pregnancy *starts to show as a gentle rounding of the stomach*

■ CHANGES IN YOU ■

■ Morning sickness may stop.
■ There will be a growing feeling of excitement and anticipation.
■ Your nipples and the surrounding skin may darken, and a dark line (the linea nigra) may appear down the center of your stomach. This fades after birth.
■ Your appetite will increase.
■ Your ordinary clothes will probably be too tight, but you may not be quite ready for maternity clothes.
■ Sleeping on your side is probably best for you and your baby from now on.

YOUR WEIGHT GAIN
The second three months
During the next three months you can expect to gain about 11–15½ lb (5–7kg), 50 to 60% of total pregnancy weight gain. Model's total weight gain at week 16: 5½ lb (2.5 kg)

60%

YOUR BABY

Length 6 in (15cm)
Weight 4¾ oz (135g)

His head *looks too large for his body*

The baby *has a neck now*

His fingers *have their own unique fingerprint pattern*

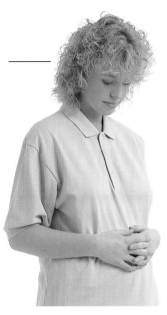

WHAT TO DO

■ Give up smoking if you have not already done so. Encourage your partner to do the same.
■ Don't use any increase in your appetite as an excuse to eat the wrong kinds of foods; eat nutritiously and watch weight gain.
■ Continue your prenatal vitamins.
■ Obstetrical visits are scheduled once a month now. An ultrasound scan and a triple screen blood test may be done if your doctor needs to pinpoint your due date or clear up any worries. Amniocentesis is also done now if there is any chance of the baby having genetic problems.

YOUR GROWING BABY

■ The eyebrows and eyelashes are growing, and the baby has fine downy hair on his face and body (known as lanugo).
■ His skin is so thin that it is transparent; networks of blood vessels can be seen underneath.
■ Joints have formed in his arms and legs, and hard bones are beginning to develop.
■ His sex organs are sufficiently mature for his sex to be evident, but this is not always detectable by an ultrasound scan.
■ The baby makes breathing movements with his chest.
■ He can suck his thumb.
■ He moves around vigorously, but you probably won't be able to feel him yet.
■ His heart is beating about twice as fast as your own; the doctor or midwife will continue to monitor it with a special listening device.
■ The baby grows rapidly during this month.

MIXED FEELINGS

YOU AND YOUR PARTNER are bound to have mixed emotions about the pregnancy, so don't be surprised if, as well as feeling elated and excited, you sometimes feel anxious or sad. Try to tolerate and understand any negative feelings; they are normal emotions.

COMMON WORRIES

The best way to dispel any worries that you may have about the baby or parenthood is to talk about them frankly with each other. It also helps to find out as much as you can about pregnancy, so you understand the changes taking place.

You

It's only natural for your feelings of excitement and anticipation to be clouded sometimes by negative thoughts. You may worry about loving the baby, but once he's born and you get to know each other, love will grow. You may also feel depressed about your changing shape, and even resent the baby for putting your body through such strains. But most major bodily changes disappear after birth, and with some gentle exercising, your shape will return.

Your partner

The baby may become a reality for the first time when you see him on the ultrasound screen. Up to now you may have felt left out, and perhaps jealous of all the attention your mate and the baby have been receiving. If you're worried about money and having enough to support your new family, try to plan ahead and budget.

Both of you

It's normal to feel excited about the new baby, yet to worry that you're not yet ready for parenthood. If you're anxious about labor and birth, learn all about them, and practice techniques, such as deep breathing, so you can feel more confident and in control when the time comes.

QUESTION & ANSWER

"How can I be sure the baby will be all right?"
The chances of the baby being abnormal are very small. Most developmental abnormalities occur in the first weeks and end in an early miscarriage. By week 13, the baby is fully formed. Make sure that your lifestyle involves nothing that could harm him.

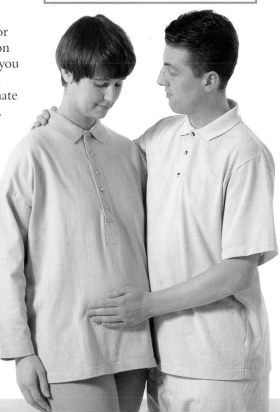

WEEK 20

YOU WILL PROBABLY have a strong sense of well-being during the middle months of pregnancy. Some women look and feel radiant, because of noticeable improvements in skin and hair. If you're feeling well, it's often a good idea to take a vacation. You should have had the excitement of hearing the fetal heartbeat and feeling the baby move by now.

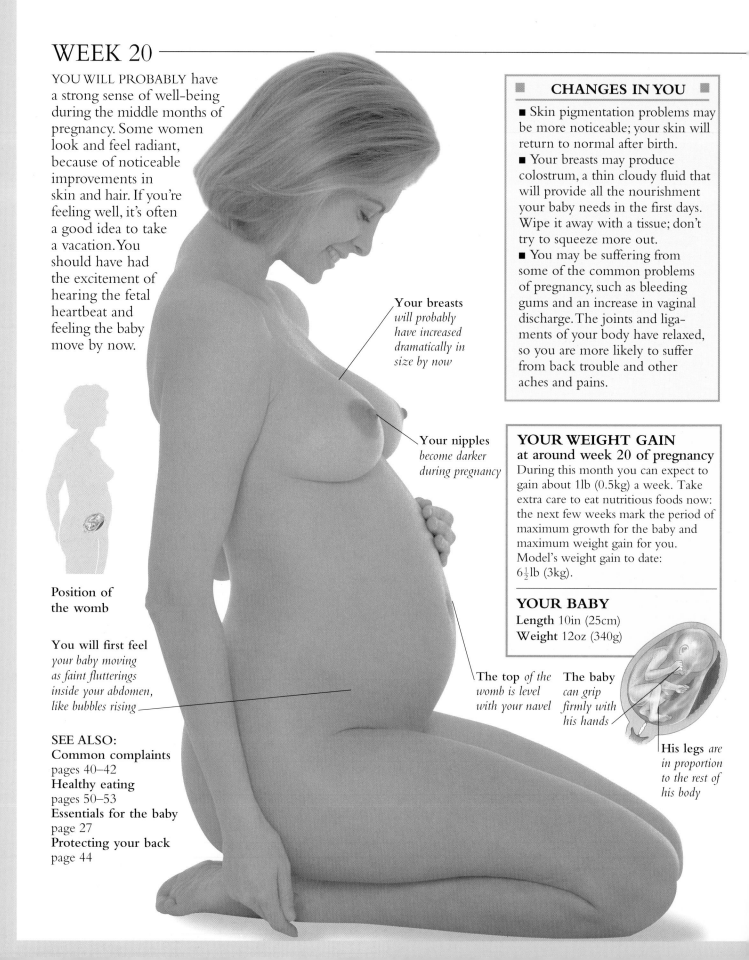

Position of the womb

You will first feel *your baby moving as faint flutterings inside your abdomen, like bubbles rising*

Your breasts *will probably have increased dramatically in size by now*

Your nipples *become darker during pregnancy*

The top *of the womb is level with your navel*

SEE ALSO:
Common complaints
pages 40–42
Healthy eating
pages 50–53
Essentials for the baby
page 27
Protecting your back
page 44

CHANGES IN YOU

■ Skin pigmentation problems may be more noticeable; your skin will return to normal after birth.
■ Your breasts may produce colostrum, a thin cloudy fluid that will provide all the nourishment your baby needs in the first days. Wipe it away with a tissue; don't try to squeeze more out.
■ You may be suffering from some of the common problems of pregnancy, such as bleeding gums and an increase in vaginal discharge. The joints and ligaments of your body have relaxed, so you are more likely to suffer from back trouble and other aches and pains.

YOUR WEIGHT GAIN
at around week 20 of pregnancy
During this month you can expect to gain about 1lb (0.5kg) a week. Take extra care to eat nutritious foods now: the next few weeks mark the period of maximum growth for the baby and maximum weight gain for you. Model's weight gain to date: $6\frac{1}{2}$lb (3kg).

YOUR BABY
Length 10in (25cm)
Weight 12oz (340g)

The baby *can grip firmly with his hands*

His legs *are in proportion to the rest of his body*

LOOKING GOOD

YOU MAY LOOK and feel your best during the middle months of your pregnancy, with lustrous hair, rosy cheeks, and smooth, healthy skin. But not everyone blooms; the high hormone levels can have less flattering effects on skin, nails, and hair, though any adverse changes usually disappear after birth.

WHAT TO DO

- Watch your posture from now on. Stand up straight and avoid straining your back. Wear low-heeled shoes.
- Take the practical steps suggested on pages 40–42 to relieve any other discomforts.
- Start to think about essential clothes and equipment for the baby, such as a crib or carriage.

QUESTION & ANSWER

"Is a long trip advisable?"
There's usually no reason you shouldn't travel during your pregnancy, but don't go alone, especially on a long car trip. Wear loose, comfortable clothes, and to help your circulation, break up a long drive by walking around for a few minutes every two hours. If you're flying or traveling by train, get up and stretch your legs in the aisles every couple of hours.

YOUR GROWING BABY

- Hair appears on the baby's head.
- Teeth are developing.
- Vernix, the white, greasy substance that protects the baby's skin in the womb, forms.
- The baby's arms and legs are well developed.
- Protective substances may be transferred to the baby through your blood to help him resist disease in the first weeks.
- The baby is very active; you should have felt his movements for the first time as a faint fluttering. He may even react to noises outside the womb, but don't worry if he doesn't move around much; it's fairly common for babies to have quiet periods.

HAIR
Thick, shiny hair is often a bonus of pregnancy. However, not all hair improves: oily hair may become more oily, and dry hair, drier and more brittle. You may lose more hair than usual. Facial and body hair also tend to darken.

Have *your hair cut into a style that is easy to take care of*

What to do If your hair is dry and ends split easily, use a mild shampoo and conditioner, and don't brush it too often or too vigorously. Wash oily hair frequently to keep it shiny. Hair is unpredictable in pregnancy, so avoid perms or having it colored.

Your *skin may become smooth and blemish-free*

SKIN TEXTURE
Your skin may improve in pregnancy: blemishes can disappear, and skin texture sometimes becomes smooth and silky. However, you may find that your skin becomes very dry, or oily, or perhaps blotchy.

What to do Cleanse thoroughly. If it is dry, gently rub moisturizer over the dry areas and add bath oil to your bath water. Use as little soap as possible.

NAILS
You may notice that your nails split and break more easily than usual.

What to do Wear gloves for household chores and gardening.

SKIN COLOR
An increase in skin pigmentation is normal during pregnancy. Moles, birthmarks, scars, and freckles usually darken and grow in size, and a brown line often appears down the center of your stomach. You may notice a brownish patch, or "butterfly mask," across your face and neck. Don't worry—this disappears soon after birth.

What to do Avoid strong sunlight because it can make pigmentation problems worse, but if you go out in the sun, use a sunscreen with maximum protection. Don't bleach the mask; if you want to disguise it, try makeup or a blemish covering stick.

WEEK 24

THIS IS OFTEN the best month of pregnancy. You will probably look well, and feel happy and contented. You should continue to gain ¾ -1lb (0.3-0.5kg) per week. You'll be visibly pregnant—finally!

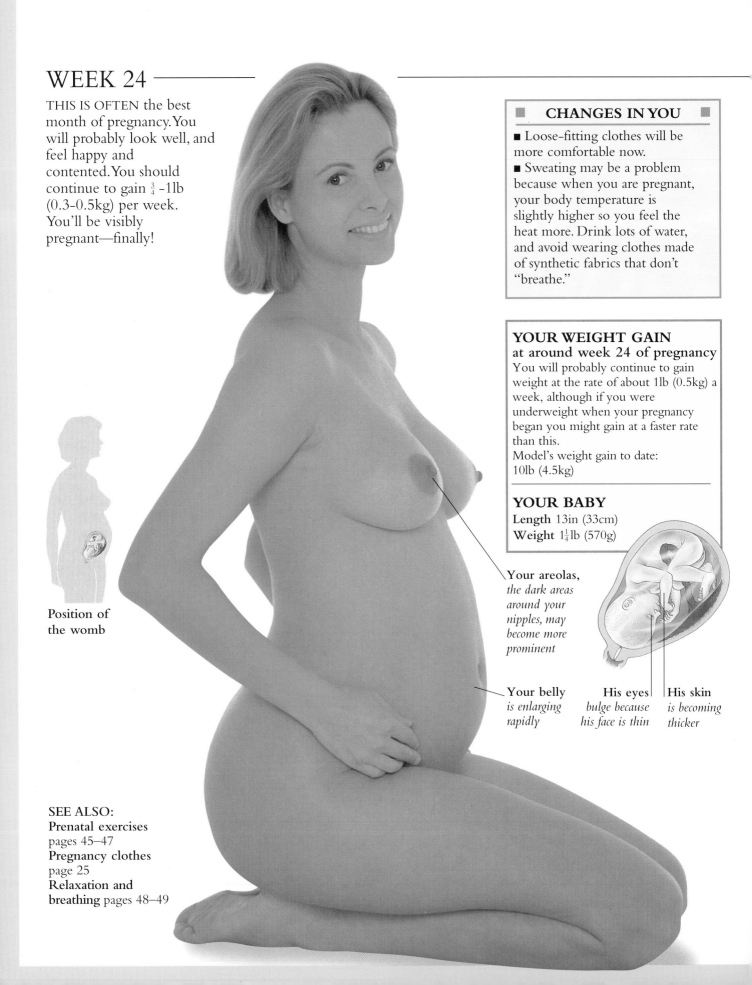

Position of the womb

SEE ALSO:
Prenatal exercises
pages 45–47
Pregnancy clothes
page 25
Relaxation and breathing pages 48–49

■ CHANGES IN YOU ■

■ Loose-fitting clothes will be more comfortable now.
■ Sweating may be a problem because when you are pregnant, your body temperature is slightly higher so you feel the heat more. Drink lots of water, and avoid wearing clothes made of synthetic fabrics that don't "breathe."

YOUR WEIGHT GAIN
at around week 24 of pregnancy
You will probably continue to gain weight at the rate of about 1lb (0.5kg) a week, although if you were underweight when your pregnancy began you might gain at a faster rate than this.
Model's weight gain to date: 10lb (4.5kg)

YOUR BABY
Length 13in (33cm)
Weight 1¼lb (570g)

Your areolas,
the dark areas around your nipples, may become more prominent

Your belly
is enlarging rapidly

His eyes
bulge because his face is thin

His skin
is becoming thicker

THE BABY IN THE WOMB

WHILE THE BABY is developing physically, he is also on the way to becoming an aware, responsive person with feelings. He lies tightly curled up in the womb, cushioned by the bag of water that surrounds him, entirely reliant on your placenta for food, oxygen, and the disposal of his waste products. However, he looks and behaves much the same as the baby he will be at birth.

WHAT TO DO

■ If you have flat or inverted nipples, you will still be able to breast-feed. Talk to your obstetrician or midwife.

■ Put your feet up as much as possible during the day. You might want to take this time to go shopping through the catalogs for maternity clothing.

■ Continue to exercise gently, but regularly. Practice relaxation and breathing exercises.

■ If you are working full-time, find a quiet spot for 15-minute breaks.

QUESTION & ANSWER

"What is the best kind of bra?"
To give your breasts the support they need in pregnancy, choose a bra (preferably cotton) with a deep band under the cups, broad shoulder straps, and an adjustable back. Check your size regularly, because your breasts will continue to grow throughout pregnancy. By the end, you might fit a cup size two sizes larger than usual. If your breasts become very heavy, wear a lightweight bra at night.

YOUR GROWING BABY

■ No fat has been put on yet, so the baby is still lean.

■ Sweat glands are forming in the skin.

■ Arm and leg muscles are well developed, and the baby tries them out regularly. He has periods of frenzied activity, when you feel him moving around, alternating with periods of calm.

■ The baby can cough and hiccup; you may feel the hiccups as a knocking movement.

SIGHT
His eyelids are still sealed, but by week 28, they become unsealed, and he may see, and open and close his eyes.

HEARING
He can hear your voice, and if he's asleep he can be awakened by loud music. He may prefer some types of music and show this by his movements. He jumps at sudden noises.

FACIAL EXPRESSIONS
He frowns, squints, purses his lips, and opens and closes his mouth.

LIFE-SUPPORT SYSTEM
The baby is nourished by the placenta and protected by warm amniotic fluid, which can change every four hours. It regulates the baby's temperature and protects against infection and sudden bumps.

MOVEMENTS
He kicks and punches, and he sometimes turns somersaults. He can make a fist.

SLEEPING PATTERNS
He sleeps and wakes randomly, and he will probably be most active when you are trying to sleep.

PERSONALITY
The part of the brain concerned with personality and intelligence becomes far more complex during the seventh month, so his personality may soon be developing.

SUCKING, SWALLOWING, AND BREATHING
He sucks his thumb and swallows the warm water (the amniotic fluid) that surrounds him, passing it out of his body as urine. You may feel his periods of hiccupping, which seem to come and go. He makes breathing movements with his chest, practicing for life outside the womb.

TASTE
His taste buds are forming, and by week 28, he can respond to sweet, sour, and bitter tastes.

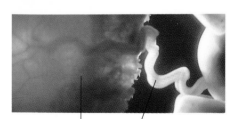

The placenta *supplies all the nutrients the baby needs; almost anything entering your body, good or bad, is filtered through to him*

The umbilical cord, *a rope of three blood vessels, links the placenta to the baby*

WEEK 28

YOU ARE NOW entering the home
stretch, with only three months to go.
The baby's activity may startle you
when he moves and your midriff
shifts dramatically. If he were
born now he would have a
good chance of survival,
given special care.

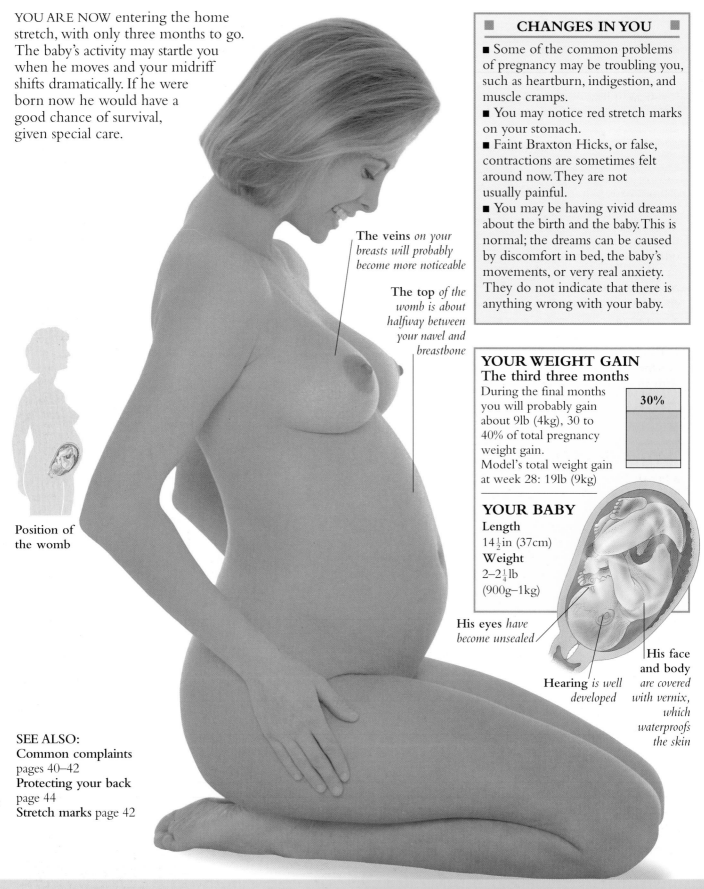

*Position of
the womb*

The veins *on your
breasts will probably
become more noticeable*

The top *of the
womb is about
halfway between
your navel and
breastbone*

SEE ALSO:
Common complaints
pages 40–42
Protecting your back
page 44
Stretch marks page 42

CHANGES IN YOU

■ Some of the common problems
of pregnancy may be troubling you,
such as heartburn, indigestion, and
muscle cramps.
■ You may notice red stretch marks
on your stomach.
■ Faint Braxton Hicks, or false,
contractions are sometimes felt
around now. They are not
usually painful.
■ You may be having vivid dreams
about the birth and the baby. This is
normal; the dreams can be caused
by discomfort in bed, the baby's
movements, or very real anxiety.
They do not indicate that there is
anything wrong with your baby.

YOUR WEIGHT GAIN
The third three months
During the final months
you will probably gain
about 9lb (4kg), 30 to
40% of total pregnancy
weight gain.
Model's total weight gain
at week 28: 19lb (9kg)

30%

YOUR BABY
Length
$14\frac{1}{2}$in (37cm)
Weight
$2–2\frac{1}{4}$lb
(900g–1kg)

His eyes *have
become unsealed*

Hearing *is well
developed*

**His face
and body** *are covered
with vernix,
which
waterproofs
the skin*

YOUR PREGNANCY WARDROBE

WHAT TO DO

■ Make sure you are getting enough rest during the day, and try to get to sleep early at night. If you are still working, put your feet up during the lunch hour and rest when you come home.

■ If you are still working full-time and you are in a job that doesn't exhaust you physically, schedule an appointment with the personnel department to discuss your future plans. Some women continue on the job until their due date, while others need a few weeks to prepare and rest at home before the birth. No matter what you and your employer decide, it's always best to clear the air.

■ Visits to the obstetrician become more frequent now. The baby's heartbeat can usually be heard with an ordinary fetal stethoscope at this point.

YOUR GROWING BABY

■ His skin is red and wrinkled, but fat is accumulating beneath it, making it more flesh-colored.

■ There have been dramatic developments in the thinking part of the brain. It's now bigger and more complex. A seven-month-old fetus can feel pain, and he responds much like a full-term baby.

■ Research has shown that the baby has more taste buds than he will have at birth, so his sense of taste is acute.

■ His lungs are still not fully mature; they need to develop a substance called surfactant, which stops them from collapsing between each breath.

■ You can feel the baby move if you put your hand on your stomach. You may even see the shape of a foot or bottom as the baby kicks and turns.

UNTIL THE FIFTH or even sixth month of your pregnancy, many of your normal clothes may be wearable if they fit loosely or you use a little creativity. However, new outfits may greatly improve your morale. You don't always have to buy special maternity wear. Look for loose-fitting clothes that are attractive, comfortable, and easy to care for from the regular departments in the stores.

Comfortable tops
Go for stretchy fabrics in soft natural fibers. Some days you may feel happier wearing a baggy sweat shirt.

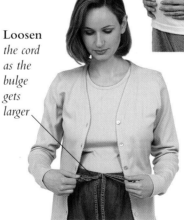

Loosen the cord as the bulge gets larger

Loose-fitting bottoms
Pants with a drawstring are comfortable and unrestricting; they are convenient because they can be adjusted to fit your expanding waistline.

Dressing up
A simple dress can look casual, but is also easy to dress up. Check that there's enough length in the hem so the dress hangs evenly as you grow larger. Maternity dresses are usually 1in (2.5cm) longer at the front to allow for this.

WHAT TO CHOOSE
You tend to feel the heat more during pregnancy, so look for lightweight, loose-fitting clothes, made of cotton or other natural fibers. If it's cold, put on layers. Avoid anything tight at the waist or that restricts blood flow in your legs, such as tight knee-high socks. Comfortable, low-heeled shoes are essential, although completely flat heels may not be as comfortable as ones with a slight lift. It may soon be difficult to lean over to tie shoes or sneakers that lace up.

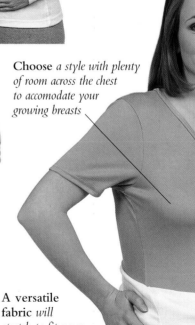

Choose *a style with plenty of room across the chest to accomodate your growing breasts*

A versatile fabric *will stretch to fit your changing shape*

WEEK 32

YOU NEED all the rest you can get, so try to lie down in the middle of the day. You will be feeling very bulky, and probably weary of your pregnant state. Now is the time to start going to childbirth classes, which will run until the end of your pregnancy. The baby is completely formed, and his body is in proportion. Fat is being deposited under his skin, so he looks plumper.

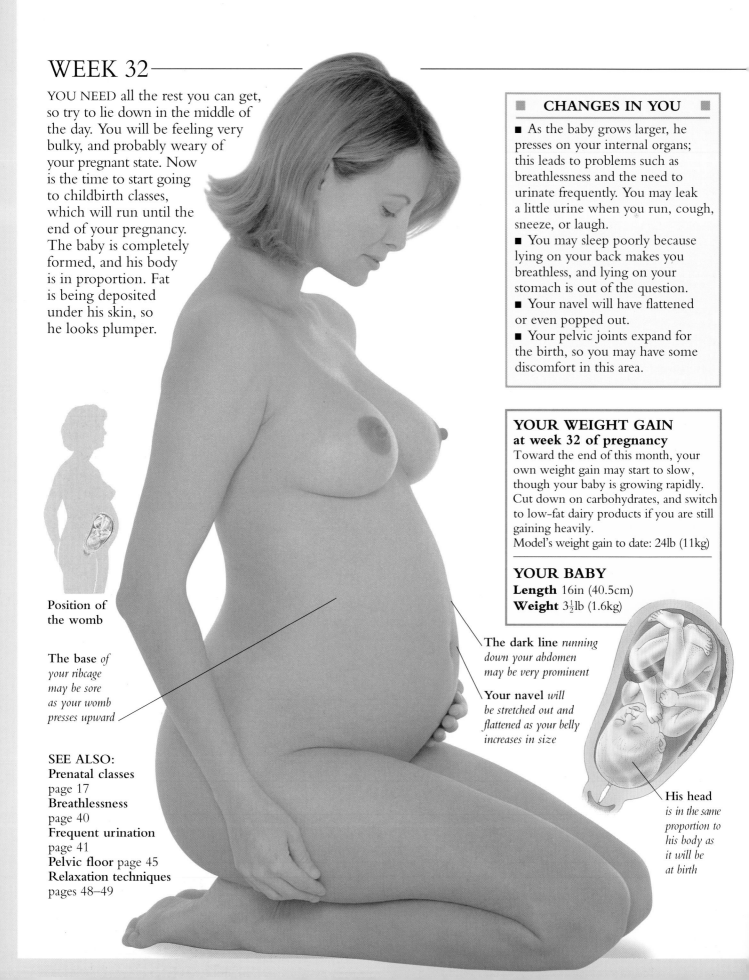

Position of the womb

The base *of your ribcage may be sore as your womb presses upward*

SEE ALSO:
Prenatal classes
page 17
Breathlessness
page 40
Frequent urination
page 41
Pelvic floor page 45
Relaxation techniques
pages 48–49

CHANGES IN YOU

■ As the baby grows larger, he presses on your internal organs; this leads to problems such as breathlessness and the need to urinate frequently. You may leak a little urine when you run, cough, sneeze, or laugh.
■ You may sleep poorly because lying on your back makes you breathless, and lying on your stomach is out of the question.
■ Your navel will have flattened or even popped out.
■ Your pelvic joints expand for the birth, so you may have some discomfort in this area.

YOUR WEIGHT GAIN
at week 32 of pregnancy
Toward the end of this month, your own weight gain may start to slow, though your baby is growing rapidly. Cut down on carbohydrates, and switch to low-fat dairy products if you are still gaining heavily.
Model's weight gain to date: 24lb (11kg)

YOUR BABY
Length 16in (40.5cm)
Weight $3\frac{1}{2}$lb (1.6kg)

The dark line *running down your abdomen may be very prominent*

Your navel *will be stretched out and flattened as your belly increases in size*

His head *is in the same proportion to his body as it will be at birth*

WHAT TO DO

- Try to take regular breaks during the day if possible.
- If you have difficulty sleeping, practice relaxation techniques before going to bed, and sleep on your side, with one leg bent and your stomach supported on a pillow. Try not to worry if you can't sleep; some insomnia is normal at this stage. All the adverse symptoms can conspire against you at night. Don't toss and turn—get up and do something.
- Keep up with your pelvic floor exercises; this is especially important if you leak urine.
- Start attending prenatal classes if you haven't already.

QUESTION & ANSWER

"I'm worried about harming the baby during intercourse. Is there any danger of this?"
This is a common worry, but an unnecessary one if your pregnancy is normal. The baby is protected and cushioned by the bag of fluid surrounding him, so he can't be harmed when you make love. The doctor will warn you if there are any dangers, such as a low placenta.

YOUR GROWING BABY

- The baby looks much the same as at birth, but his body still needs to fill out more.
- He can now tell the difference between light and dark.
- Because there is less room in the womb, he may have turned into a head-down position by now, ready for birth.

ESSENTIALS FOR YOUR BABY

BUY THE FOLLOWING basic items for your new baby.

EQUIPMENT
You will need:
- a carriage, crib, or bassinet for your baby to sleep in
- appropriate bedding
- a soft blanket
- bottle-feeding equipment if you are going to bottle-feed
    - baby bathtub
    - two soft towels
    - changing mat or table
    - diaper-changing equipment and diapers
    - an infant car seat, if you have a car; some double as infant seats.
And be sure there is a smoke detector in your home, if you don't already have one.

Choose a style of suit with snaps up the front and around the thighs and crotch

CLOTHES
These should be marked "newborn." You will need:
- six undershirts
- eight stretchsuits
- two sweaters
- two infant sleeping or drawstring gowns
- two pairs of soft socks or bootees
- sun hat or woolen hat.

ENJOYING SEX

MAKING LOVE is often particularly enjoyable during pregnancy. Some women become aroused more easily as a result of the increase in hormone levels. And there are no worries about contraception.

OTHER WAYS OF LOVING
There may be times when you lose interest in sex, especially in the first and last weeks. This doesn't mean that you have to stop loving each other physically. Even if you feel too tired or heavy to make love, find other ways to show your affection, such as kissing, cuddling, stroking, and touching.

A CHANGE OF POSITION
In the last weeks of pregnancy, you may find the traditional man-on-top position difficult. Experiment with other positions; perhaps try sitting on your partner's lap, kneeling with him behind, or both lying side by side.

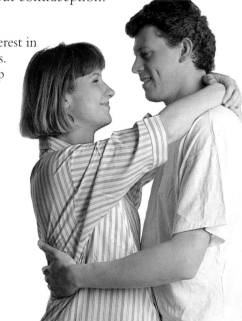

WEEK 36

BY NOW you should have started to wind your life down in preparation for the birth. You may be longing for the pregnancy to be over, yet feeling apprehensive about labor, birth, and becoming a parent. In fact, your emotions can swing wildly. The baby takes up all the space in the womb, so he kicks and punches, rather than shifting his body.

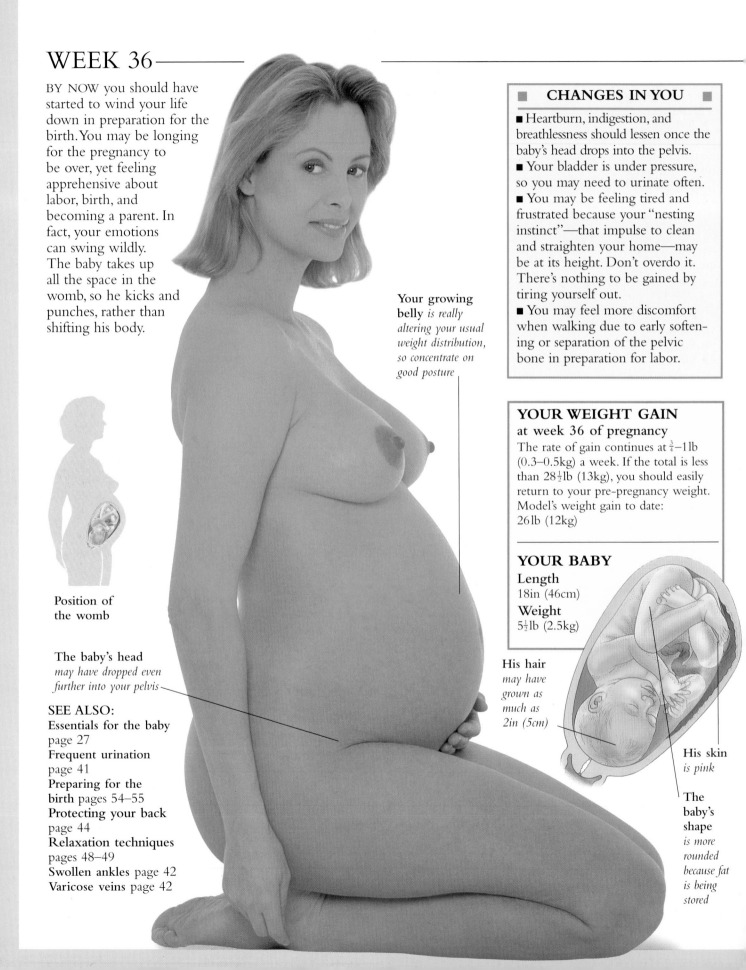

Position of the womb

The baby's head *may have dropped even further into your pelvis*

SEE ALSO:
Essentials for the baby page 27
Frequent urination page 41
Preparing for the birth pages 54–55
Protecting your back page 44
Relaxation techniques pages 48–49
Swollen ankles page 42
Varicose veins page 42

Your growing belly *is really altering your usual weight distribution, so concentrate on good posture*

■ CHANGES IN YOU ■

■ Heartburn, indigestion, and breathlessness should lessen once the baby's head drops into the pelvis.
■ Your bladder is under pressure, so you may need to urinate often.
■ You may be feeling tired and frustrated because your "nesting instinct"—that impulse to clean and straighten your home—may be at its height. Don't overdo it. There's nothing to be gained by tiring yourself out.
■ You may feel more discomfort when walking due to early softening or separation of the pelvic bone in preparation for labor.

YOUR WEIGHT GAIN
at week 36 of pregnancy
The rate of gain continues at $\frac{3}{4}$–1lb (0.3–0.5kg) a week. If the total is less than $28\frac{1}{2}$lb (13kg), you should easily return to your pre-pregnancy weight. Model's weight gain to date: 26lb (12kg)

YOUR BABY
Length
18in (46cm)
Weight
$5\frac{1}{2}$lb (2.5kg)

His hair *may have grown as much as 2in (5cm)*

His skin *is pink*

The baby's shape *is more rounded because fat is being stored*

—RESTING IN LATER PREGNANCY—

DURING THE LAST WEEKS, you will probably become tired very easily. You may not be sleeping as well as usual, and you will also feel exhausted by the extra weight you have been carrying around. It's important not to fight this tiredness, but to rest and relax as much as possible.

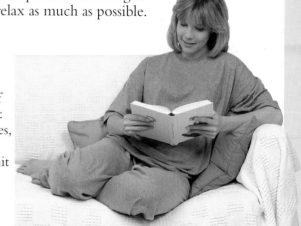

TO AVOID TIRING YOURSELF

Put your feet up whenever you need to during the day. Think of quiet things to do while you rest: practice gentle relaxation exercises, listen to soothing music, read a book or magazine, or perhaps knit something for the baby. It also helps if you try to do things at a slower pace than usual, so that you don't become overtired.

WHAT TO DO

- Put your feet up whenever you can to guard against swollen ankles and varicose veins.
- Doctor visits may be once a week now.
- If you are having your baby in the hospital, make sure you take a tour of the delivery room and maternity area.
- Buy your nursing bras.
- Go food shopping and stock up on all the basics so they'll be there for your return. If you have a freezer, fill it with easy meals.
- Pack your suitcase.
- Lie on your side: it is more comfortable for you and better for your baby as it raises placental blood flow.

QUESTION & ANSWER

"Should I have my partner with me during labor?"
Most hospitals and childbirth experts actively encourage this. Labor can be a long process and a lonely one unless you have someone close to share it with. The natural choice is your baby's father. But if he really doesn't want to be there, it's unfair to put too much pressure on him. It's quite acceptable to have a relative or a good friend there instead.

YOUR GROWING BABY

- If this is your first baby, his head will probably have descended into the pelvis, ready for birth.
- Soft nails have grown to the tips of his fingers and toes.
- In a boy, the testicles should have descended.
- The baby will gain about 1oz (28g) every day for the remaining four weeks in the womb.

—YOUR NURSING BRA—

IF YOU WANT to breast-feed your baby after birth, you will need at least two front-opening nursing bras. To make sure these are the right size, it's best to buy them no earlier than week 36.

WHAT TO LOOK FOR

There are two main types of bra: one has flaps, which open to expose the nipple and surrounding breast; the other fastens in front between the cups, so you can expose the whole breast. The front-opening kind is best, because it allows the baby to feel and touch as much of the breast as possible. This helps your milk let-down reflex (see pages 93 and 96). Look for plain cotton and wide straps.

MEASURING YOURSELF

Take the measurements while wearing one of your ordinary pregnancy bras.

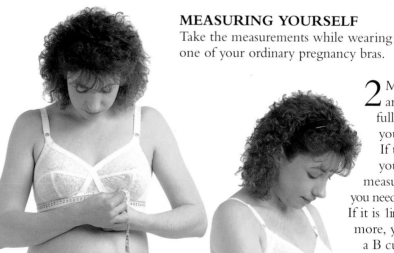

1 Measure around your body below your breasts. Add 5in (12cm) to get your final chest measurement.

2 Measure around the fullest part of your breasts. If this equals your chest measurement, you need an A cup. If it is 1in (2.5cm) more, you need a B cup. If it is 2in (5cm) more, you need a C cup.

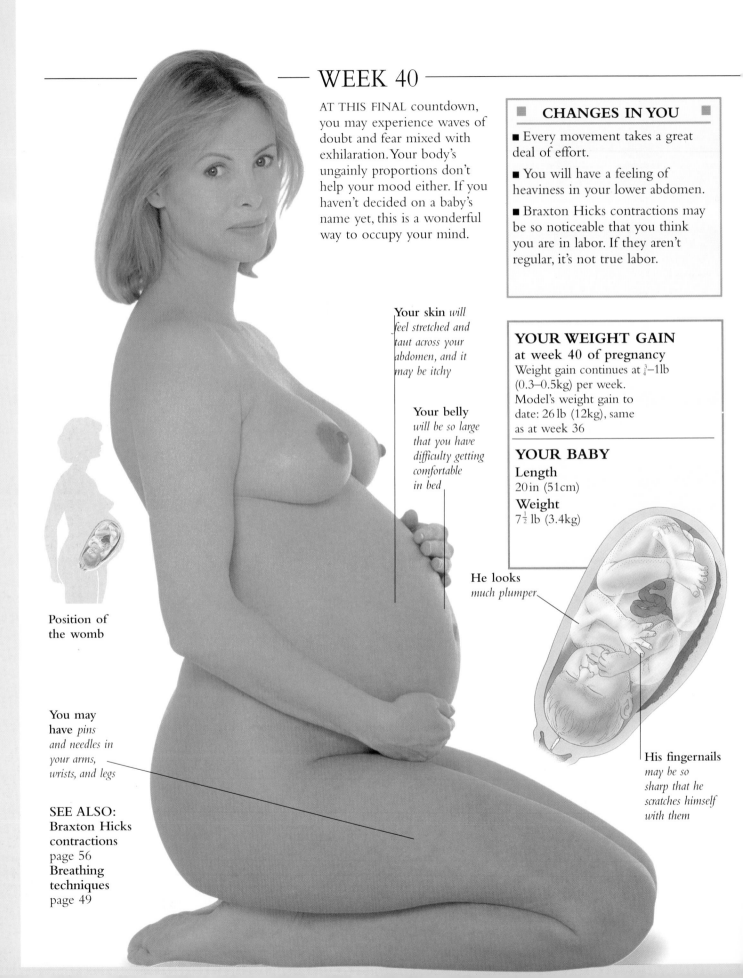

— WEEK 40 —

AT THIS FINAL countdown, you may experience waves of doubt and fear mixed with exhilaration. Your body's ungainly proportions don't help your mood either. If you haven't decided on a baby's name yet, this is a wonderful way to occupy your mind.

■ CHANGES IN YOU ■

■ Every movement takes a great deal of effort.

■ You will have a feeling of heaviness in your lower abdomen.

■ Braxton Hicks contractions may be so noticeable that you think you are in labor. If they aren't regular, it's not true labor.

Your skin *will feel stretched and taut across your abdomen, and it may be itchy*

Your belly *will be so large that you have difficulty getting comfortable in bed*

YOUR WEIGHT GAIN

at week 40 of pregnancy
Weight gain continues at $\frac{3}{4}$–1lb (0.3–0.5kg) per week. Model's weight gain to date: 26 lb (12kg), same as at week 36

YOUR BABY

Length
20 in (51cm)
Weight
$7\frac{1}{2}$ lb (3.4kg)

He looks *much plumper*

His fingernails *may be so sharp that he scratches himself with them*

Position of
the womb

You may have *pins and needles in your arms, wrists, and legs*

SEE ALSO:
Braxton Hicks contractions
page 56
Breathing techniques
page 49

AFTER THE BIRTH

AFTER ALL the weeks of preparation and planning, you can now hold your baby in your arms. You may feel overwhelmingly protective yet tentative toward this tiny person, so dependent on you for everything.

THE FIRST WEEKS

Life in the early weeks revolves around your baby and can be absolutely topsy-turvy and exhausting. Once you get to know each other, and you become more adept at handling him, he will settle down, and your life will fall into a routine.

■ BEFORE BIRTH ■

■ Rest as much as possible, and enjoy these last baby-free days.
■ If you don't feel at least ten movements from your baby during the day, ask your doctor or midwife to check his heart because he may be in distress.
■ If you're having Braxton Hicks contractions, use them to practice breathing techniques.
■ Remember, it's a "due month"; it's perfectly normal for a baby to be born two weeks on either side of the expected delivery date.

TOTAL WEIGHT GAIN

The average amount of weight gain during pregnancy varies from 26 to 30lb (12 to 14kg). The total weight gain is made up of:

fetus	7.5 lbs
placenta	1.5 lbs
amniotic fluid	2 lbs
uterus and breasts	4.5 lbs
blood and fluids	6.5 lbs
fat	4 – 8 lbs

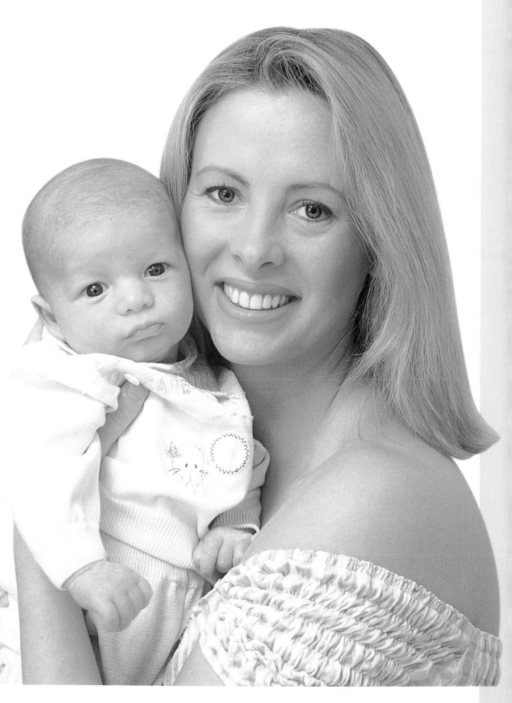

■ YOUR GROWING BABY ■

■ Most of the lanugo hair (see page 19) has disappeared, though there may still be a little on his shoulders, arms, and legs.
■ He may still be covered in vernix, or just have traces left in his skin folds.
■ A dark tar-like substance called meconium has been gathering in the baby's intestines; this will be passed in his first bowel movements after birth (see page 146).

PRENATAL CARE

Taking good care of yourself and your growing baby during pregnancy is critical. Soon after you miss your first period or your pregnancy is confirmed using an at-home test kit, your prenatal care should begin. This modern system of regular visits to the physician or midwife who will eventually deliver your baby offers mothers-to-be reassuring checks, tests, and a

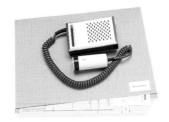

constant source of answers to those troubling questions. Some women stay with their regular physician, others want to find a new specialist. Talk to friends who have recently given birth and ask for recommendations. The more information you can gather, the better your birth experience will be. The important thing is to start your prenatal care early.

WHERE TO HAVE YOUR BABY

ONE OF THE FIRST DECISIONS you will need to make is where to have your baby. Most babies today are born in a hospital. Some hospitals now feature birthing rooms, which are more homelike than typical labor and delivery settings. There are also childbirth centers usually staffed by midwives. And, occasionally it is possible to have your baby at home, providing your obstetrician or midwife is agreeable.

HOSPITAL BIRTH

A hospital offers all the equipment and expertise available for giving pain medication, for monitoring the baby's progress, for intervening in the birth to help you and the baby, if necessary, and for providing emergency care to you both.

There are level one (primary), level two (secondary), and level three (tertiary) hospitals, each designed to provide a certain level of care. A level one hospital is a community hospital designed to handle uncomplicated cases and routine procedures. A level two hospital can do more complicated procedures and has a nursery to care for sick babies, but not very sick babies. A level three hospital is usually a large medical center, staffed by specialists in many fields; it will have a neonatal intensive care unit and perinatalogists on staff.

You and your doctor should discuss which type of hospital you should plan to use. The decision will be based on the course of your pregnancy and whether or not any complications or

special problems are expected. In all cases, the hospital you go to should have some means—say, a helicopter—to transport you and/or the baby to a level three hospital if serious unexpected problems develop.

After the birth, a few days in the hospital may give you the rest you need to cope at home later. The average stay is 24–48 hours for vaginal birth and up to four days for C-sections. If you are a first-time mother, you may also find the support of staff and other mothers reassuring.

Take a hospital tour

Because hospital policies regarding labor and delivery vary tremendously across the country, some women decide to tour nearby medical centers before arranging their first prenatal visit with an obstetrician. Not all doctors are on staff or affiliated at all hospitals in a geographical area. Call ahead and ask if you and your mate can see the obstetrical unit to learn all about family-centered births, special labor and

delivery rooms, and visiting hours for husbands or siblings. Seek recommendations from women who have recently become mothers. After you settle on a hospital, you can gather the names of physicians whose patients deliver there.

Birthing rooms

In a traditional hospital birth, a woman labors in one room, and immediately before birth, she is moved to a special delivery or operating room. In recent years, more hospitals have realized that moving a patient at the critical moment in giving birth is not always appropriate and now almost all hospitals offer birthing rooms. Some hospitals offer LDRP (labor, delivery, recovery, post partum) rooms, where women do everything in one room. Designed for women who are in a low-risk category and expect to deliver their babies normally, these rooms are often more homelike than typical operating rooms, and expectant couples can

remain together in an informal setting. A birthing bed, one with a split frame that separates the bottom half from the head of the bed at the time of delivery, is often available, too. Ask about these options; sometimes if you don't inquire, you won't be put on a birthing room reservation list.

BIRTHING CENTERS

These are small out-of-hospital facilities where normal, low-risk births can be handled. They are fairly new on the American childbirth scene and are staffed by midwives and nurses, with obstetricians usually on call for special assistance. Checkups, childbirth classes, and some routine prenatal tests as well as normal childbirth are available at these centers. For the one nearest you, contact the American College of Nurse Midwives, 1522 K Street NW, Suite 1000, Washington, D.C. 20005. Send a self-addressed stamped envelope to speed your reply.

CHOOSING AN OBSTETRICIAN

The American College of Obstetricians and Gynecologists can provide you with a list of specialists in your area. Their resource center is located at 409 Twelfth Street SW, Washington, D.C. 20024. There are other physicians who can manage your pregnancy, too, such as family practitioners. If possible, choose a physician or midwife and hospital affiliated with your HMO. What is crucial for you is to find someone you feel comfortable with and who really understands your needs. Go to an initial appointment with a written list of questions and be prepared to participate in your prenatal care. Ignorance is never bliss when it comes to having a baby.

PRENATAL-CARE OPTIONS

Group practices Some physicians prefer to work in a group. They relieve each other in a specialty that can demand full concentration 24 hours a day. This may mean that you will see various doctors during your pregnancy. Even if the same doctor treats you at each prenatal visit, try to get to know all the group members. There are group practices as small as two and as large as six or even eight obstetricians.

Hospital midwife programs Midwives, graduate registered nurses who have completed training programs and are certified by the American College of Nurse Midwives, are becoming more popular. Some are associated with hospital maternity units. They handle low-risk cases and an obstetrician is

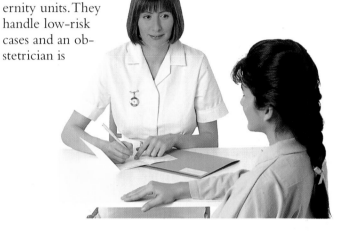

generally on call for backup assistance. If you have no signs of complications, a midwife may be able to monitor your pregnancy and deliver your baby. The letters C.N.M. alongside the name, indicate the professional qualifications.

QUESTIONS TO ASK

HOSPITAL POLICIES vary, so discuss any issues that are important to you with your obstetrician. It's natural to have preconceived ideas about labor and birth, but the reality is often quite different. Even though you may be opposed to pain medication, for example, keep an open mind. In an emergency or under severe strain, you may need it. This list covers some of the questions you might like to ask.

ABOUT LABOR

Can my partner or a friend stay with me throughout labor? Will he or she ever be asked to leave the delivery room? **Will** I be able to move around during labor? **What** is the hospital policy on pain medication, routine fetal monitoring, and drugs to induce labor (see pages 64, 65 and 66)? **What** kind of pain relief will I be offered; are epidural anesthesia or tranquilizers (see pages 64 and 65) available?

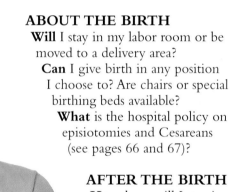

ABOUT THE BIRTH

Will I stay in my labor room or be moved to a delivery area?
Can I give birth in any position I choose to? Are chairs or special birthing beds available?
What is the hospital policy on episiotomies and Cesareans (see pages 66 and 67)?

AFTER THE BIRTH

How long will I stay in hospital after the delivery?
Is "rooming-in" available?
What are the visiting hours?
Is there a special care baby unit? If not, where will my baby be taken if special treatment is needed?

A TYPICAL PRENATAL VISIT

YOUR FIRST VISIT to the obstetrician should take place soon after you miss your period. You will probably be going once a month until 28 weeks. Visits become more frequent after this, usually every two weeks until you are 36 weeks pregnant, and every week in the last month. Routine tests are carried out by the doctor or midwife at every visit, to make sure that the pregnancy is progressing normally.

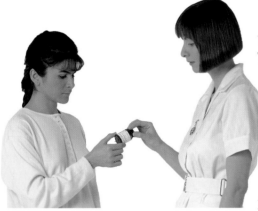

URINE SAMPLE every visit

This will be tested for:
■ traces of sugar, which, if found, could be a sign of diabetes (see page 38)
■ traces of protein, which could indicate that your kidneys are not working properly. If protein is found in you urine later in pregnancy, this could be a sign of preeclampsia (see page 38).

HEIGHT first visit

Your height will be measured, as this is a guide to the size of your pelvis; a small pelvis can sometimes mean a difficult delivery.

INITIAL APPOINTMENT

At the first visit, the doctor or midwife will ask you some questions about you and your partner, to find out whether there is anything that could affect the pregnancy or your baby. Routines and procedures vary from place to place, but you can usually expect to be asked about:

■ personal details, such as your date of birth and what you and your partner do

■ your ethnic background, because some forms of anemia are inherited and affect certain ethnic groups (see Blood Tests, opposite)

■ your health: serious illnesses or operations you may have had, whether you are being treated for any disease, and whether you have any allergies or are taking any medications

■ your family's medical history: whether there are twins or any inherited illnesses in your family or your partner's family

■ the type of contraceptives you and your partner used before you became pregnant, and when you stopped using them

■ your periods: when they began, whether they are regular, when the first day of your last period was, and how long your cycle is

■ any previous pregnancies, including miscarriages and abortions.

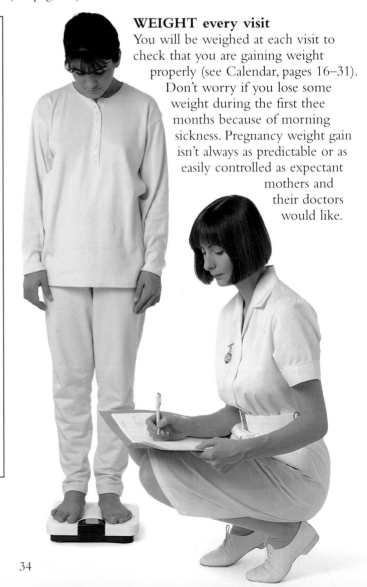

WEIGHT every visit

You will be weighed at each visit to check that you are gaining weight properly (see Calendar, pages 16–31). Don't worry if you lose some weight during the first thee months because of morning sickness. Pregnancy weight gain isn't always as predictable or as easily controlled as expectant mothers and their doctors would like.

BLOOD TESTS first visit

Some blood will be taken from your arm to check:
- your blood type and your rhesus, or Rh, factor (see page 38)
- that you are not anemic (see page 38)
- that you are immune to German measles (see page 10), toxoplasmosis, and hepatitis B
- that you do not have a sexually transmitted disease, such as syphilis, which must be treated before week 20 if it is not to harm the baby
- that you are not HIV positive
- for sickle cell trait, if you and your partner are of African or West Indian descent; for thalassemia, if your families come from the Mediterranean or the Middle and Far East. These forms of anemia are inherited and could put the baby's health at risk.

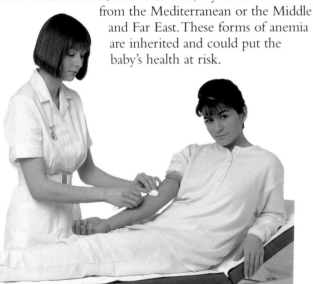

- for Tay-Sachs disease if your families are Jewish or French-Canadian.

BLOOD PRESSURE every visit

Your blood pressure is slightly lower in pregnancy, and it is measured regularly to detect any sudden rises and keep them under control. Normal blood pressure is about 120/70, and there will be cause for concern if your blood pressure rises above 140/90.

Raised blood pressure can be a sign of a number of problems, including preeclampsia (see page 38). However, the stress of a prenatal examination, and waiting for test results, can also cause a higher-than-normal reading, so your blood pressure may be taken again later on during the visit. Ask the doctor or nurse to tell you what your blood pressure is, if she does not automatically do so. It should be written on your chart.

GENERAL EXAMINATION first visit

The doctor or midwife will examine you physically and listen to your heart and lungs. Your breasts will be checked for lumps and inverted nipples (see page 23). A Pap smear and cultures of the cervix are done to check for abnormal cells or infection.

ASKING QUESTIONS

There are bound to be things that puzzle or worry you, or even just interest you, during your pregnancy. Your prenatal visits are your chance to ask about them. It is a good idea to write down any questions before seeing the doctor. Under pressure, it is easy to forget them. Not all doctors are good at explaining medical matters in nonmedical terms, so if you don't understand the answer you have been given, ask again, and again if necessary, to clear up any anxieties you may have.

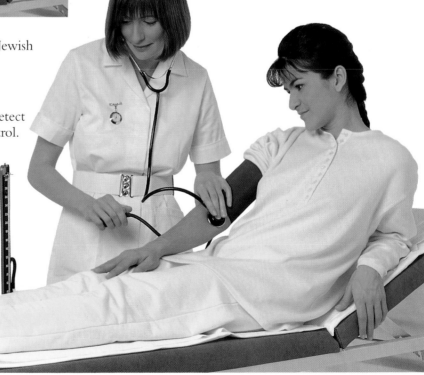

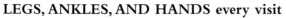

LEGS, ANKLES, AND HANDS every visit
The doctor or midwife will look at your lower legs, ankles, and hands, and feel them to check that there is no swelling or puffiness (edema). A little swelling in the last weeks of pregnancy is normal, especially at the end of the day, but if it's excessive it may be a sign of preeclampsia (see page 38). Your legs will also be checked for varicose veins (see page 42).

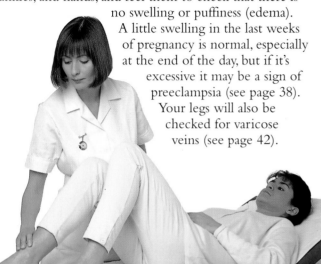

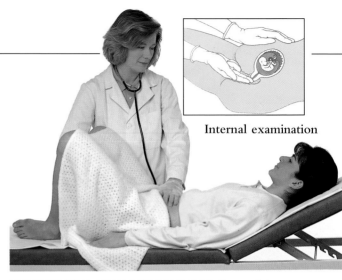

Internal examination

INTERNAL EXAMINATION first visit
The doctor may give you an internal examination, to confirm the stage of the pregnancy, to check your pelvis for abnormalities, and to make sure that the entrance to the womb (the cervix) is tightly closed. You may also have a cervical Pap smear at the same time to check for abnormal cells; ask for the result at your next visit.

The examination won't hurt you or the baby and needn't be uncomfortable if you relax. You will be asked to lie on your back with your legs bent and your knees comfortably apart. The doctor will put two fingers of one hand into the vagina and press your abdomen gently with the other hand.

LISTENING TO THE BABY'S HEARTBEAT every visit (after week 12)
From early in pregnancy, this may be done with an electronic instrument (see below), which amplifies the baby's heartbeat so you can hear it, too. After week 20, the doctor or midwife may listen with a standard stethoscope.

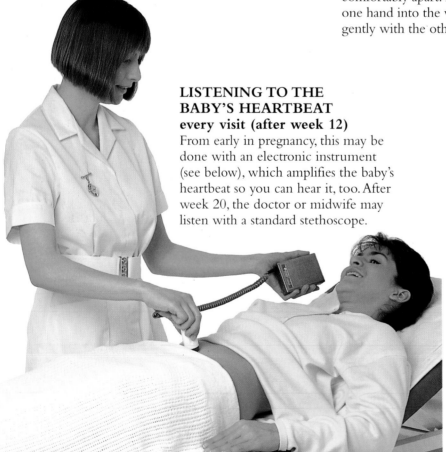

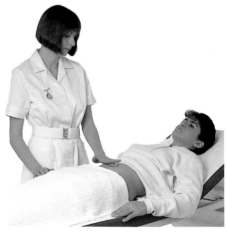

FEELING THE ABDOMEN every visit
Your abdomen will be felt gently to check the position of the top of the womb, which provides a good clue to the rate of the baby's growth. Later in pregnancy, these physical examinations can tell the position of the fetus. In the final weeks, the doctor will want to see if the head is dropping into the pelvis (engaging).

EXTRA TESTS

SOME PRENATAL TESTS are offered only in certain circumstances, such as a sonogram if you are bleeding early in pregnancy. Women over 35 or at high risk because of family history may be offered early biochemical screens for genetic abnormalities. When problems are detected early enough, intervention may be a possible option.

FIRST TRIMESTER SCREENING weeks 11–14

This test combines a limited ultrasound scan of the back of the fetus's neck and a blood test measuring the levels of human chorionic gonadotropin (HCG) and pregnancy-associated plasma protein A (PAPP-A) in the mother's bloodstream. The screen is used to detect fetal cardiac problems and chromosomal abnormalities. Women who have this test still need to have an Alpha Fetoprotein test between weeks 16 and 18.

CHORIONIC VILLUS SAMPLING (CVS) weeks 10–12

Some inherited disorders can be detected very early in pregnancy by examining a small piece of the growing placenta. The sample is removed through the entrance to the womb or through the abdomen.

The advantage of CVS is that it can be done in the first trimester of pregnancy. The miscarriage rate for the test is about one woman in 150.

ALPHA FETOPROTEIN (AFP) TEST weeks 14–18

This blood test measures the amount of alpha fetoprotein, a substance that is produced by the baby in the womb and passes into your bloodstream. A higher-than-normal level of AFP can indicate twins, a more advanced pregnancy than you thought, or a fetal abnormality. The most common abnormality causing a raised AFP level is a neural tube defect, such as spina bifida. Mothers with a low AFP level are at an increased risk for having a baby with Down syndrome. Many obstetricians do quadruple screening for levels of AFP, estriol (uE3), human chorionic gonadotropin (HCG), and inhibin-A in the mother's blood.

When results are screen positive (indicating an increased risk), further tests, such as an ultrasound or amniocentesis, are offered.

ULTRASOUND SCAN week 16 (and sometimes later)

This is an exciting test, because it enables you and your partner to "see" your baby, often moving around, for the first time. Ultrasound does not always show the baby's sex, but it can be used to:

■ make sure the fetus is growing and developing normally;
■ determine the fetus's age and expected delivery date;
■ check the position of the baby and the placenta before amniocentesis, or later in pregnancy, to make sure the placenta isn't blocking the womb's neck;
■ detect certain abnormalities, such as brain and spinal problems; and
■ find out whether you are carrying more than one baby.

If you're having the test early in your pregnancy, you will be asked to drink plenty of water and arrive with a full bladder, so that the womb is clearly visible on the screen. The safe, painless test takes 20 to 30 minutes.

AMNIOCENTESIS weeks 16–18 (and sometimes later)

Amniocentesis can be used to detect some abnormalities in the baby, such as Down syndrome and spina bifida. It is not offered routinely, as there is a risk of miscarriage in about one woman in 200. Your doctor may suggest the test if you:

■ are over 35 (the risk of having a baby with Down syndrome rises with age);
■ have a family history of inherited disease; or
■ have an abnormal AFP level.

After an ultrasound to check the position of the baby and the placenta, a hollow needle is inserted through the abdominal wall into the womb, and a sample of the fluid that surrounds the baby and contains some of his cells is taken. The cells are then tested for abnormality. Results take 14 to 21 days.

PERINEAL CULTURE week 36

This is a check to see if you carry group-B streptococcus bacteria, which can infect your newborn during labor. It is easily treated with antibiotics.

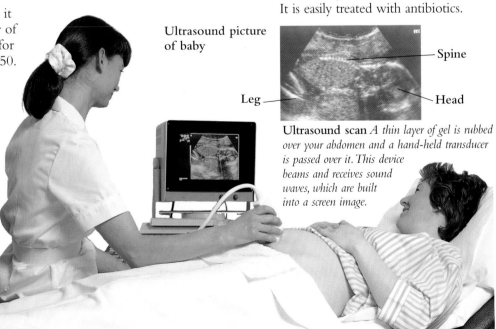

Ultrasound picture of baby

Spine

Leg

Head

Ultrasound scan *A thin layer of gel is rubbed over your abdomen and a hand-held transducer is passed over it. This device beams and receives sound waves, which are built into a screen image.*

HIGH-RISK PREGNANCIES

THE MAJORITY OF PREGNANCIES are straight-forward, but occasionally there are circumstances that alert your doctor to possible complications. You might have a general medical condition that puts you into a high-risk category. Or sometimes symptoms develop that warn the doctor that special care is needed.

ANEMIA

Many women are slightly anemic before they become pregnant because they lack iron. Anemia simply means that you do not have enough red blood cells. It is especially important to correct this imbalance, so that you can cope with the increased demands of pregnancy. Being anemic can make you feel tired.

Treatment Try to prevent the problem by eating a varied diet, with plenty of iron-rich foods (see page 52). If blood tests show you are anemic, your physician can prescribe iron supplements. Take iron tablets directly after meals, with plenty of fluid, particularly fruit juice, because they can irritate the stomach and cause constipation, diarrhea, or nausea. Milk interferes with iron absorption.

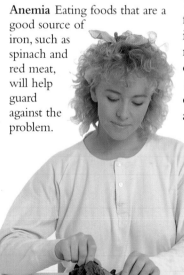

Anemia Eating foods that are a good source of iron, such as spinach and red meat, will help guard against the problem.

DIABETES

Diabetes must be carefully controlled during pregnancy and your blood sugar level constantly monitored. The better your diabetes is controlled, the lower your baby's risk for a congenital anomaly. Some women develop a mild form of diabetes for the first time during pregnancy. This nearly always disappears soon after the birth of the baby.

Treatment To keep your blood sugar level stable, your doctor may adjust your insulin intake during the pregnancy. Pay special attention to diet. Your doctor may also recommend more frequent visits and a special ultrasound scan, called a fetal echogram, to check your baby's heart.

RHESUS NEGATIVE MOTHER

Your blood is tested at the first prenatal visit to see if it is rhesus positive or rhesus negative. About 15 percent of people are rhesus, or Rh, negative, and if you are one of these, you will only have a problem in your pregnancy if you give birth to an Rh positive baby. When blood types are incompatible like this, it seldom harms a first baby, but could cause complications in later pregnancies.

Treatment if you're an Rh negative mother, you will be given an injection of Rhogam at 28 weeks. The obstetrician will also give an injection after the birth if the baby is Rh positive. These injections stop your immune system from creating antibodies that could hurt your baby.

INCOMPETENT CERVIX

In a normal pregnancy, the cervix (neck of the womb) stays closed until labor begins. If miscarriages occur frequently after the third month of pregnancy, the reason could be that the neck of the womb is weak. Under the pressure of a growing pregnancy, the cervix opens up and expels the baby.

Treatment Your doctor may suggest minor surgery to stitch the cervix closed at the start of the pregnancy. The stitch is removed near the end of pregnancy, or as you go into labor.

PREECLAMPSIA

A common—and serious—problem in late pregnancy, preeclampsia is a combination of the following symptoms: blood pressure above 140/90; excessive weight gain; swollen face or hands; and traces of protein in the urine. If you develop any of these, the doctor will monitor you very carefully.

If blood pressure rises untreated, it could progress to the extremely dangerous condition of eclampsia, where convulsions may occur, putting you and your baby at risk.

Treatment Delivery is the treatment. Your doctor will probably advise bed rest. You may be given a drug to prevent convulsions. If the signs are severe, you will be admitted to the hospital, even though you might be feeling healthy. Labor may be induced (see page 66).

EMERGENCY SIGNS

Call for emergency help immediately if you have:
- a severe headache that won't go away
- misty or blurred vision
- severe, prolonged stomach pains
- vaginal bleeding
- a leakage of fluid, which suggests that your water has broken early
- frequent, painful urination (drink plenty of water in the meantime)

Consult your physician immediately if you have:
- swollen hands, face, and ankles and visual disturbances
- severe, frequent vomiting
- a temperature of 100.4°F (38°C)
- no movement, or fewer than 10 kicks, from you baby for 12 hours after week 28

MISCARRIAGE (SPONTANEOUS ABORTION)

A miscarriage is the ending of a pregnancy before 20 weeks. It may happen to one in five pregnancies. Most miscarriages occur in the first 12 weeks, often before the woman has realized she is pregnant, and usually because the fetus is not developing normally. Bleeding from the vagina is usually the first sign. Call your doctor immediately and lie down. If you are Rh negative, Rhogam should be administered after the miscarriage.

Threatened abortion

A small amount of bleeding may not be predictive of a miscarriage. Your doctor will probably recommend bed rest, the bleeding may stop, and if you take it easy for a few days, the pregnancy may proceed without any increased risk of abnormality in the baby. You may be given another pregnancy test or an ultrasound scan (see page 37) to confirm that all is well.

Incomplete abortion (miscarriage)

If the bleeding is heavy and you are in pain, it probably means that the baby was not developing normally. You may have to go into the hospital for a D & C, dilation and curettage, during which your womb is cleaned out.

Your feelings

Even if you miscarry early in pregnancy, you will feel an intense sense of loss. Other people don't always understand that you feel a need to mourn your baby. Worrying about whether you can even have a normal, healthy baby is common. You may feel guilty too, though you should never blame yourself; it really isn't your fault. It's quite safe to try to get pregnant again. Some doctors suggest waiting until at least two menstrual cycles have passed. Unless you have had three or more miscarriages, there is no reason why you shouldn't have a successful pregnancy next time.

VAGINAL BLEEDING

If you notice bleeding from your vagina, call your doctor without delay and go lie down. Before 20 weeks of pregnancy, it can be a sign of an impending miscarriage. After 20 weeks, it may mean that the placenta is bleeding. This can happen if the placenta has started to separate from the wall of the womb (placental abruption) or if the placenta is too low in the womb and covering, or partially covering, the cervix (placenta previa).

Treatment The placenta is the baby's lifeline, so if the doctor thinks there is any risk to it, you will probably be admitted to the hospital immediately, where the position of the placenta can be checked. You may then stay in the hospital until after the birth. If you have lost a lot of blood, you may be given a blood transfusion, and the baby will probably be delivered as soon as possible, by inducing labor or by Cesarean section. If bleeding is slight and occurs several weeks before the baby is due, the doctor may wait for labor to start naturally, while observing you closely.

"SMALL FOR DATE" BABIES

A baby who doesn't grow properly in the womb and is small at birth is called a "small for date" baby. This is not a premature baby and it may happen because the expectant mother smokes or eats a poor diet or because the placenta isn't working properly. (A general medical condition, such as underlying hypertension or a viral infection, may also be the cause.)

Treatment If tests during pregnancy show your baby is small, you will be monitored very closely to check his health and to watch the flow of blood to the placenta. If the baby stops growing or appears to be distressed in any way, he will be delivered early either by inducing labor or Cesarean birth (see pages 66 and 67).

TWINS

Your pregnancy and labor will progress normally, although you will have two second stages in labor, and you may go into labor prematurely. There is a greater likelihood of complications, such as anemia, preeclampsia, and the babies lying abnormally in the womb. You may also find that all the common disorders of pregnancy are exaggerated, especially in the last few months.

Treatment Regular prenatal visits are essential if you are expecting twins, so that any complications can be spotted immediately. A multiple pregnancy puts great strain on your body so watch your posture and rest as much as possible, especially in the last few weeks. To avoid digestion problems, eat small amounts of fresh, unprocessed food at frequent intervals.

Twins You may find this position comfortable to rest in.

COMMON COMPLAINTS

You may suffer from a variety of discomforts in pregnancy that unnerve and exasperate you, but your aches and pains are probably perfectly normal. Many are caused by hormonal changes, or because your body is under extra pressure. A few symptoms, however, should be taken more seriously. Call the doctor if you have any of the signs listed in the box on page 38.

■ COMPLAINT ■	■ SYMPTOMS ■	■ WHAT TO DO ■
Bleeding gums The gums become softer and more easily injured in pregnancy. They may be inflamed, allowing plaque to collect at the base of the teeth. This can lead to gum disease and tooth decay.	Bleeding from the gums, especially after brushing your teeth.	▲ Brush and floss your teeth thoroughly after eating. ▲ See your dentist—but only have X rays if it is absolutely essential.
Breathlessness The growing baby puts pressure on the diaphragm and prevents you from breathing freely. The problem is often relieved about a month before the birth, when the baby's head descends into the pelvis. Breathlessness can also be caused by anemia.	Feeling breathless when you exert yourself, or even when you talk.	▲ Rest as much as possible. ▲ Try crouching if there's no chair around and you feel breathless. ▲ At night, use an extra pillow. ▲ If the problem is severe, consult your doctor or midwife.
Constipation The pregnancy hormone progesterone relaxes the muscles of the intestine, which slows down bowel movements, making you more likely to become constipated.	Passing hard, dry stools at less frequent intervals than usual.	▲ Eat plenty of high-fiber foods and drink lots of water. Go to the bathroom often. ▲ Exercise regularly. ▲ Take any prescribed iron supplements on a full stomach, with plenty of fluid. ▲ See your doctor if the problem persists. Avoid laxatives.
Muscle cramps Cause is unknown.	Painful contractions of muscles, usually in the calves and the feet, and often at night. Commonly started by a leg stretch with the toes pointed down.	▲ Massage the affected calf or foot. ▲ Be sure you are taking in enough calcium and phosphorus. ▲ Walk around once the pain has eased to improve your circulation. ▲ Stretch calf muscles while pushing against a wall.
Feeling faint Oxygen to the brain may be altered during pregnancy.	Feeling dizzy and unstable. Needing to sit or lie down.	▲ Try not to stand still for too long. ▲ If you feel faint, sit down and put your head between your knees. ▲ Get up slowly from a hot bath, or when sitting or lying down. Turn to one side first when you are getting up after lying on your back. ▲ Be sure you are drinking enough water and other fluids.

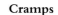

Breathlessness
 Crouching helps if you suddenly feel out of breath halfway up the stairs. Hold on to the banister.

Cramps
 Pull your foot up toward you with your hand, and massage the calf vigorously, to help relieve painful cramps.

Backache see page 44
 Skin pigmentation see page 21

■ COMPLAINT ■	■ SYMPTOMS ■	■ WHAT TO DO ■
Frequent urination Caused by the womb pressing on the bladder. The problem is often relieved in the middle months of pregnancy.	You need to urinate often.	▲ If you find yourself getting up in the night to go to the bathroom, try drinking less in the evenings. ▲ See your doctor if you feel any pain because you could have an infection.
Heartburn The valve at the entrance to your stomach relaxes in pregnancy because of hormonal changes, so stomach acid passes back into the esophagus (the tube leading to your stomach).	A strong burning pain in the center of the chest.	▲ Avoid large meals, highly spiced or fried foods. ▲ At night, use extra pillows to raise your head. ▲ See your doctor, who may advise medication to treat stomach acidity.
Leaking urine Caused by weak pelvic floor muscles (see page 45), and the growing baby pressing on your bladder.	Leakage of urine whenever you run, cough, sneeze, or laugh.	▲ Urinate often. ▲ Practice pelvic floor exercises regularly. ▲ Avoid heavy lifting, and try to avoid becoming constipated.
Morning sickness One of the first signs of pregnancy, nausea is usually worse in the morning, but it can occur at any time of the day. It usually disappears after week 12, but may continue throughout the pregnancy.	Feeling sick, often at the smell of certain foods or cigarette smoke. Most women find there is a particular time of day when this happens.	▲ Try eating small, frequent meals throughout the day. ▲ Avoid foods and smells that make you feel sick. ▲ Consult your doctor, who may prescribe safe medication to maintain nutrition.
Hemorrhoids Pressure from the baby's head causes swollen veins around the anus. Straining to empty the bowels will make the problem worse. Mild hemorrhoids usually disappear, without treatment, after the baby is born.	Itching, soreness, and possibly pain or bleeding when you empty your bowels.	▲ Avoid becoming constipated. ▲ Try not to stand for long periods. ▲ An ice pack held against the hemorrhoids may ease itching. ▲ If hemorrhoids persist, tell the doctor or midwife. He or she may recommend an ointment.
Rash Usually occurs in women who are overweight and who perspire freely. Can be caused by hormonal changes.	Red rash, which usually develops in sweaty skin folds under the breasts or in the groin.	▲ Wash and dry these areas often. Use unperfumed soap. ▲ Expose area to air. ▲ Wear loose cotton clothes.
Sleeping difficulty You may have a problem because the baby is kicking, you have to go to the bathroom frequently, or the sheer size of your baby makes it difficult to get comfortable in bed.	Having trouble going to sleep in the first place, and finding it hard to get to sleep after waking. Some women find they have very frightening dreams about the birth or the baby. Don't worry about dreams; they do not reflect what will happen.	▲ Reading, gentle relaxation exercises, or a warm bath before bedtime may help. ▲ Experiment with extra pillows. If you sleep on your side, put a pillow under your top thigh.

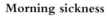

Heartburn and sleeplessness
This piled-up arrangement of pillows is comfortable if you suffer from heartburn, or are unable to sleep.

Morning sickness
To counteract nausea, try eating dry crackers, toast, or fruit. Eliminate fried or highly seasoned foods and drink lots of water. Ginger snaps or ginger ale may be helpful.

■ COMPLAINT ■	■ SYMPTOMS ■	■ WHAT TO DO ■
Stretch marks These form if your skin stretches beyond its normal elasticity. Excess weight gain can also cause them. The marks may disappear, but are more likely to fade to thin silvery streaks.	Red marks that sometimes appear on the skin of the thighs, stomach, or breasts during pregnancy.	▲ Try not to put on weight too rapidly. ▲ Rubbing moisturizer into the skin may feel cool and soothing, although creams and ointments won't prevent or heal stretch marks.
Sweating This is caused by hormonal changes, and because blood flow to the skin increases in pregnancy.	Perspiring after very little exertion, or waking up in the night feeling hot and sweaty.	▲ Wear loose cotton clothes. Avoid man-made materials. ▲ Drink plenty of water. ▲ Open a window at night.
Swollen ankles and fingers Some swelling (edema) is normal in pregnancy, because the body holds extra water. This is usually no cause for concern.	Slight swelling in the ankles, especially in hot weather and at the end of the day. This shouldn't cause pain or discomfort.	▲ Rest often with your feet up. ▲ Drink plenty of fluids and reduce salt intake. ▲ See your doctor or midwife. Marked swelling could be a warning sign of preeclampsia (see page 38). ▲ Watch your weight.
Yeast infections Hormonal changes during pregnancy increase the chances of developing yeast infections. Washing with some soaps can worsen the problem.	A thick white curd-like vaginal discharge and severe itching. There may also be soreness and pain when you urinate.	▲ Keep the genital area as dry as possible. ▲ Wear only cotton or cotton-crotch underpants. ▲ Avoid panty hose, tight jeans, and vaginal deodorants. ▲ See your doctor, who may be able to advise treatment.
Tiredness This is caused by the extra demands that pregnancy makes on your body, and may also be the result of worry.	Feeling weary, and wanting to sleep in the day. Needing to sleep longer at night.	▲ Rest as much as possible and practice relaxation exercises. ▲ Go to bed earlier. ▲ Don't overexert yourself.
Vaginal discharge You may notice some increase in the amount of mucus produced by the vagina because of the hormonal changes during pregnancy.	Slight increase in clear or white discharge, without soreness or pain.	▲ Avoid vaginal deodorants and perfumed soap products. ▲ See your doctor if you have any itching, soreness, colored, or foul-smelling discharge.
Varicose veins You are more likely to develop these in a second or third pregnancy, if you are overweight, or they run in your family. Standing for too long, or sitting cross-legged, can worsen them.	Aching legs; the veins in the calves and the thighs become painful and swollen.	▲ Rest often with your feet up. Try raising the foot of your bed with pillows under the mattress. ▲ Support stockings may help. Put them on before getting up in the morning. Be sure the stockings do not constrict the lower legs. ▲ Exercise your feet.

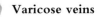

Swollen ankles and varicose veins
Gently circle your ankles and feet to improve circulation.

Varicose veins
Rest with your feet well elevated on at least two cushions if you suffer from this problem. Tuck another cushion into the small of your back.

KEEPING FIT AND RELAXED

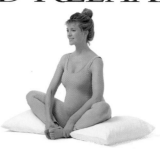

Pregnancy, labor, and birth will place great demands on your body, so the more you can prepare yourself physically, the better you will feel. You will also find it easier to get back into shape when the baby is born. Learning relaxation exercises is important too; they will help you calm down and cope far more effectively in labor, and they are invaluable for relieving stress and for increasing blood flow to the placenta. Even if you normally hate the idea of exercise, try the exercises on the following pages. They are specially designed to make your joints and muscles more supple, in preparation for labor and birth. You can begin special prenatal exercises as soon as the pregnancy is confirmed, or earlier if you wish. Practice at home or sign up for an exercise class designed for expectant mothers. Don't worry though if you are well into pregnancy before you begin; it's never too late to start. Build up gradually until you are exercising for about 20 minutes every day.

EXERCISING SENSIBLY

If you're athletic and have always been so, pregnancy shouldn't slow you down. But there are cautions:

■ Pregnancy is not a time to launch into a fitness blitz; just continue with what your body is used to. If you want to keep on going to your dance or exercise class, make sure the teacher knows you are pregnant.

■ Don't exercise to the point where you feel very tired or out of breath.

■ Be sure not to become overheated or dehydrated. Discuss guidelines with your doctor.

■ Discuss potentially hazardous sports, such as skiing, water-skiing, and riding, with your doctor or midwife.

■ Be extra careful in the first and last weeks of pregnancy, because you may overstretch ligaments.

Swimming
This is excellent and perfectly safe, since the water supports your body.

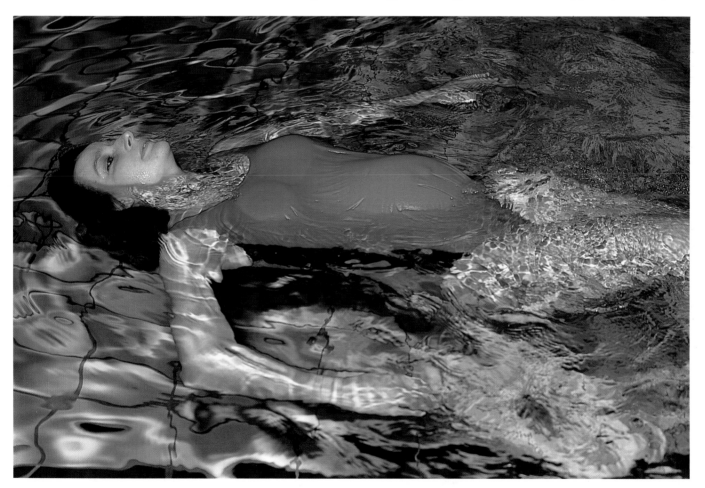

TAKING CARE OF YOUR BODY

DURING PREGNANCY, your posture can make a real difference in your overall health. You're far more likely to suffer from backache because the weight of the baby pulls you forward, and you'll have a tendency to lean slightly backward to compensate. This strains the muscles of the lower back and pelvis, especially toward the end of pregnancy.

Be aware of your body, whatever you are doing. Avoid heavy lifting, and try to keep your back straight whenever possible. Wear low heels; high heels throw your weight even further forward.

PROTECTING YOUR BACK

To avoid back trouble, it's equally important to be aware of how you use your body when doing everyday activities such as gardening, lifting a child, or carrying heavy bags. The hormones of pregnancy stretch and soften the muscles of the lower back, so these are more easily strained if you bend over, get up too suddenly, or lift something awkwardly or in the wrong way.

Lower yourself
Do as much as you can at floor level, kneeling down to garden, clean, make a bed, or dress a child, instead of bending over.

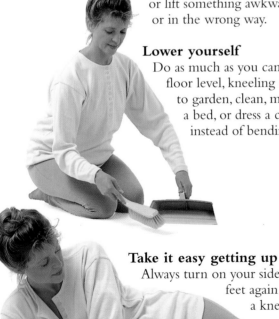

Take it easy getting up
Always turn on your side when getting up and on your feet again after lying down. Move into a kneeling position. Use your thigh strength to push yourself up; keep your back straight.

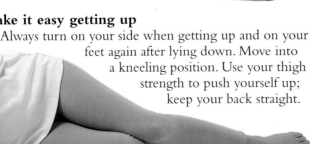

Drop *your shoulders and keep them back*

Hold *your back straight*

Tuck in *your bottom*

Lift *your chest and ribs*

Tighten *your stomach muscles*

Bend *your knees slightly*

Stand *with your feet a little way apart*

STANDING TALL
Take a good look at the way you normally stand in front of a full-length mirror. Straighten your back, so that the weight of the baby is centered and supported by your thighs, buttocks, and stomach muscles. This will help prevent backache, and tone up your abdominal muscles, making it easier for you to regain your figure after the birth.

Poor posture
This is common during pregnancy. As the baby grows, its weight throws you off-balance, so you may overarch your back and thrust your abdomen forward.

Lifting and carrying
When lifting an object, bend your knees and keep your back as straight as possible, bringing the object close in to your body. Try not to lift something heavy from up high, because you may lose your balance. If you're carrying heavy bags, divide the weight equally on each side.

Keep *your back straight*

Position *your weight around the object, and face it squarely*

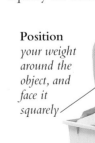

THE PELVIC FLOOR

THIS IS A HAMMOCK of muscles that supports the bowel, bladder, and womb. During pregnancy, the muscles go soft and stretchy, and this, together with the weight of the baby pushing down, weakens them, making you feel heavy and uncomfortable. You may also leak a little urine whenever you run, sneeze, cough, or laugh. To avoid these problems, it's essential to strengthen the pelvic floor.

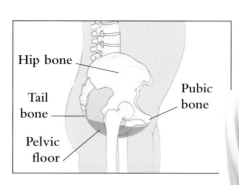

The pelvic floor
This forms part of the pelvis, a bony area, which cradles and protects the baby in the womb. The baby has to pass through it at birth.

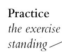

Practice the exercise standing

Practice the exercise sitting

DO THIS WHEN:
- waiting for a bus or train
- ironing or cooking
- watching TV
- having intercourse
- you have *emptied* your bladder.

STRENGTHENING THE PELVIC FLOOR
Practice this exercise at least three or four times a day: you can do it anytime, anywhere—lying down, sitting, or standing. You will find it useful in the second stage of labor. Knowing how to relax the muscles reduces the risk of a tear, because you can ease the passage of the baby through the pelvis without pushing too fast or frantically.

Lie on your back, with your knees bent and your feet flat on the floor. Now tighten the muscles, squeezing as if stopping a stream of urine. Imagine you are trying to pull something into your vagina, drawing it in slightly, then pausing, then pulling, until you can go no further. Hold for a moment, then let go gradually. Repeat ten times.

PELVIC TILT

THIS EXERCISE helps you move the pelvis with ease, which is good preparation for labor. It also strengthens the stomach muscles and makes the back more flexible. It is especially helpful if you suffer from backache, and when you are in this all-fours position, your partner can rub the base of your back to soothe any pain. You can do the tilt in any position; remember to keep your shoulders still.

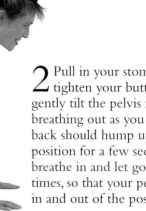

1 Kneel on the floor on your hands and knees. Make sure that your back is flat. (At first it helps to use a mirror to check this.)

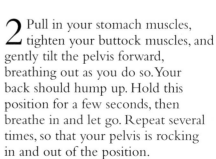

2 Pull in your stomach muscles, tighten your buttock muscles, and gently tilt the pelvis forward, breathing out as you do so. Your back should hump up. Hold this position for a few seconds, then breathe in and let go. Repeat several times, so that your pelvis is rocking in and out of the position.

DO THIS WHEN:
- lying on your back
- standing
- sitting
- kneeling
- listening to music.

TAILOR SITTING

THIS STRENGTHENS the back and makes your thighs and pelvis more flexible. It also improves blood flow in the lower part of the body, and will encourage your legs to fall apart naturally at birth. The main position below is easier than it looks, because your body is more supple in pregnancy.

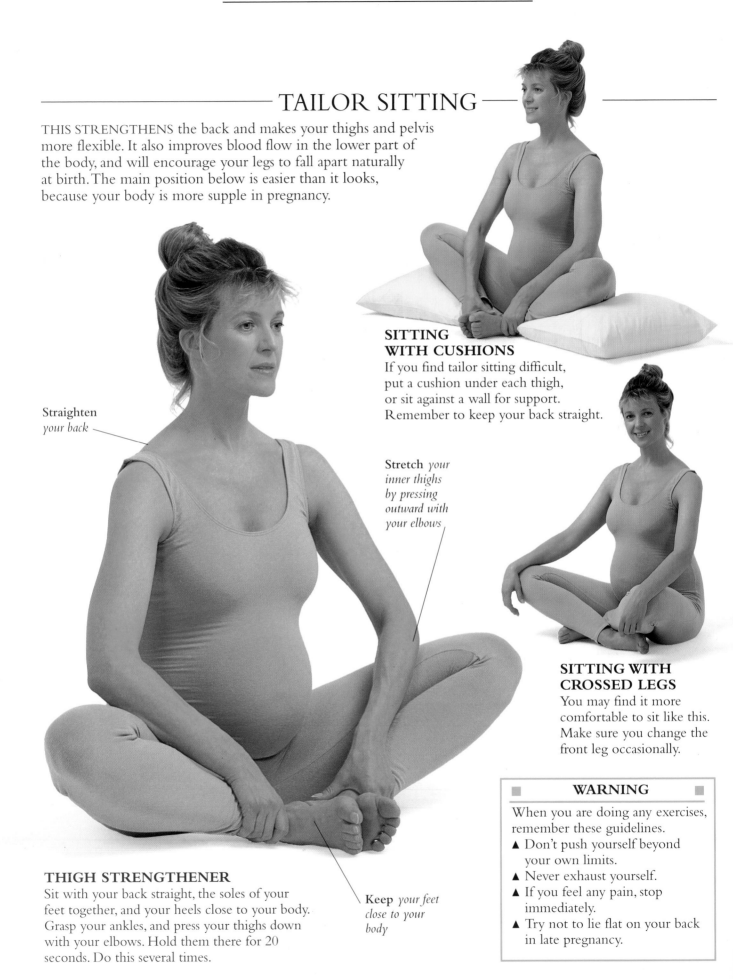

Straighten *your back*

Stretch *your inner thighs by pressing outward with your elbows*

SITTING WITH CUSHIONS

If you find tailor sitting difficult, put a cushion under each thigh, or sit against a wall for support. Remember to keep your back straight.

SITTING WITH CROSSED LEGS

You may find it more comfortable to sit like this. Make sure you change the front leg occasionally.

THIGH STRENGTHENER

Sit with your back straight, the soles of your feet together, and your heels close to your body. Grasp your ankles, and press your thighs down with your elbows. Hold them there for 20 seconds. Do this several times.

Keep *your feet close to your body*

■ WARNING ■

When you are doing any exercises, remember these guidelines.
▲ Don't push yourself beyond your own limits.
▲ Never exhaust yourself.
▲ If you feel any pain, stop immediately.
▲ Try not to lie flat on your back in late pregnancy.

SQUATTING

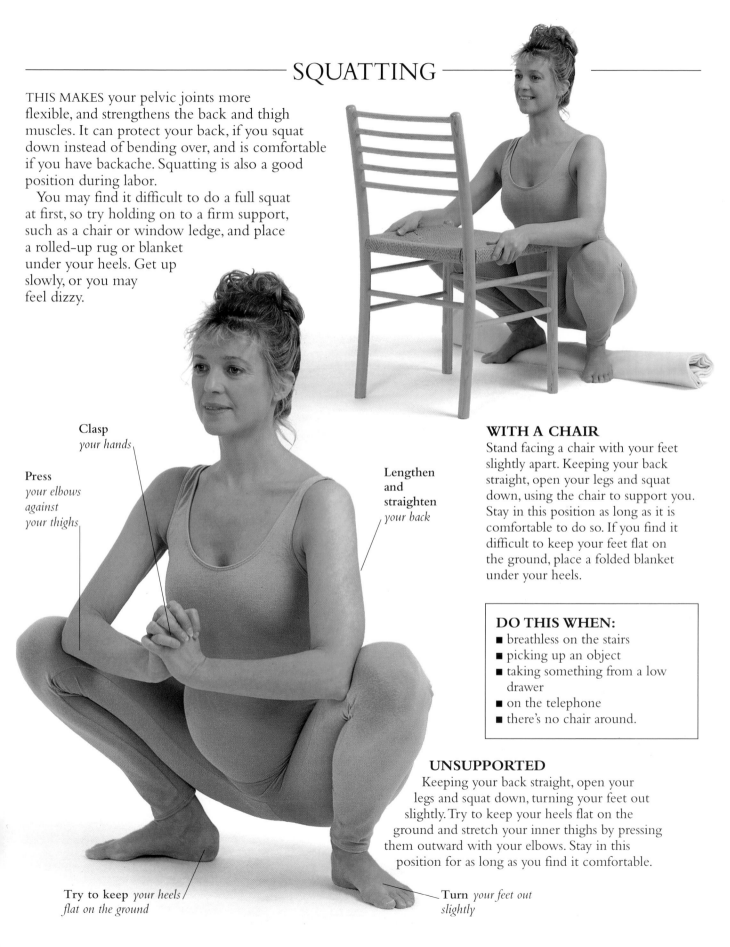

THIS MAKES your pelvic joints more flexible, and strengthens the back and thigh muscles. It can protect your back, if you squat down instead of bending over, and is comfortable if you have backache. Squatting is also a good position during labor.

You may find it difficult to do a full squat at first, so try holding on to a firm support, such as a chair or window ledge, and place a rolled-up rug or blanket under your heels. Get up slowly, or you may feel dizzy.

Clasp *your hands*

Press *your elbows against your thighs*

Lengthen and straighten *your back*

Try to keep *your heels flat on the ground*

Turn *your feet out slightly*

WITH A CHAIR
Stand facing a chair with your feet slightly apart. Keeping your back straight, open your legs and squat down, using the chair to support you. Stay in this position as long as it is comfortable to do so. If you find it difficult to keep your feet flat on the ground, place a folded blanket under your heels.

DO THIS WHEN:
- breathless on the stairs
- picking up an object
- taking something from a low drawer
- on the telephone
- there's no chair around.

UNSUPPORTED
Keeping your back straight, open your legs and squat down, turning your feet out slightly. Try to keep your heels flat on the ground and stretch your inner thighs by pressing them outward with your elbows. Stay in this position for as long as you find it comfortable.

RELAXATION AND BREATHING

THESE EXERCISES are among the most useful you can learn. They are invaluable during labor, when knowing how to breathe properly and relax the muscles of your body will help you cope with contractions and save vital energy. Practice them regularly so that they become a natural response during labor. Relaxation will also help you unwind at any time you feel tense or anxious.

HOW TO RELAX
Practice these exercises in a warm room where you won't be disturbed. Later you should find it easy to relax anywhere.

Relax your body
Lie on your back, fully propped up by pillows, or on your side, with one leg bent and supported on cushions. Now tense and relax the muscles of each part of your body in turn, starting with the toes and working upward. After doing this for eight to ten minutes, let your body go limp. Try to feel heavy, as though you are sinking into the floor. Now tighten your forehead, then relax. Try to tighten any muscle in the body without tightening the forehead.

Lying on your side
Try lying on your side with one leg bent and supported on cushions. You will be more comfortable and this position is better for your baby as it raises placental blood flow. Don't place too many pillows under your head, because this is bad for your spine.

WARNING

Don't lie flat on your back in the late stages of pregnancy. You can restrict the flow of oxygen to the baby in this position, and you yourself may feel faint.

Tilt *your head from side to side, then hold still*

Screw up *your eyes, open, then close*

Pull in *your stomach muscles, then relax*

Arch *the small of your back, then let go*

Clench *your hands, then open*

Squeeze *your buttock muscles, then let go*

BREATHING FOR LABOR

Practice the different levels of breathing with a partner or friend, so that you are relaxed and calm during labor, and can even control your body during contractions.

Light breathing

This level of breathing will help you at the height of a contraction. Breathe in and out of your mouth, taking air into the upper part of your lungs only. A partner or friend should put her hands on your shoulder blades and feel them move. Practice making the breaths lighter and lighter, but take an occasional deeper breath when you need one.

Deep breathing

This has a calming effect, helpful at the beginning and end of contractions. Sit comfortably and as relaxed as possible. Breathe in deeply through the nose, right to the bottom of your lungs. Your partner or friend should place his or her hands just above your waistline and feel your ribcage move. Now, concentrate on breathing slowly and gently out. Let the next in-breath follow naturally.

Panting

After the first stage of labor, you will want to push, even though the cervix may not be fully opened. You can resist this by taking two short breaths, and then blowing a longer breath out: say "huff, huff, blow" to yourself.

Tighten *your thigh muscles, then let the tension go*

Bend *your feet at the ankles, then let go*

Relax your mind

While relaxing your body, try to calm and empty your mind. Breathe slowly and evenly, sighing each breath out gently. Do not breathe too hard.

Alternatively, repeat a word or sound silently to yourself, or concentrate on some pleasant or peaceful image. Try not to follow any thoughts that arise.

Tense *your calf muscles, then relax*

Curl *your toes, then relax*

EATING FOR A HEALTHY BABY

A baby has only one source of food—you. During pregnancy, more than at any other time, it is essential that you have as varied and balanced a diet as possible. You do not need to plan this specially, nor do you have to eat for two. You only need to eat 300 extra calories a day during pregnancy. All you have to do is eat a variety of fresh, unprocessed foods from the selection below, to ensure that you get all the nutrients you need. Once you are, or know you want to become, pregnant, think about how many healthy foods you eat regularly. Do you eat or drink ánything that might harm the baby? Increase your intake of raw vegetables and fresh fruit, and cut down on sugary, salty, and processed foods.

ESSENTIAL NUTRIENTS

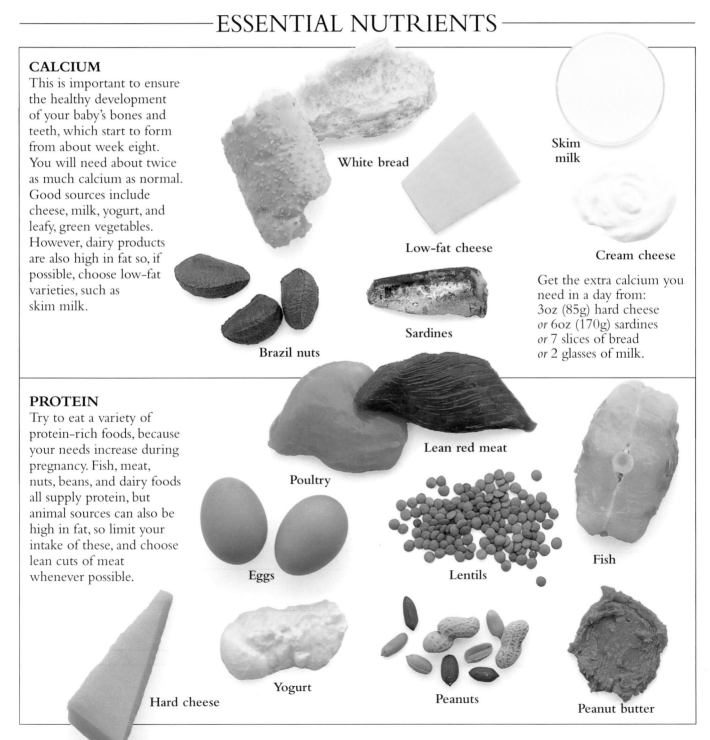

CALCIUM

This is important to ensure the healthy development of your baby's bones and teeth, which start to form from about week eight. You will need about twice as much calcium as normal. Good sources include cheese, milk, yogurt, and leafy, green vegetables. However, dairy products are also high in fat so, if possible, choose low-fat varieties, such as skim milk.

White bread

Low-fat cheese

Skim milk

Cream cheese

Brazil nuts

Sardines

Get the extra calcium you need in a day from:
3oz (85g) hard cheese
or 6oz (170g) sardines
or 7 slices of bread
or 2 glasses of milk.

PROTEIN

Try to eat a variety of protein-rich foods, because your needs increase during pregnancy. Fish, meat, nuts, beans, and dairy foods all supply protein, but animal sources can also be high in fat, so limit your intake of these, and choose lean cuts of meat whenever possible.

Lean red meat

Poultry

Eggs

Lentils

Fish

Hard cheese

Yogurt

Peanuts

Peanut butter

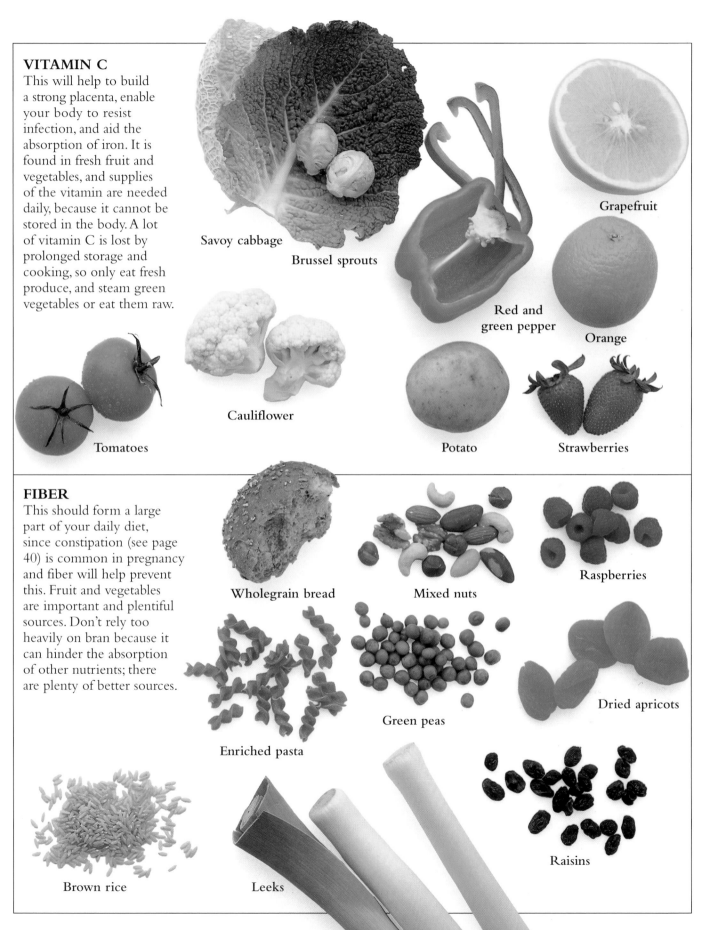

VITAMIN C

This will help to build a strong placenta, enable your body to resist infection, and aid the absorption of iron. It is found in fresh fruit and vegetables, and supplies of the vitamin are needed daily, because it cannot be stored in the body. A lot of vitamin C is lost by prolonged storage and cooking, so only eat fresh produce, and steam green vegetables or eat them raw.

Savoy cabbage

Brussel sprouts

Grapefruit

Red and green pepper

Orange

Cauliflower

Tomatoes

Potato

Strawberries

FIBER

This should form a large part of your daily diet, since constipation (see page 40) is common in pregnancy and fiber will help prevent this. Fruit and vegetables are important and plentiful sources. Don't rely too heavily on bran because it can hinder the absorption of other nutrients; there are plenty of better sources.

Wholegrain bread

Mixed nuts

Raspberries

Enriched pasta

Green peas

Dried apricots

Brown rice

Leeks

Raisins

FOLIC ACID

This is needed for the development of the baby's central nervous system, especially in the first few weeks. The body cannot store this nutrient, and in pregnancy excretes several times the normal amount, so it's essential to have a daily supply. Fresh dark green, leafy vegetables are a good source of folic acid, but steam or eat them raw because a lot of the vitamin is destroyed by cooking.

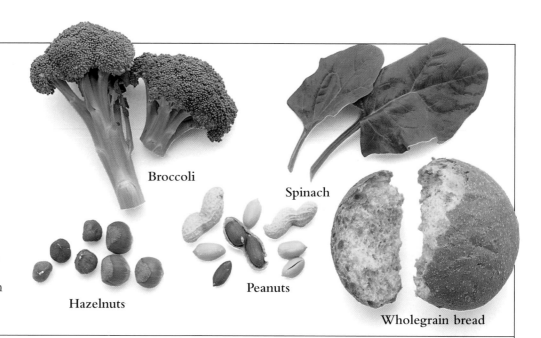

Broccoli

Spinach

Hazelnuts

Peanuts

Wholegrain bread

IRON

The baby will need to build up stores of iron for after the birth, and the extra blood your body produces needs iron to carry oxygen. Iron from animal sources is absorbed more easily than that from foods such as beans and dried fruit, so if you do not eat meat, combine iron-rich foods with those rich in vitamin C to maximize absorption. Although liver is a good source of iron, it also contains high levels of vitamin A. Because excess vitamin A may damage the developing baby, liver or liver products should not be eaten during pregnancy.

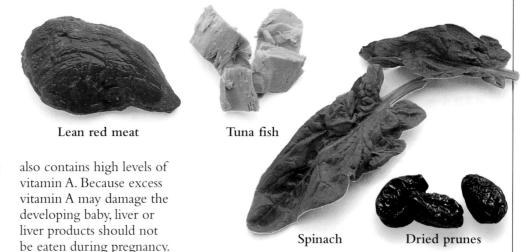

Lean red meat

Tuna fish

Spinach

Dried prunes

VEGETARIAN DIET

If you eat a variety of protein-rich foods and fresh fruit and vegetables every day, you should provide the baby with all that he needs. The only nutrients you may lack are iron and vitamin B12; the body has great difficulty absorbing iron that comes from plant sources, so you may be given supplements of the mineral to compensate. If you are vegan, and don't eat dairy foods, you may also be prescribed calcium, and vitamins D and B12.

SALT

Most people have far too much salt in their diet. During pregnancy, it is even more important to reduce the amount of salt you eat, because too much can exacerbate swelling.

FLUID

This is essential during pregnancy for keeping your kidneys healthy and avoiding constipation. Water is best. You should drink at least 2 quarts (about 8 glasses) of water a day.

TOP FOODS

These foods are excellent sources of at least one nutrient. Try to eat some of them every day:
■ Cheese, milk, yogurt: calcium, protein.
■ Dark green, leafy vegetables: vitamin C, fiber, folic acid.
■ Lean red meat: protein, iron.
■ Oranges: vitamin C, fiber.
■ Poultry: protein, iron.
■ Raisins and prunes: iron.
■ Fish such as flounder, tuna, or salmon: protein.
■ Wholegrain bread: protein, fiber, folic acid.
■ Enriched pasta and brown rice: fiber.

TAKING SUPPLEMENTS

Folic acid supplements are recommended in the first three months. Iron supplements may be prescribed if you are anemic, and some doctors also recommend them routinely. Try to eat a varied diet with lots of fresh foods, and follow any advice your doctor may have on vitamin supplements.

PROTECTING YOUR BABY

ALMOST EVERYTHING you consume during your pregnancy—both good and bad—can make its way to your baby via the placenta

PROCESSED FOODS

Avoid processed convenience foods, such as canned foods and packet mixes. Processed foods often have sugar and salt added, and they may contain a lot of fat, as well as preservatives, flavorings, and colorings. Read labels carefully and choose additive-free products.

Eat *a variety of fresh, unprocessed foods*

PREPARED FOODS

Avoid hot cafeteria foods, pre-cooked supermarket meals, and ready to eat poultry (unless prepared piping hot). These foods may contain bacteria that can be passed to the baby and put his life at risk.

CHEESE

Soft matured cheese, such as Brie, made from both pasteurized and un-pasteurized milk products can be harmful, so it's best to avoid them.

Unpasteurized goat's milk and goat's milk products should be avoided too, because they may contain a parasite called toxoplasma.

COFFEE, TEA, AND HOT CHOCOLATE

Reduce your intake to no more than one cup of caffeine-containing drinks a day. Cut them out altogether, if possible, and drink plenty of mineral water instead.

HERBAL TEAS

Certain herbal teas have pharmaceutical effects that can be harmful during pregnancy. Limit your intake to fruit-flavored noncaffeinated teas, such as raspberry and lemon.

SUGAR

Sugary foods, such as cakes, cookies, candies, sodas, and cola drinks, are low in essential nutrients, and can cause excess weight gain. Get your energy from starchy carbohydrates, such as whole-grain bread, and cut down on sweet things. Although aspartame (Nutrasweet) has no proven harmful effects, it is advisable to use it in moderation.

CRAVINGS

It's common in pregnancy to find that you suddenly develop a taste for certain foods, such as pickled onions or ice cream. If you long for a particular food, go ahead and indulge yourself within reason, provided it isn't fattening and doesn't cause indigestion.

DON'T DRINK YOUR CALORIES

Two quarts of water plus one quart of milk provide all the fluids a pregnant woman needs. Don't drink your calories in, for example, high-calorie fruit juices.

ALTERNATIVES TO ALCOHOL

Any alcohol that you drink during pregnancy is passed through the placenta into your baby's bloodstream, and can be harmful. So it's best to cut out alcohol altogether and make your own soft drinks using pure, additive-free ingredients.

Even beers and wines that claim to be alcohol free or low in alcohol may not necessarily be free from additives and chemicals that may harm your baby. Check with your obstetrician before regularly including them in your diet.

Sparkling orange Orange juice diluted with sparkling water or club soda is a simple but refreshing drink. Remember that fruit juices are very high in calories, and it is best to eat the natural fruit instead.

Banana milkshake This tastes delicious and is high in calcium and protein. Make it by mixing together a banana and 2 cups of milk. A blender or food processor works best.

PRACTICAL PREPARATIONS

About a month before your delivery date, make sure that everything is ready for your baby's homecoming. For instance, go food shopping and start planning for meals and other essentials that will make your life easier after the birth. It's not too soon to pack for your trip to the hospital or birthing center either. Put your open suitcase on the floor of your bedroom and start assembling the things you'll want when you are away from home. Some hospitals or doctors offer mothers-to-be a list of what to bring. Buy or borrow the equipment for your new baby.

HELPFUL THINGS FOR LABOR

ALL THE ITEMS below may be useful in labor and immediately after birth. Don't put them into your suitcase. Pack them separately, because you will want them during labor.

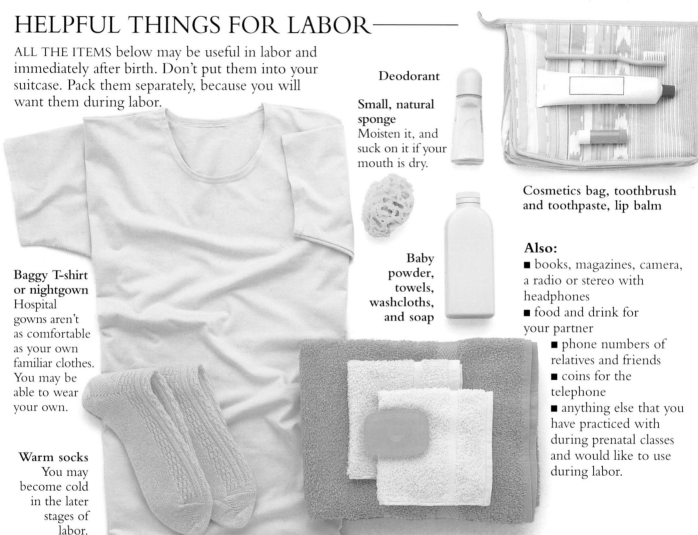

Deodorant

Small, natural sponge
Moisten it, and suck on it if your mouth is dry.

Cosmetics bag, toothbrush and toothpaste, lip balm

Baby powder, towels, washcloths, and soap

Also:
- books, magazines, camera, a radio or stereo with headphones
- food and drink for your partner
- phone numbers of relatives and friends
- coins for the telephone
- anything else that you have practiced with during prenatal classes and would like to use during labor.

Baggy T-shirt or nightgown
Hospital gowns aren't as comfortable as your own familiar clothes. You may be able to wear your own.

Warm socks
You may become cold in the later stages of labor.

GOING TO THE HOSPITAL WHEN YOU ARE IN LABOR
It's always a good idea to make trial runs to the hospital or birthing center long before you feel those first pains of labor. When you and your partner are under the stress of imminent childbirth or you are counting contractions, you certainly don't want to get lost or stuck in unfamiliar territory. Knowing which door to enter when you arrive at the hospital and where you'll be headed inside can be a relief. Ask about the preliminary papers you'll need to fill out. And, if you'll be using a big city hospital, you ought to have a good idea of what rush hour traffic conditions might be like.

In the last few weeks of pregnancy, make sure your car always has enough gas to get you there. Put money or tokens for road tolls or emergency calls in your car ahead of time.

If you aren't going to be driving in your own car, keep the name and phone number of a 24-hour taxi service posted by the telephone. Or if someone has volunteered to drive you to the hospital, make sure that they will be expecting a call and will be able to respond to it instantly at any hour of the day or night. Post their phone number in a handy location by your telephone where you can find it quickly and easily.

FOR AFTER THE BIRTH

THIS CHECKLIST will help you as you pack; if you go into labor unexpectedly and haven't packed your suitcase, these are the items your partner should assemble. The hospital will probably provide all the essentials for the baby during your stay.

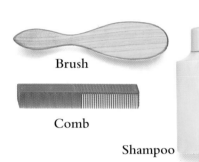

Brush

Comb

Shampoo

Breast pads
Slip these inside your bra to absorb leaking milk. Shaped ones are best.

Nipple cream
This relieves sore nipples.

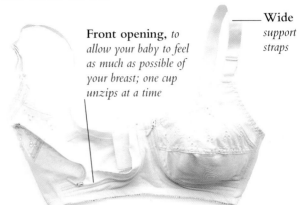

Front opening, *to allow your baby to feel as much as possible of your breast; one cup unzips at a time*

Wide *support straps*

Two or three nursing bras

Also:
■ tissues
■ hairdryer
■ note paper and pen
■ hand mirror for freshening up at bedside.

Two boxes of belt-free sanitary pads
One box should be super-absorbent for the first few days; the hospital may supply these

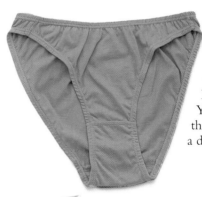

Six pairs of underpants
Buy cotton pants. You may go through several pairs a day so pack a pile.

Two to three machine-washable nightgowns and a bathrobe
These should be made of cotton because it is the most comfortable fiber.

Front opening, *with buttons that undo well below the breasts, if breast-feeding*

Low-heeled slippers

COMING HOME
Choose an outfit for your partner to bring when it's time for you to be discharged. Don't pick anything too tight fitting; you will not be back to your pre-pregnancy size. The baby needs clothes for coming home, too, so set aside:
■ two diapers, a pin, and waterproof pants if you're not using disposables (most hospitals provide diapers, so check first)
■ undershirt
■ stretchsuit or nightgown
■ sweater and hat
■ receiving blanket or a warm blanket for cold weather.

LABOR AND BIRTH

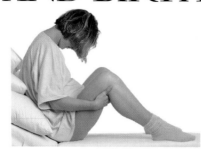

At last the long weeks of waiting are over. Labor and delivery are the culmination of your pregnancy, and the moment when you first see your baby is now only a matter of hours away. You may be excited, yet apprehensive about how well your labor will go. If you have prepared yourself and understand what is happening to your body and your baby at each stage, it won't be so frightening. Stay calm and you'll save energy. The pain of labor can be intense or mild, but you should never be made to feel like a failure. There are no perfect standards for having a baby, so even as you practice your breathing and relaxation techniques, don't be too hard on yourself. This is not a race you are going to win or lose but a little human being you are bringing into the world.

KNOWING YOU ARE IN LABOR

EVERY WOMAN'S EXPERIENCE is different, but first-time mothers often worry that they won't recognize true labor. In late pregnancy, you may be plagued by short, irregular pains, called Braxton-Hicks contractions, and there's always the possibility of confusing these with the real thing.

SIGNS OF LABOR
A show
The plug of thick, blood-stained mucus that blocks the neck of the womb in pregnancy usually passes out of the vagina before or during early labor.
What to do The show may happen a few days before you go into labor, so wait until you start to feel regular pains in your abdomen or back, or your water breaks, before calling the doctor.

Your water breaks
The bag of fluid that surrounds the baby can break at any time during labor. It may be a sudden flood, but it's far more common to notice a trickle of fluid. If the baby's head descends into the pelvis, it may stem the tide.
What to do If your water breaks, you should go to the hospital to be examined. The doctor or midwife will check the position of the baby and the location of the umbilical cord. Meanwhile, wear a sanitary napkin.

Contractions
These may start off as a dull backache or as a feeling of indigestion, or you may have shooting pains down your thighs. As time goes by you will have contractions in your abdomen, rather like bad menstrual cramps.
What to do When the contractions seem to be regular, time them. If you think you are in labor, call the doctor. Unless contractions are coming every five minutes or are very painful, there is no need to go to the hospital immediately, especially if your water hasn't broken. A first labor usually lasts about 12 to 14 hours, and it is often better to spend several hours of this time at home. Move around gently. Try taking a shower, if your water hasn't broken. The hospital will probably suggest that you wait until the contractions are quite strong and occurring every five minutes or so before you leave home.

FALSE STARTS
Throughout pregnancy, the womb contracts. In the last weeks, these Braxton-Hicks contractions become stronger, so you may think you are in labor. However true labor contractions occur very regularly and grow stronger and more frequent, so you should be able to tell when the real thing begins.

If you are able to talk to someone through your contractions, you are not in real labor yet.

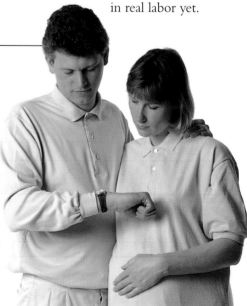

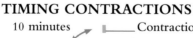

TIMING CONTRACTIONS

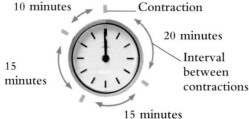

10 minutes — Contraction
20 minutes — Interval between contractions
15 minutes
15 minutes

Time contractions for an hour, noting when each one starts and ends. They should become stronger and more frequent, and last for at least 40 seconds. The diagram shows intervals between contractions in early labor.

THE FIRST STAGE

DURING THIS STAGE, the muscles of your womb contract to open up the cervix (neck of the womb) to allow the baby to pass through at birth. It usually takes an average of 10 to 12 hours for a first baby, but may take considerably longer.

Don't be surprised if at some time in the first stage you suddenly feel panic-stricken. However well prepared you are, the feeling that your body has been taken over by a process that you can't control can be frightening. Stay calm and try to go with your body. It is now that you will most appreciate having your partner or a good friend by your side, especially if they understand labor and have gone to prenatal classes.

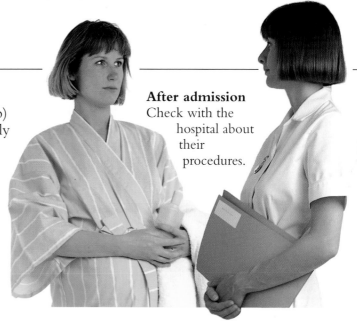

After admission
Check with the hospital about their procedures.

ADMISSION TO THE HOSPITAL

It's useful to have a partner alongside you all the way. He or she can act as a kind of intermediary between you and the medical staff, which will help when you don't feel like talking.

Once you reach the hospital, a nurse or technician will carry out several routine admission procedures.

Checking you

After you have changed into the hospital gown or the clothes you brought for the birth, the nurse may take your blood pressure, temperature, and pulse, and give you an internal examination to check how far the neck of the womb has opened. You will also be asked to give a urine sample which will be tested for traces of protein and sugar.

Checking the baby

The nurse will check the baby's position by feeling your abdomen, and she will listen to his heartbeat with an obstetric stethoscope or a special instrument (see page 65).

The nurse or doctor may also attach a machine to electronically monitor the baby's heartbeat. It will indicate how much oxygen your baby is getting during contractions.

Optional hospital routines

Some hospitals routinely administer enemas to women in labor to clear out the lower bowel in preparation for pushing when the time comes.

Another "prep" that some hospitals do is shaving the pubic area of the expectant mother.

INTERNAL EXAMINATIONS

The doctor may give you regular internal examinations to check the position of the baby and to determine how much the cervix is dilating (opening up). Ask for progress reports if you are not told. It is encouraging to find that the cervix is widening, but it may not happen at a steady rate.

The doctor may want to examine you either during or between contractions, so tell the nurse if you feel one coming. You may be asked to lie on your side, propped up with pillows. Relax as much as possible. Don't pressure yourself to be perfect. Getting through labor can be tough.

THE CERVIX IN LABOR

This is normally kept closed by a ring of muscles. Other muscles run from the cervix up and over the womb. These contract during labor, drawing the cervix into the womb, and then stretching it so it is wide enough for the baby's head to pass through.

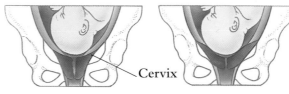

Cervix

1 The tough cervix is gradually softened by hormonal changes.

2 Gentle contractions then efface (thin) the cervix.

3 Once it is fully effaced, stronger contractions dilate it.

POSITIONS FOR THE FIRST STAGE

Try a variety of positions in the first stage. Different positions will probably be comfortable at different times. Practice these positions beforehand, so that you can follow your body's natural cues with ease.

You may find that you want to lie down during the first stage. Rest on your side, not your back, with your head and upper thigh supported by cushions.

Staying upright

During early contractions, support yourself on a nearby surface, such as a wall, chair seat, or the hospital bed. Kneel down if necessary.

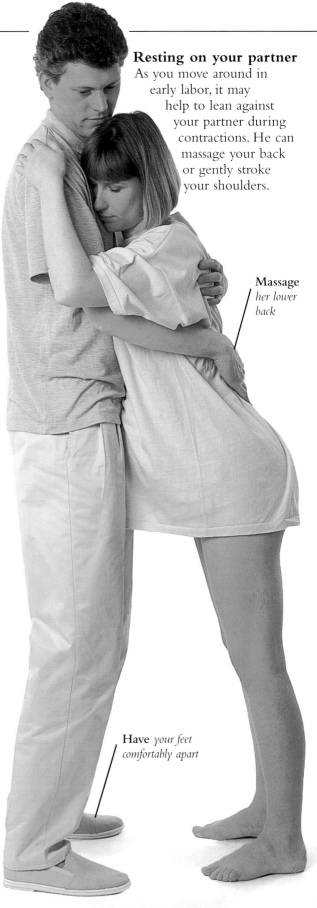

Resting on your partner
As you move around in early labor, it may help to lean against your partner during contractions. He can massage your back or gently stroke your shoulders.

Massage *her lower back*

Sitting forward

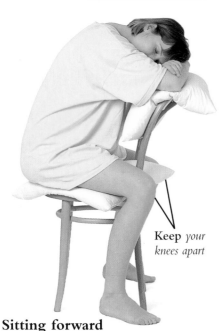

Keep *your knees apart*

Cushion the seat of a chair and sit on it, facing its back. Put a pillow over the chair back and lean on it. Rest your head on your folded arms. A "birthing ball" is a more comfortable alternative to a chair.

WHAT YOUR PARTNER CAN DO

■ During contractions, give her plenty of praise, comfort, and support.
■ Remind her of the relaxation and breathing techniques she has learned (pages 48–49).
■ Mop her brow, give her ice chips, hold her hand, massage her back, suggest a change of position, or do anything else that helps. Learn beforehand where and how she likes to be touched and massaged.
■ Act as a mediator between your partner and the hospital staff. Support her decision, for example, on pain medication.

Have *your feet comfortably apart*

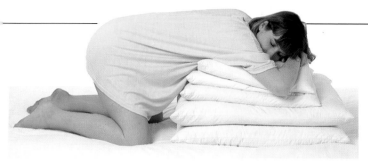

Kneeling forward
Kneel down, legs apart, and relax forward on a pile of pillows or a birthing ball. Stay as upright as possible because you want the baby to move down. Sit to one side between contractions.

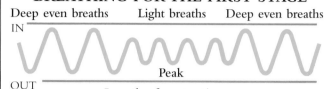

BREATHING FOR THE FIRST STAGE

Deep even breaths   Light breaths   Deep even breaths

IN

Peak

OUT

Length of contraction

At the beginning and end of a contraction, breathe deeply and evenly, in through the nose and out of the mouth. When the contraction peaks, try a lighter, shallower kind of breathing. Both in and out breaths should be through your mouth. Don't do this for too long, because you will feel dizzy.

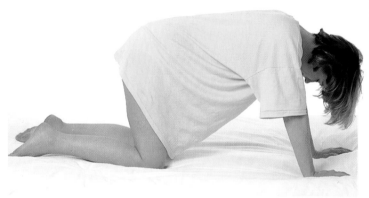

On all fours
Kneel down on your hands and knees on the floor (you may find a mattress more comfortable), and tilt your pelvis up and down. Do not arch your back. Between contractions, relax forward and rest your head in your arms.

BACK LABOR
When the baby is facing toward your abdomen, instead of away from it, his head tends to press against your spine, causing backache. To relieve pain:
■ lean forward with your weight supported, such as on all fours, to take the baby's weight off your back, and rock your pelvis up and down (as shown above); move around between contractions
■ ask your partner to massage your back, or hold a hot-water bottle to the base of your spine between contractions.

WAYS TO HELP YOURSELF
■ Keep moving between contractions; this helps you cope physically with the pain. During contractions, take up a comfortable position.
■ Try to stay as upright as possible, so the baby's head sits firmly on the cervix, making your contractions stronger and more effective.
■ Concentrate on your breathing, to calm you and take your mind off contractions.
■ Relax between contractions (see pages 48–49) to save energy for when you need it.
■ Purse your lips and breathe at a slow and steady pace.
■ Look at a fixed spot or object to help take your mind off a contraction.
■ Take one contraction at a time, and consider the contractions to follow. Think of each contraction as a wave, which you have to ride over to reach the baby.
■ Urinate often, so a full bladder doesn't get in the way of the baby.

Lower back massage
This may relieve backache, and calm and reassure you. Your partner should massage you at the base of the spine, using the heel of his hand to make firm, circular movements.

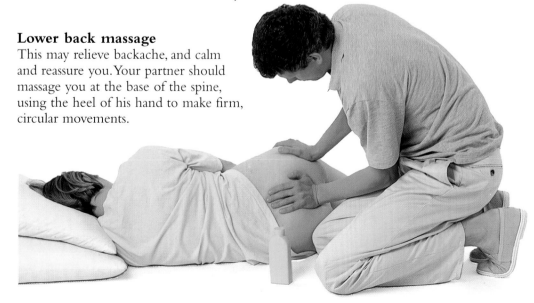

TRANSITION

THE MOST DIFFICULT time in labor is often at the end of the first stage, when contractions are strongest. They last about a minute, with only 2–3 minutes between contractions, so there is little time to rest after one before the next is upon you. This phase, which often lasts about half an hour, is known as transition. You will be tired, and you may feel disheartened, tearful, excitable, or just bad-tempered. You will probably lose all sense of time and doze off between contractions. Nausea, vomiting, and shivering are common.

   Eventually, you may have a strong urge to push. If you do this too early, the cervix can become swollen. Tell the doctor you are ready to push. She may examine you to determine whether your cervix is fully dilated.

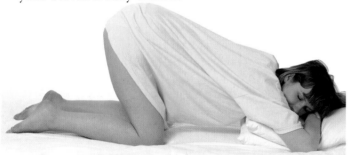

To stop yourself pushing
If the doctor says you are not fully dilated but you feel the urge to push, adopt this position and say "huff, huff, blow" to yourself (see above).

Kneel down, and lean forward, resting your head in your arms; stick your bottom in the air. This reduces the urge to push, and also makes pushing more difficult.

BREATHING FOR TRANSITION

Short breaths   Short breaths   Short breaths

IN

OUT

Blow   Blow   Gently out

If you want to push too early, say "huff, huff, blow" to yourself, taking two short in- and out-breaths, and blowing a longer breath out. When the need to push fades, give a slow even breath out.

WHAT YOU CAN DO AS A PARTNER

■ Try to relax her, encourage her, and wipe away any perspiration; if she doesn't want to be touched, stay back.
■ Breathe with her through contractions.
■ Put thick socks on her legs if they start to shake, and hold them still.
■ If she wants to push, call the doctor at once.

THE CERVIX IN LABOR

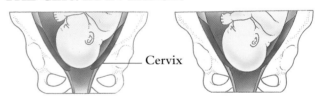

Cervix

At 2¾ in (7cm), the doctor can feel the cervix stretched out around the baby's head.

When the doctor can't feel the cervix—at about 4in (10cm) dilated—you are fully dilated.

THE SECOND STAGE

ONCE THE CERVIX has dilated and you can push, the second stage of labor has begun. You can now add your own efforts to the powerful contractions of the womb and help push the baby out. If the baby is lying in a slightly different position, you may not feel this urge to push, but the midwife will guide and encourage you so that you push when it is most need-ed. Together with your partner, she will help you find the most comfortable position in which to push.

   In a first pregnancy, this stage averages 1–2 hours. In subsequent pregnancies, it is much shorter, about 20 minutes. With an epidural, this stage may last 3 hours.

BREATHING FOR THE SECOND STAGE

Deep breaths   Deep even breaths   Even breaths

IN

Push   Push

OUT

When you want to push (this may happen several times during a contraction), take a deep breath and hold it for a short time as you bear down with your chin on your chest. It's important to do what your body tells you. Between pushes, take a few deep calming breaths. Relax slowly as the contraction fades.

POSITIONS FOR DELIVERY

Try to be as upright as possible when pushing, so you are working with gravity, rather than against it.

Sitting upright

You may find it comfortable to relax in this position between contractions. Rest propped up by pillows at a 45-degree angle.

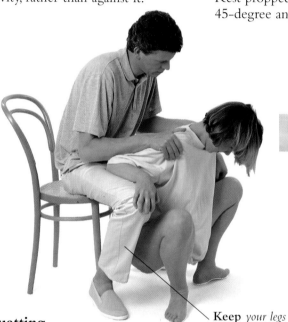

Squatting

This is a good pushing position because it opens the pelvis wide and uses gravity to help push out the baby. But squatting can increase the risk of perineal tears during delivery, and unless you've practiced it before-hand (see page 47), it can get tiring.

If your partner sits on the edge of the chair, with his legs apart, you can squat between his knees, resting your arms on his thighs for support.

Keep *your legs comfortably apart*

Kneeling

This may be less tiring than squatting, and is also a good pushing position. A helper on each side will make you feel more stable. You may also find kneeling down on all fours comfortable; keep your back straight.

WHAT CAN YOU DO AS A PARTNER

■ Try to relax her between contractions and continue to give support.
■ If she is interested, tell her what you can see as the baby's head emerges, but don't be surprised if she doesn't seem to notice you.

WAYS TO HELP YOURSELF

■ Push smoothly and steadily during a contraction.
■ Try to relax the muscles of your pelvic floor, so you feel as if you are letting go completely.
■ Keep your face relaxed.
■ Don't worry about trying to control your bowels, or about any leakage of water from the bladder.
■ Rest as much as possible between contractions, so you save all your energy for pushing.

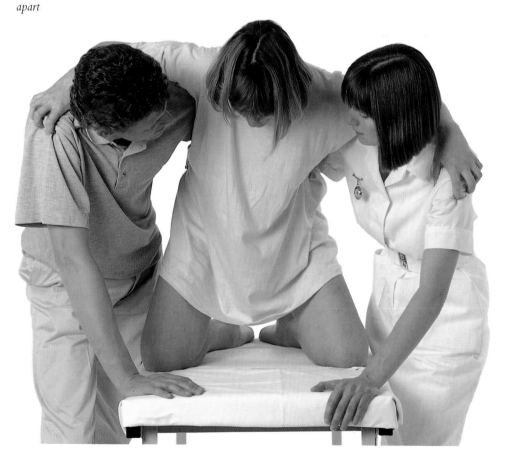

THE BIRTH

THE CLIMAX of labor has now arrived, and your baby is about to be born. After all your hard work, you can actually touch your baby's head for the first time as it emerges, if you want to.

Your partner's company may calm you and give you confidence during the long hours of labor and delivery. If you have both been to childbirth classes, you have trained together for this moment. Your partner can coach and support you and remind you of breathing and relaxation techniques. The sheer force of the muscular contractions can make you feel that your body has been taken over and rendered powerless. You experience physical sensations that are completely new to you. Your partner can rub your back, sponge your brow, and count you through the contractions so that you can push with them. His involvement will help him to feel that he is a more integral part of the birthing process. If your partner is not able to be there, you will appreciate the help of a close friend or relative.

You will hold your baby very soon and will probably feel a great sense of physical relief, but there may also be wonder, emotional tears of joy, or perhaps a feeling of great tenderness toward your baby. Exhausting, painful, and emotionally overwhelming, the birth of your baby will certainly be one of the most memorable and extraordinary experiences of your life.

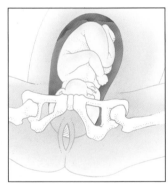 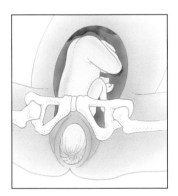 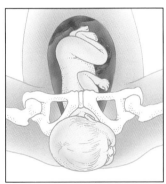 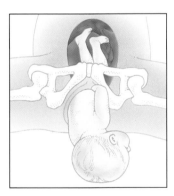

1 The baby's head moves nearer to the vaginal opening, until eventually there is a bulge where it is pressing against the pelvic floor. Soon the head itself will be seen, moving forward with each contraction, and perhaps slipping back slightly as the contraction fades. Don't be discouraged if this happens; it is a perfectly normal part of the process.

2 When the head "crowns" (the top is visible), the doctor may ask you not to push, because if the head is born too quickly, your skin might tear. So, relax and pant for a few seconds. If there is a risk of a serious tear, or the baby is distressed, you will have an episiotomy (see page 66). As the head widens the vaginal opening, there will be a stinging feeling, but this only lasts for a short while and is soon followed by numbness because the tissues have been stretched so much.

3 The head may be born face down. The doctor will probably check the umbilical cord, to make sure it isn't looped around the baby's neck. (If it is, the cord can usually be slipped over the head when the body is delivered.) Then the baby turns her head to one side so that it is in line with her shoulders. The doctor cleans her eyes, nose, and mouth, and if necessary, sucks out any fluid from her upper air passages using a tube.

4 The body comes sliding out. The doctor may clear the baby's airways again to make sure she can breathe easily. Your baby will probably look rather blue at first. She may be covered in vernix, a sticky, grayish-white substance, and streaks of blood. She may be crying. The umbilical cord is usually clamped and cut at this point.

"I'm very worried about damaging the skin or muscles of my vagina during birth. Is there danger of this?"
You won't damage yourself push-ing. The vaginal walls are elastic and made of folds, so they can stretch to allow the baby through.

"Should I breast-feed my baby immediately after the birth?"
The baby needs to be stabilized in a warmer first. After the Apgar scores are known, then, if you are not too tired, you can try to place the baby to your breast.

THE APGAR SCORE
Immediately after birth, the nurse will assess the baby's breathing, heart rate, skin color, movements, and response to stimulation, and give her an Apgar score of between 0 and 10. The score tells the doctor whether or not there is need for resuscitation if the baby is in trouble. Apgar scores of 7 or above at 5 minutes after birth are considered good.

THE THIRD STAGE
Your birth experience is not complete until the placenta is also delivered. It may take only a few seconds for it to separate spontaneously from the wall of your uterus and contractions will reduce it in size dramatically. Or, it might take up to half an hour. You may lose a little blood as this happens. You may also have to push a bit to rid your body of it, but the pushes will be nothing compared to what you have just gone through. The doctor may push down gently on your abdomen and massage your uterus. Occasionally, oxytocin is administered to speed up this third stage. Your physician will make sure the placenta is complete because if pieces of it remain in your uterus, they can cause excessive bleeding later.

AFTER THE BIRTH
You will be cleaned up, and the obstetrician will stitch any tears or surgical cuts you've sustained (see page 66). In most hospitals a nurse will examine the baby and quickly rule out any abnormalities. Sometimes, the baby is given vitamin K at this time to prevent a rare bleeding disorder.

   Babies are often not hungry immediately after birth since they have been fed right until the moment the umbilical cord is cut.

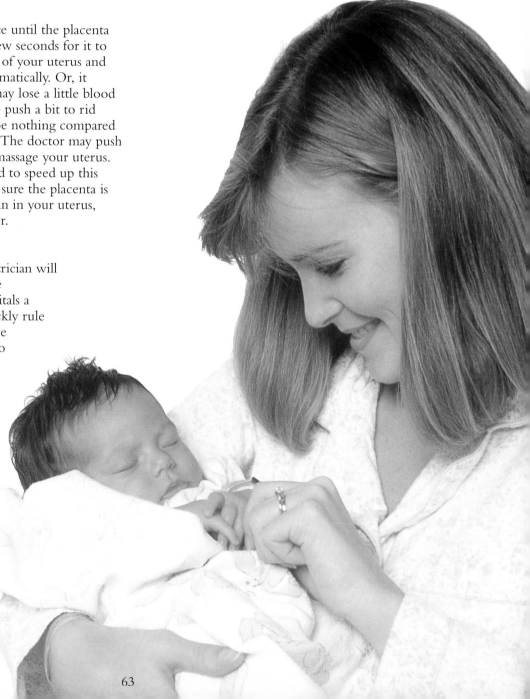

Becoming a family
After the birth, you can relax and spend a few quiet moments alone gently cuddling your new baby.

PAIN RELIEF

ALTHOUGH LABOR is not pain-free, the pain does have a purpose: every contraction brings you one step nearer to the birth of your baby. At the start you may be determined to have a completely natural birth with no pain medication, but keep an open mind. Whether you need it or not depends very much on your labor and your ability to deal with pain—and pain is always worse if you try to fight it. You may be able to cope using the self-help methods on pages 59 and 61. But if the discomfort is more than you can bear, ask for pain medication, and don't feel like a failure.

EPIDURAL

An epidural is a type of anesthesia that relieves pain by temporarily numbing the abdomen. It can be especially good for back labor. Not all hospitals offer epidurals, and they are always administered by a specially trained anesthesiologist.

Epidural, or spinal, anesthetics have improved dramatically over the years. They have become much lighter so that you keep some sensation, while all pain is blocked. With newer epidurals, you should feel pressure, but not pain, and should be able to push successfully, with a minimal chance of needing forceps. However, you should know that very small amounts of epidural may cross the placenta and affect the fetal heart rate. If given before you are dilated about 2 in (4–5cm), epidurals have been shown to increase the chance of a forceps or Cesarean delivery.

An epidural may lower your blood pressure, but this should not affect your baby. Although it can take some time to wear off, it may also be exactly what you need to get you through a physically exhausting experience. Talk to your physician about the pros and cons, especially if either of you anticipates a difficult labor and delivery.

An epidural may take about 20 minutes to start working. You will be asked to sit up or to curl up in a ball with your knees tucked under your chin, so your back is as round as possible. The anesthesia is injected into the epidural space through a catheter inserted in your lower back. A tube may be taped in place, so that you can be given additional medication at a later stage.

Giving the anesthesia
A tiny plastic catheter is inserted between the vertebrae of your spine. A fine tube is passed through the needle, and local anesthetic is fed into this.

Vertebra
Hollow needle
Spinal cord
Epidural space

You will be hooked up to an intravenous (IV) line in your arm and monitored continually so movement is restricted.

If the epidural works properly, you should have no pain and remain aware of what is happening. Some women feel faint and have a headache after epidural delivery.

DEMEROL

Also called meperidine, this is a synthetic narcotic that may be used in the hospital during labor.

With small dosages, you may feel drowsy but can be awakened to participate in all aspects of the birth. With an average dose it takes about 20 minutes for the relaxation to come over you, but it will last up to three hours and it gives some women the strength or willpower to stay on top of difficult contractions. In that brief interval between contractions, you can actually nap. However, some women report that they end up feeling nauseated or disoriented by Demerol. Unfortunately, narcotics like Demerol do cross the placenta and end up in the baby's system, just like the epidural drugs. At birth, this narcotic may inhibit the newborn's ability to breath deeply, but this effect can be minimized by keeping the dosages small. Medication is always available in the delivery room to handle any infant suffering from a drug-induced side effect such as this.

LOCAL ANESTHESIA

These pain inhibitors may be used at various times during labor and delivery. The pudendal block works on the nerves that supply the vagina and perineum, or that space between the vagina and the rectum. A pudendal block may be administered at delivery because your doctor has decided to use forceps. If you've had an episiotomy, you'll also have local anesthesia when the surgical cut is stitched up.

GENERAL ANESTHESIA

In years past, women in labor were just put to sleep and drugs such as sodium pentothal were given at delivery. This is no longer common medical practice. Unless your baby is suddenly in distress and you are being rushed in for an emergency Cesarean, you won't have general anesthesia. When this happens, the doctor needs to deliver the baby immediately and can't wait the 20 to 30 minutes necessary for an epidural to take effect. When C-sections can be planned in advance, many mothers now choose to be awake for the delivery.

LAMAZE METHOD

In 1951, a method for a drug-free birth using a type of self-hypnosis was introduced by Dr. Ferdinand Lamaze in France. This psychoprophylactic approach to the birthing process incorporates massage, relaxation, and breathing techniques as well as the continuous emotional support of the husband (or other coach) and nurse working as a "team."

Lamaze International (1-800-368-4404) provides certified childbirth educators and is the only organization that certifies Lamaze childbirth educators (LCCEs). Lamaze childbirth education classes are comprehensive. They begin in the third trimester and utilize strategies that reduce the mother's fear, which can exacerbate the pain associated with childbirth. Lamaze classes also allow women to make more informed decisions about the methods of pain relief available to them during the birthing process.

MONITORING

THROUGHOUT LABOR your baby's heartbeat will be monitored so that any signs of distress can be detected as early as possible. This will be done either with a hand-held standard obstetric stethoscope, an external monitor attached to your abdomen, or an internal fetal monitor attached to the baby's head.

OBSTETRIC STETHOSCOPE

A nurse or doctor may place the instrument on your abdomen at regular intervals throughout labor to listen to the baby's heartbeat. This type of monitoring requires a nurse at your bedside at all times.

ELECTRONIC FETAL MONITORING (EFM)

This is a way of recording the baby's heartbeat and your contractions using sophisticated electronic equipment. Some hospitals monitor only at intervals. Others do so throughout labor because
- your labor was induced,
- you are having an epidural,
- you have a problem or condition that puts you or the baby at risk, or
- the baby is distressed at any time.

External or internal EFM is not usually painful, but it does restrict your freedom to move around, which may make your contractions more uncomfortable. In recent years, routine electronic fetal monitoring has come under fire because of incidences where readings have been inaccurately interpreted. If the doctor suggests continual monitoring for no obvious reason, ask if it's really necessary.

What happens

You will probably be asked to lie on the hospital bed with your trunk supported by pillows, and small pads will be attached to your abdomen to monitor the baby's heartbeat and to measure your contractions. These appear on a paper printout attached to the monitor. Later in labor, when your water has broken, the baby's heartbeat can be measured directly by clipping an electrode to his head. This internal method is the most accurate way to monitor fetal well-being. Fetal heart rate monitors detect abnormalities in the baby's heart rate and check that the fetus is getting enough oxygen.

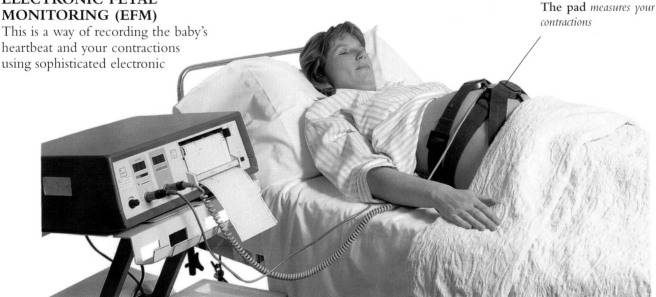

The pad *measures your contractions*

SPECIAL PROCEDURES

■ EPISIOTOMY ■	■ ASSISTED DELIVERY ■	■ INDUCTION ■
This small cut widens the vaginal opening and prevents a tear. Some obstetricians perform episiotomies more often than others, so speak to your obstetrician about routine practices.	Sometimes the baby has to be helped out with forceps or by vacuum. Neither forceps or vacuum extractor are used until the cervix is fully dilated, and the baby's head has descended into the pelvis. The cervix must be fully dilated for any operative vaginal delivery, otherwise you will probably need a C-section.	If you are induced, labor is started artificially. Various methods may be used to speed up labor if it is going slowly.
When used An episiotomy may be needed if: ■ the baby has a big head ■ you have an assisted delivery (forceps) ■ the skin around your vaginal opening hasn't stretched enough.	**When used** You may have an assisted delivery if: ■ you cannot push the baby out, perhaps because he has a big head ■ you are exhausted or the baby shows signs of distress during the labor	**When used** Labor may be induced if: ■ you are beyond 42 weeks and the baby shows signs of being distressed or the placenta starts to fail ■ you have high blood pressure, or another problem or condition that puts you or the baby at risk.
What happens Your pelvic floor area will probably be numbed with an injection of local anesthesia. Then, a small cut is made from the bottom of the vagina at the peak of a contraction. Sometimes there is no time for an injection, but the stretching of the tissues also numbs them, so you shouldn't feel any pain. Stitching up after an episiotomy or a tear may take some time, because the different layers of skin and muscle have to be carefully sewn together. It can be painful, too, so ask for more anesthesia if you need some. The stitches will dissolve so they won't have to be removed.	**What happens** ■ **Forceps** You will probably be given an injection of local anesthesia into your pelvic floor area, and an episiotomy. The doctor positions the forceps on either side of the baby's head and gently pulls to deliver it. You can help by pushing. The rest of the body is delivered normally. **Forceps** These form a cage around the baby's head, protecting it from pressure and damage. ■ **Vacuum** A small plastic or, rarely, metal cup, connected to a vacuum pump, is passed into the vagina and attached to the baby's head. The baby is gently pulled through the birth canal as you push.	**What happens** Induction is always planned in advance, and you will be asked to go into the hospital. Labor may be induced in either of two ways: **1** Giving you a hormone–Pitocin (oxytocin)—which makes the womb contract. This is fed through an IV in your arm at a controlled rate. Ask for the needle to be inserted into the arm you use least. Sometimes, the drug is administered to speed up a labor that has slowed considerably or stopped altogether. The amount given can be electronically calculated with the intravenous drip. **2** Breaking your water, or amniotomy. The doctor makes a small hole in the bag of fluid surrounding the baby, using a special instrument that passes through the cervix. Most women don't feel any pain. Contractions nearly always start soon afterward.
Effects Some discomfort and soreness is normal after an episiotomy, but pain can be severe if an infection develops. The wound should heal within 10 to 14 days, but if you are sore after this time, ask your doctor. A big tear hurts more than a small episiotomy.	**Effects** ■ The forceps may leave pressure marks or bruises on either side of the baby's head, but these are harmless and disappear within a few days. ■ The vacuum cup will cause slight swelling, and later a bruise, on the baby's head. This gradually subsides.	**Effects** ■ Amniotomy is usually painless and labor ordinarily begins soon after the membranes have been broken. ■ An artificial hormone–Pitocin (oxytocin)–is administered slowly in an IV drip and gradually increased until labor is in full force.

CESAREAN BIRTH

BREECH BIRTH

A breech baby is born bottom or, occasionally, feet first. About three in 100 births are breech, During a normal vaginal delivery, the baby's head puts tremendous pressure on the birth canal, forcing it to dilate. The head itself decreases in diameter, making it easier to emerge at birth. That's why so many newborns have elongated or misshapen heads at first.

In a breech presentation, however, the baby's bottom or feet are delivered first and the aftercoming head may or may not fit through the mother's pelvis, depending on the size of the baby and the size of the mother's pelvis. In most cases of breech presentation, obstetricians consider a Cesarean delivery to be safer than a vaginal birth.

TWINS

There is always an increased risk of complications when twins are on the way, so they should be born at a hospital. Sometimes they arrive prematurely or the stress of carrying them brings on preeclampsia (see page 38). One of the babies may be in a breech or some other awkward position.

A woman carrying twins will go through the first stage but have two second stages, as she pushes first one baby out and then the other. The second twin is usually born 10 to 30 minutes after the first.

WITH A CESAREAN birth, the baby is delivered abdominally. You may know you are going to have a Cesarean, or C-section, in advance, or it may be an emergency operation because of a problem in labor. If a Cesarean is planned, you can have an epidural, or spinal (see page 64), so you are awake throughout and can hold your baby right away. This may also be possible if you are told in labor that a Cesarean is imminent. In a real emergency, however, general anesthesia is often necessary so the doctor can deliver the baby quickly.

Some mothers may feel disappointed with a Cesarean birth, but a decision for such a procedure is made in the best interests of the baby. You should also remember that a vaginal birth is often possible in subsequent pregnancies.

WHAT HAPPENS

Your pubic hair will be shaved and you will be hooked up to an IV in your arm. A catheter will also be inserted into your bladder to keep it empty during the surgery. If the Cesarean section was planned, you may have opted for an epidural so you can be awake during the procedure. If it's an emergency because of something that has come up during your labor, you may have to be given general anesthesia that will put you to sleep. There are two types of incisions: a vertical cut from your navel to your pubic hairline or a horizontal ("bikini") cut made near the top of your pubic hairline. The baby's head is delivered first and mucus may be suctioned from his mouth even before his feet are visible.

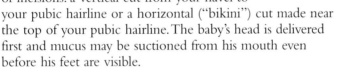

The incision
The "bikini" cut is usually made horizontally, just above the pubic hairline, and it is almost invisible when it heals.

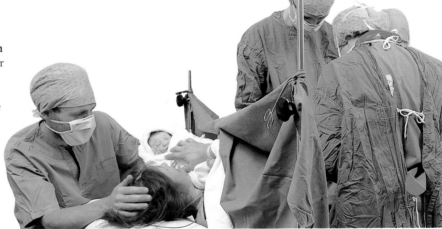

Stitching the incision
You or your partner can look at the baby before she goes to the nursery to be stabilized.

AFTER THE OPERATION

You will be encouraged to walk soon after the birth. The incision will be painful for a few days, so ask for pain medication. Moving around won't open it up. Stand tall and cup your hands over the wound. You may find that it helps to hold your abdomen when you laugh, sneeze, or cough. Try using a footstool when you are getting in or out of bed. Check with your doctor before starting any exercise routines (see page 72). The stitches will be removed several days later, unless they're the soluble type, and you will feel much better after a week. Don't strain yourself for at least six weeks. The scar fades, usually within six months.

YOUR NEW BABY

Don't let very first impressions of your newborn shock you. Your baby may look dramatically different from the cherubic pictures of infants you've seen in books. His head may be misshapen from having been elongated to fit through the birth canal. His arms and legs may be a little blue, and he may be covered with a white, greasy substance called vernix. His body is not working efficiently yet, so you may notice spots, blotches, and changes of color, which are perfectly normal. Ask your pediatrician if you are worried. He can put your mind at ease. You may love your baby immediately. But if you don't feel this way at first, give yourself time. Once you get to know each other as you care for him, and find that he responds to your touch and the sound of your voice, love will grow naturally.

FIRST IMPRESSIONS

VERY FEW BABIES look picture perfect at birth. In fact, blotchy skin, pointy heads, swollen genitals, lots of downy body hair, and the grayish-white vernix covering their little bodies may make you want to delay those first formal portrait sittings.

HEAD
A strange pointed shape is caused by the pressure of birth. The head should look normal in two weeks.
On the top of the head is a soft spot (fontanelle), where the bones of the skull have not yet joined together. They should fuse by the time the child is 18 months.

EYES
Eye color varies at birth. True eye color may not develop until the baby is about six months old.
Puffy eyelids are usually caused by the pressure of birth, but ask the doctor or midwife to check your baby's eyes, as there is sometimes an infection.
Squinting is common. The baby may look cross-eyed at times in the first months.

TONGUE
This may seem anchored to the floor of the mouth, so that the tip looks slightly forked when the baby sticks it out. The tip will grow forward in the first year.

HANDS AND FEET
These may be bluish because the baby's circulation is not working properly. If you move your baby into another position, they should turn pink.
The fingernails are often long at birth.

BREASTS
Your baby's breasts may be swollen and even leak a little milk as a result of maternal hormones. This is normal in both sexes. The swelling should go down within a few weeks; do not massage or squeeze the milk out.

GENITALS
These look large on both male and female babies.
A baby girl may have discharge from her vagina. This is caused by the mother's hormones and will soon disappear.
The testicles of a baby boy are often pulled up into his groin.

The **fontanelle** *cannot be damaged through everyday handling*

Your baby *may have a good head of hair, or he may be bald*

His hands *will be clenched*

Red marks *are caused by pressure from the birth, or because the baby's skin is still immature*

The umbilical cord *stump drops off in about ten days*

The baby can see *you at birth if you hold him about 8in (20cm) away from your face*

SKIN

Spots and rashes are very common, and should vanish of their own accord.

Peeling skin, especially on the hands and feet, should disappear in a couple of days.

Downy body hair (lanugo) may be noticeable, especially if the baby was born early. This rubs off within two weeks.

Greasy white vernix is the substance that protects the baby's skin in the womb and may cover him completely. It can be easily wiped off.

Birthmarks usually vanish. These include:

■ red marks, often found on the eyelids, forehead, and at the back of the neck; they take about a year to go away

■ strawberry birthmarks, which can be worrisome as they gradually increase in size. However, they may disappear by the time the child is five

■ blue patches, often found on the lower backs of babies with dark skin

■ port wine stain, a bright-red or purple mark, which is permanent

STOOL

A newborn baby's first bowel movement contains a dark, sticky substance called meconium. Once he is feeding, the stool changes.

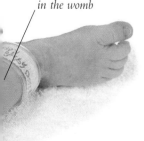

The baby's legs
often look bowed because he has been curled up in the womb

CHECKS ON THE BABY

YOUR BABY will be examined many times in the first week. The obstetrician or midwife will do a quick and immediate check right there on delivery while your baby is lying on your abdomen or in your arms. If you've arranged for your own pediatrician to be at the hospital, that's who will begin the careful weighing, measuring, and reassuring that all is normal.

GENERAL EXAMINATION

The pediatrician will check the baby from head to toe to ensure nothing is abnormal.

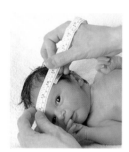

1 The doctor measures the head, and looks for abnormalities. He checks the fontanelle, and feels the roof of the mouth to make sure it is complete.

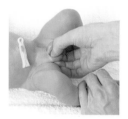

2 He listens to the heart and lungs to see if they are normal. An irregular heartbeat is common among newborn babies, and does not usually indicate a defect.

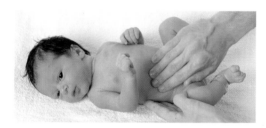

3 By putting his hands on the baby's tummy, the doctor checks that the abdominal organs are the right size. He also feels the pulses in the baby's groin.

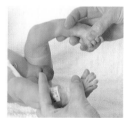

4 The genitals are checked for abnormality. If you have a boy, the doctor will be looking to see if both testicles have descended.

5 He gently moves the baby's limbs back and forth, and checks that the lower legs and feet are aligned, that the legs are the right length, and that his reflexes are normal.

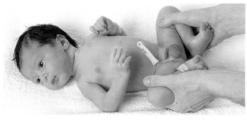

6 The doctor checks the hips for any dislocation by bending the baby's legs up and gently circling them.

SPECIAL TESTS

A blood test is done during your hospital stay to check for conditions such as thyroid deficiency and PKU (phenylketonuria), a rare but treatable metabolic disorder. It involves a small prick on the baby's heel. PKU can cause mental disabilities if it's not detected early in life.

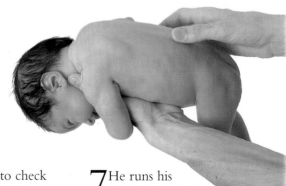

7 He runs his thumb down the baby's back, making sure that all the vertebrae are in place along the spine.

SPECIAL CARE BABIES

SOME BABIES need special care after birth. When an infant is born prematurely (born before 37 weeks), or is "small for date" (see page 39), she may spend the first days of her life in the intensive care unit because of problems with breathing, feeding, and keeping warm. Life with a baby under intensive care is bound to be hard. Not only will you be separated from her before you have gotten to know her, but you will see her surrounded by the intimidating array of equipment that is keeping her safe. This can be frightening at first. Helping the hospital staff take care of your baby will calm you and make this difficult bonding a little easier.

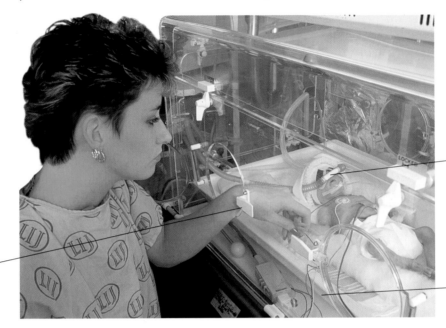

The baby in the incubator
Your baby needs just as much love and attention as any normal, healthy baby.

Feeding tube, *which passes into the baby's stomach; you can express your own milk to be fed to the baby*

Portholes, *so you can touch your baby and talk to her*

Tilting ray, *to help with respiration and feeding*

GETTING TO KNOW YOUR BABY

It's important to spend as much time with your baby as possible; many hospitals have special rooms you can stay in, so you are near to your baby and can take part in her daily care. At first, she may look so small and vulnerable that you worry about touching her. But, all babies respond to loving handling. And even if she can't be taken out of the incubator and cuddled, you can still talk to her and stroke her through the portholes in the side. You may even be able to help with changing her diapers and dressing her.

ASKING QUESTIONS

Ask the doctor or nursing staff about anything that worries you. Often parents don't ask questions because their baby looks so frail that they are afraid of the answers. But with modern medical technology, even babies born before 28 weeks can survive.

FEEDING

If the baby can suck, you may be able to feed her normally. Otherwise, she will be fed through a tube, which is passed through her nose or mouth and down into her stomach.

JAUNDICE

Jaundice usually becomes noticeable one to three days after birth. It turns the baby's skin and the whites of the eyes slightly yellow. This happens because a baby's liver is still immature, and bilirubin, a pigment which occurs as a result of the normal breakdown of red blood cells, accumulates in the blood faster than the liver can dispose of it.

Jaundice usually clears up in a few days of it own accord. Sometimes jaundice has to be treated with a special light (phototherapy). This can usually be done in the newborn nursery. In a few severe cases, the baby is transferred to intensive care.

STILLBIRTH

Very rarely, a baby is born dead; this is commonly called a stillbirth. Because of modern medical techniques and fetal monitoring, an infant isn't likely to die during labor or delivery. But positive statistics won't make it any easier for you to bear if you baby is stillborn. Don't turn away physically from your dead baby; hold him, give him a name, and grieve for him. Don't carry the burden single-handedly, involve the baby's father, and find someone with whom you can talk frankly, whether it's an individual therapist or a self-help group.

GETTING BACK TO NORMAL

For the first few weeks after delivery, try to sleep whenever you can. Don't be tempted to use free moments to catch up on housework or errands. Your postpartum checkup isn't usually scheduled until four to six weeks after the birth, but you should not hesitate to call your obstetrician before that if you have any problems, even what you might consider minor. Your baby's pediatrician can be a storehouse of answers. Get to know him; your worries should never be discounted. You may be aghast when you first see your body after birth. Your familiar belly will be gone, though your stomach will be far from flat. Your breasts will be large, and the tops of your legs will feel heavy. If you feel good and the doctor says okay, start your postnatal exercises from the first day after birth.

HOW YOU WILL FEEL

YOU WILL have some discomfort, and even pain, in the first days after birth. Speak to your doctor or the hospital staff if anything worries you.

AFTERPAINS
The cramping pains in your stomach, especially when breast-feeding, mean the womb is contracting back to its prepregnant size. This is a good sign that your body is returning to normal. These afterpains may last several days.
What to do If contractions are severe, ask your doctor to recommend a mild pain-killer to ease them.

BLADDER
It's normal to urinate often in the first days, as the body eliminates the extra fluid gained in pregnancy.

What to do Urinating may be difficult at first, because of soreness, but try to do so as soon as possible after birth.
■ Get up and move around to encourage the flow.
■ Take a long shower as soon as you feel steady on your feet. The warm water will relax your muscles.
■ If you have stitches, try pouring warm water over them as you urinate to stop your skin from stinging.

BLEEDING
You may have vaginal bleeding for anywhere from two to six weeks. The bright red discharge is heavy at first, but over the next few days it changes color, and gradually becomes brownish. Often the discharge will continue until your first menstrual period.

What to do Wear sanitary pads; don't use internal tampons at this time, as they can cause infection.

BOWELS
You may not need to empty your bowels for a day or more after the birth.
What to do Get up and move as soon as you can: walking around will start your bowels working.
■ Drink plenty of water and eat high-fiber foods to stimulate your bowels.
■ When you need to move your bowels, do so at once, but don't strain or push.
■ It is most unlikely that any stitches will tear when you move your bowels, but holding a clean sanitary pad against the area while you do so may feel good and give you confidence.
STITCHES
These may be very sore until you are healed. Most dissolve in about a week; external ones may fall out.
What to do The following suggestions will help.
■ Practice pelvic floor exercises as soon as possible after birth to speed up healing.
■ Keep stitches clean by relaxing in a warm bath. Dry the area thoroughly afterward.
■ Soothe soreness by applying an ice-pack or a local anesthetic to the area.
■ Lie down to take pressure off the stitches, or sit on a rubber ring.

COPING WITH THE BLUES
Many women feel low a few days after delivery, usually when their breast milk comes in. One cause is the sudden change in hormone levels, another is the feeling of anticlimax that inevitably occurs after birth. These postnatal blues usually vanish. If you feel depressed for more than four weeks, or your depression is very severe, see your obstetrician or talk to your midwife.

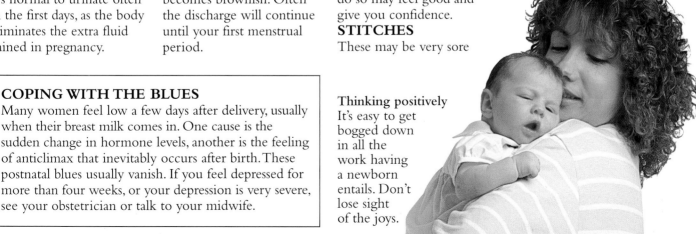

Thinking positively
It's easy to get bogged down in all the work having a newborn entails. Don't lose sight of the joys.

SHAPING UP AFTER BIRTH

WITH SOME GENTLE EXERCISING every day, your figure can return to normal again in as little as three months after the birth, although your stomach muscles may not be as firm as before. Build up slowly at first, because your ligaments are still soft and stretchy, and always stop if you feel pain or tiredness. It's best to exercise in short but frequent spurts.

> ### ■ WARNING ■
>
> If you have had a Cesarean, you won't be ready to start the exercises for your stomach muscles until much later after birth. When you're ready, begin with the week one routine. Check with your doctor first before practicing any exercises, and stop if you feel pain.

WEEK ONE
You can begin to strengthen the stretched, and possibly weakened, muscles of your pelvic floor and stomach from the first day after birth. The pelvic floor and foot pedaling exercises are also good several weeks after a Cesarean.

PELVIC FLOOR EXERCISE from day one
Practice gentle squeezing and lifting exercises (see page 45) as often as possible every day to stop yourself from leaking urine involuntarily. It's important to do this before you go on to the exercises in week two. If you have had stitches, strengthening the pelvic floor will help heal them.

FOOT PEDALING from day one
This will stop swelling in the legs and improve circulation. Bend your feet up and down at the ankle. Practice hourly if you can find the time.

STOMACH TONER from day one
A gentle way to strengthen these muscles is to pull them in as you breathe out, hold them in for a few seconds, then relax. Try to do this as often as possible.

From day five after birth, if you feel alright, practice the following exercise twice a day:

1 Lie on your back with your head and shoulders supported on two pillows, and your legs bent and slightly apart. Cross your arms over your stomach.

2 Lift your head and shoulders, and as you do this, breathe out and press gently on each side of your stomach with the palms of your hands, as if pulling the two sides together. Hold this position for a few seconds, then breathe in, and relax. Repeat three times.

WEEK TWO
After about a week, try the following exercises as a daily routine, and continue for at least three months. Repeat each exercise as many times as is comfortable. Begin with the curl-downs, and when you can do these easily, move on to the other exercises. If you find that new exercises strain you, practice the curl-downs for a few days longer. Remember to keep practicing the exercise for your pelvic floor.

CURL-DOWNS
1 Sit up, with your legs bent and slightly apart, and your arms folded in front of you.

2 Breathe out while gently tilting your pelvis forward, and gradually lean back until you feel the muscles of your stomach tighten. Hold for as long as you comfortably can while breathing normally. Then breathe in and sit up straight.

SIDE BENDS

1 Lie flat on your back with your arms by your side and the palms of your hands resting on the outsides of your thighs.

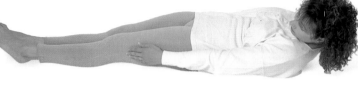

2 Lift your head slightly, and bending to the left, slide your left hand down your leg. Lie back and rest for a moment, then repeat on your right side. As this becomes easy, try bending to each side two or three times before you lie back and rest.

CURL-UPS

1 Lie flat on your back on the floor, with your knees bent and your feet slightly apart. Rest your hands on your thighs.

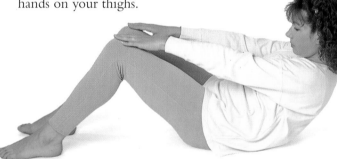

2 Breathe out, and lift your head and shoulders, stretching forward to touch your knees with your hands. Don't worry if you can't reach far enough at first, you will succeed with practice. Breathe in and relax.

WHEN THIS IS EASY, TRY:

■ lifting yourself up more slowly and holding the position for longer
■ placing your hands on your chest as you lift your head and shoulders
■ clasping your hands behind your head as you lift yourself up.

CHECKING YOUR PELVIC FLOOR

By three months after birth, these muscles should be strong again. Test them by skipping. If any urine leaks, practice the pelvic floor exercises for another month and try again. If leaking is still a problem after four months, see your doctor.

HOW YOUR BODY RECOVERS

YOUR BODY won't be fully recovered for at least six months after the birth, but by the time you have your six-week checkup, it should be getting back to normal. Your womb may have shrunk back to its prepregnant size, and you may have started your periods again. If you have been exercising regularly, your muscles should be in far better shape.

YOUR CHECKUP

Your postpartum checkup with the obstetrician or midwife is usually set four to six weeks after delivery. The visit is a chance to relive the happy moments of the birth, so do ask about aspects you may have missed. These memories are important.

What Happens

■ Your blood pressure, weight, and a sample of urine will be checked.
■ Your breasts and stomach will be examined. The doctor will make sure that any stitches have healed.
■ You will have an internal examination to check the size and position of the womb, and may be given a cervical Pap test.
■ The doctor will discuss contraception; if you wish it, you may be fitted for a diaphragm or IUD.

YOUR PERIODS

The first menstrual period after birth is often longer and heavier than usual. If you are breast-feeding, your periods may not start until after your baby is weaned. If you are bottle-feeding, a period usually comes four to six weeks after the birth.

QUESTIONS & ANSWERS

"When can we resume our sex life?"
The best time to start making love again is when your vagina has healed and you are both ready. For most women, it takes four weeks. But you may feel too sore and tender to resume sex until after your checkup.
  When you do resume your sex life, take it slowly. Relax as much as you can, and use extra lubrication, because your vagina may be sore and drier than normal.

"I'm breast-feeding my baby; do we still have to use contraception?"
Even if you are breast-feeding or haven't started your periods again, you need to use contraception. The doctor or midwife can discuss this with you soon after the birth. If you want to go on the pill, or if you previously used a diaphragm, you need to discuss these forms of contraception with your doctor or midwife.

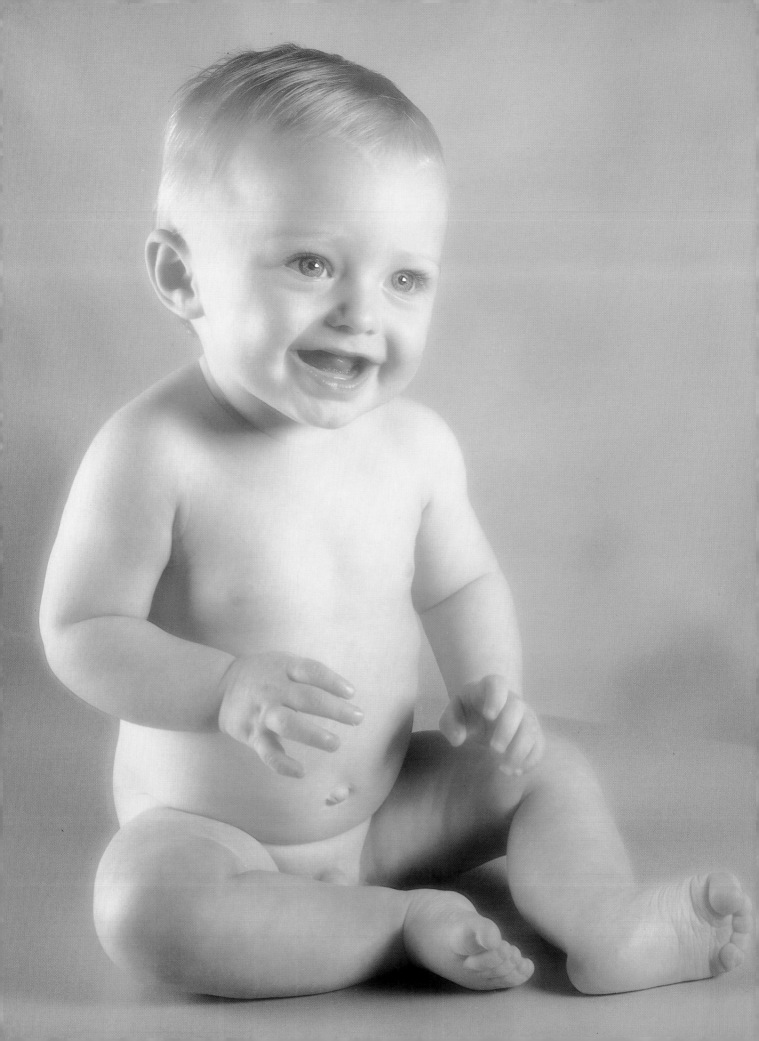

2
BABY CARE

■ ■ ■ ■ ■

A step-by-step, practical guide to
caring for your baby,
from birth to three years.

THE FIRST WEEKS OF LIFE

Nothing can really prepare you for the reality of having a child. The first weeks in the life of your baby can seem like a chaotic whirlwind of new experiences and sensations as you get to know this new person in your lives and adapt to the feeling of being a parent. You have so much to learn: how to feed and nourish your baby, how to dress her and care for her skin, what she likes and what she doesn't like. Looking after a new baby involves a combination of warmth, attention, and physical stamina. Although some of this will be instinctive, at other times you may feel lost. In fact, you'll learn new skills: before long, eating with one hand while nursing or holding a bottle with the other will come naturally. The early phase of adjustment and chaos doesn't have to last long. This chapter tells how one couple and their new baby, Amy, coped in the first few weeks. Life may be even more stressful for a single parent, but it is important to remember that every baby is different, and you will soon find your own way of managing.

"The first weeks weren't easy. You think you're a capable, confident person, then you have a helpless baby to look after and you feel like jelly!"

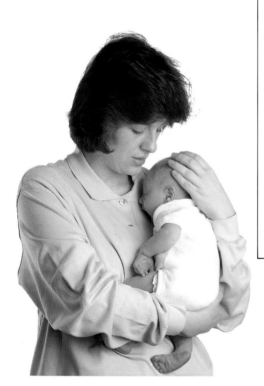

First days at home
Life with your new baby will take you by surprise. Her apparent vulnerability produces new, powerful feelings within you, while a turmoil of emotions makes you burst into tears for no reason, or become distressed by, say, the news. Don't fight your feelings; concentrate on the new life you are nurturing.

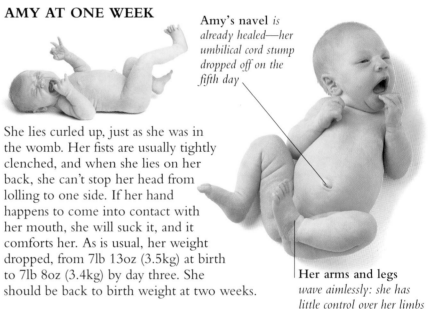

AMY AT ONE WEEK

Amy's navel is already healed—her umbilical cord stump dropped off on the fifth day

She lies curled up, just as she was in the womb. Her fists are usually tightly clenched, and when she lies on her back, she can't stop her head from lolling to one side. If her hand happens to come into contact with her mouth, she will suck it, and it comforts her. As is usual, her weight dropped, from 7lb 13oz (3.5kg) at birth to 7lb 8oz (3.4kg) by day three. She should be back to birth weight at two weeks.

Her arms and legs *wave aimlessly: she has little control over her limbs*

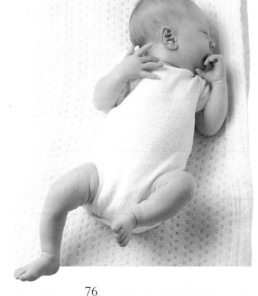

Amy asleep
Newborn babies sleep an average of 16 hours a day, but Amy rarely manages that much sleep. Some days she sleeps as little as 10 or 11 hours in total, with a long, stormy period from late afternoon to late at night when she only dozes for short periods. During her times of deep sleep, she is totally oblivious to her surroundings. Within five weeks she adopts a more sociable pattern, sleeping longer at night and going to bed earlier.

Becoming a family

Now there are three of you (or two of you if you are a single parent), and everything changes. Your partner is no longer just your lover, he's your companion and ally in this new adventure of parenthood—and she's as much his baby as yours. Your tried and tested family relationships will subtly change too: You're not just a son or a daughter any more. You're a parent, with a new life depending on you. No matter how topsy-turvy your life seems at this time, try to make time for your partner. Often the new father is shell-shocked in the days immediately following the birth, and he needs your support as much as you need his. Let him share in the care of the baby: He may be more nervous than you when handling her floppy body, but, with practice, he will grow more confident.

"The first days were such a tangle of conflicting feelings—elation and overwhelming pride at being a father, anxiety about Ruth, exhaustion from the round-the-clock demands of our new baby, even a tiny regret that our happy, carefree life together seemed to be at an end."

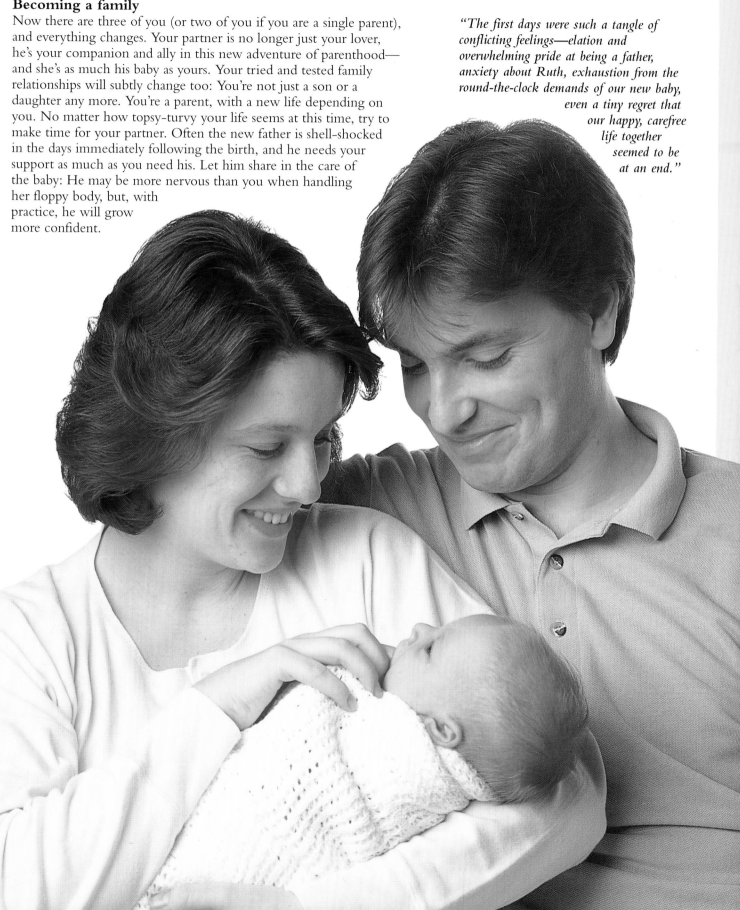

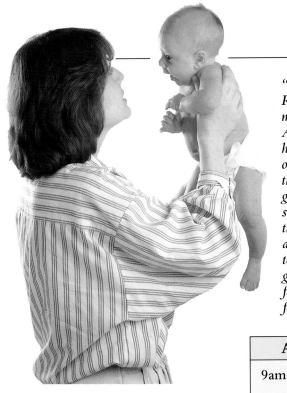

AMY'S DAY

"Amy seemed insatiably hungry. Ruth was good at expressing her milk, so in the evenings when Amy was at her fussiest, for hours at a stretch, I could take over with a bottle. I took over the diaper-changing too, to give Ruth a break. I was surprised to find I even loved that—it was one way Amy and I built a closeness together. We would play little games, or I would make funny faces, or introduce her to her feet and hands."

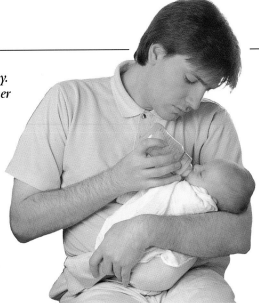

Building a loving relationship

Right from the beginning, your relationship with your new baby is an intense, two-way one that will grow into a real and lasting love. As you bring her up close to talk and coo to her, she will gaze raptly at your face—and eye contact plays a big part when you are falling in love. She will reward your efforts to calm her by quieting down at the sound of your voice when you sing and talk to her. And when she's miserable, she wants you to comfort her.

A TYPICAL DAY AT AROUND THREE WEEKS OF AGE★

9am	**Ruth is awakened** by Amy crying in the small crib next to her. She had nursed her at 5 am, and they had both fallen asleep again. Amy is breast-fed again.	1pm	**Amy cries** so Ruth nurses her, and afterward they both doze off.
10am	**Ruth takes Amy** into the bathroom to change her diaper and clothes and sponge bathe her. Then she puts Amy in the infant seat and chats to her while she dresses herself.	3:30pm	**A friend** ringing the doorbell wakes Ruth. She has some advice on how to relieve Ruth's sore nipples. Then together they wake Amy and chat to her.
11am	**Amy falls asleep.** Ruth puts the dirty laundry in the washing machine and straightens up. Then, she puts her feet up.	4pm	**Her friend** leaves, but Amy is cranky from being awakened, so Ruth feeds her to soothe her.
12:30pm	**Ruth has** some lunch.	5:30pm	**Ruth puts Amy** in the baby carriage. Then she walks to the station to meet Tim. The fresh air and movement put Amy to sleep.

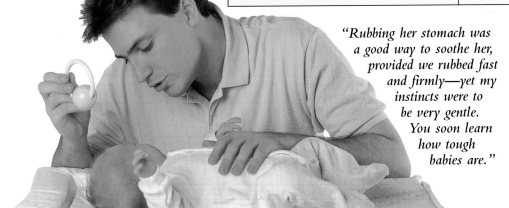

"Rubbing her stomach was a good way to soothe her, provided we rubbed fast and firmly—yet my instincts were to be very gentle. You soon learn how tough babies are."

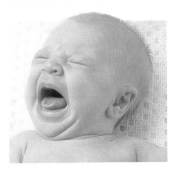

Amy crying

Crying is your baby's way of expressing her need for love and comfort. Always respond—don't ignore her.

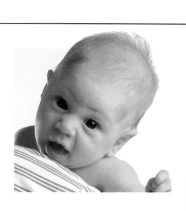

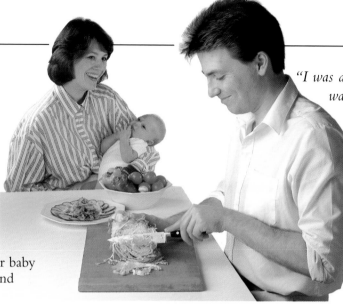

Amy wakeful
Held against your shoulder, your baby has a good view of the world, and will enjoy her wakeful times.

"I was astonished at how difficult it was to get any small job finished during the day. Once Tim got home from work it was up to him to get the supper ready—sometimes I wouldn't even be dressed! It was odd for me to be so disorganized. I wasn't used to having so little time for myself."

6:15pm	**Home again,** and May starts to cry. Ruth feeds her, changes her, then rocks her in her arms. Feeding is the only thing that really soothes Amy at this time of day, but Ruth is sore, so it's painful. Tim catches some sleep.	10pm	**Amy is still crying:** she will be soothed for a while, then cry again. Tim and Ruth let her suck, walk her around, or push her in a carriage.
8:30pm	**Time wakes up** and he and Ruth take turns carrying Amy around and preparing some food. Amy dozes off for a few minutes at a time, then wakes and cries—so dinner is an erratic affair with Tim trying to bottle-feed and then Ruth breast-feeding Amy.	2am	**Amy falls asleep** at last. Tim and Ruth go to bed, exhausted.
		4am	**Amy wakes** and cries, so Ruth nurses her. Tim wakes up, too, and helps rock Amy back to sleep after she's been fed.
		7am	**The alarm goes off** and Time gets up to go to work—he's had four hours' sleep, plus two hours earlier.

*Although this schedule provides some indications of a typical day, you should remember that newborns usually nurse 8 to 12 times a day. For more on typical newborn feeding patterns, see page 88. For typical urine and stool patterns in newborns, see page 146.

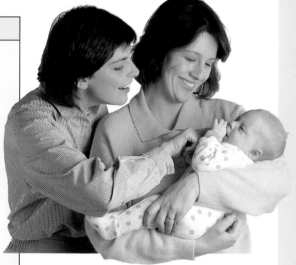

Involving other family members
Your parents, sisters, and brothers will all be eager to meet the new baby; but don't feel guilty about limiting visitors if you want to.

Getting plenty of rest
Every new mother has to learn to cope with too little sleep. Plenty of rest whenever you can catch it is the only answer—and it's especially important if you're breast-feeding. Rest whenever your baby sleeps, even if you don't sleep. Your body isn't strong enough yet for strenuous work, and the housework can go undone for now.

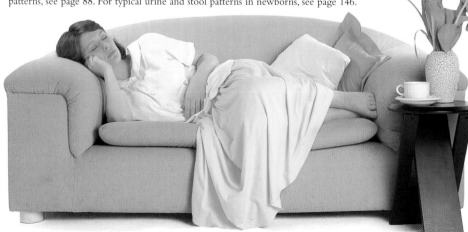

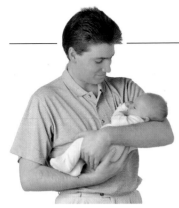

SIX WEEKS OLD

"By six weeks Amy was a real person—nothing like the greedy, screaming bundle of only weeks before. She responded to each of us in her own way: her first, crooked smiles were just for me, usually when I changed her, but at times only Ruth would do. We were lucky, Amy was very perky and she helped us to love her; and you certainly learn fast when you have a new baby reliant on you for every need."

PREMATURE BABIES

Your baby's first six weeks at home may be especially difficult if she was born prematurely. She may cry more than the average baby, be difficult to comfort, or be very sleepy and reluctant to nurse. In addition to your natural anxiety about your baby, you may feel rejected by her: she doesn't make you feel she loves you, so it's that much harder to love her in return. Your pre-term baby will need extra care from you. She loses heat quickly, so you need to keep your home warm for her, especially when bathing or changing her, and she will need frequent feedings to help her grow. Even though she may have a small appetite and be a trouble-some eater, offer her the breast or a bottle as often as every two hours, letting her take as much as she wants. Concentrate on giving the physical and emotional care she needs. In time she will grow more responsive to you, and you will learn to understand her better.

AMY AT SIX WEEKS

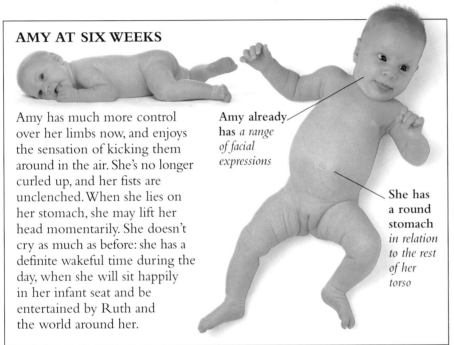

Amy has much more control over her limbs now, and enjoys the sensation of kicking them around in the air. She's no longer curled up, and her fists are unclenched. When she lies on her stomach, she may lift her head momentarily. She doesn't cry as much as before: she has a definite wakeful time during the day, when she will sit happily in her infant seat and be entertained by Ruth and the world around her.

Amy already has *a range of facial expressions*

She has a round stomach *in relation to the rest of her torso*

AMY'S SIX-WEEK CHECKUP

The one-month or six-week checkup is usually the first of the major development exams for a new baby. Your pediatrician or family practitioner will do it in a friendly atmosphere.

1 **General assessment** The doctor discusses Amy's general well-being and demeanor with Ruth. She wakes Amy and talks to her to assess how she responds to the stimulus of a new face. The doctor is looking for that magical early smile, a sure sign that Amy is developing a normal, sociable personality. She checks Amy's sight by moving a rattle across her field of vision. Amy follows it with both eyes, demonstrating healthy eyesight with no sign of a squint.

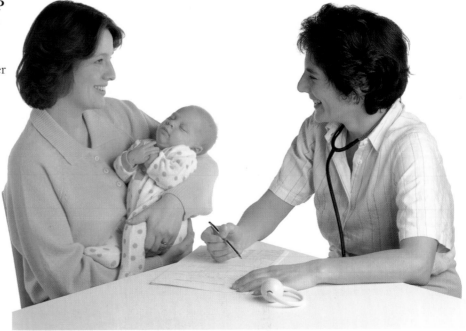

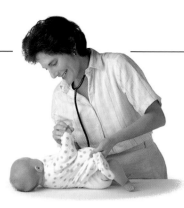

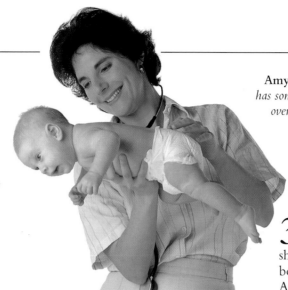

Amy already has some control over her neck muscles

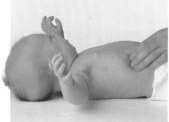

2 Limbs and muscle tone The doctor undresses Amy herself, so she can observe her muscle tone and how she moves her limbs.

3 Control of head The doctor holds Amy in the air to see that she holds her head in line with her body. Then she watches as she pulls Amy into a sitting position.

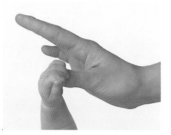

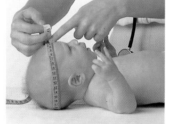

4 Grasp reflex A baby at birth can grasp hold of a finger put into her palm and hold on strongly. By six weeks it's normal for her birth reflexes to begin to disappear, as Amy's have.

5 Head circumference Amy has her head measured, to check for normal growth. Her head is now 15in (38cm).

6 Heartbeat The doctor listens to Amy's heart with a stethoscope: about 120 beats a minute is normal for the first year.

7 Internal organs A good feel around Amy's stomach reassures the doctor that her liver, stomach, and spleen are all growing normally, and none is too big or the wrong shape.

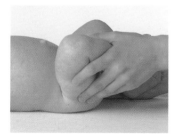

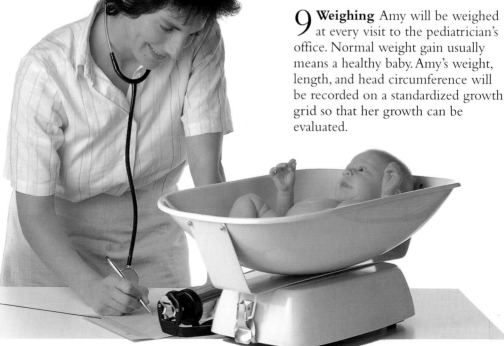

8 Hip check Hip dislocation is a possibility still, so the doctor tests the action of the joints with her middle fingers, as she manipulates Amy's legs.

9 Weighing Amy will be weighed at every visit to the pediatrician's office. Normal weight gain usually means a healthy baby. Amy's weight, length, and head circumference will be recorded on a standardized growth grid so that her growth can be evaluated.

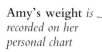

Amy's weight is recorded on her personal chart

HANDLING YOUR BABY

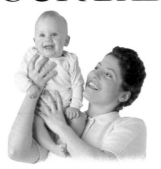

From an early age, your baby needs closeness and comfort as well as food, warmth, and sleep. To begin with, you will probably feel quite nervous about handling and cuddling him. Your hands seem so clumsy, his limbs so floppy, his head and neck so fragile. Your normal, careful handling won't hurt him; even the soft fontanelle on the top of his head has a tough membrane to protect it. But you may startle him if you pick him up suddenly, making him fling his limbs out.

It frightens him when he senses he may fall. It won't be long before you're both much more confident around each other. As your baby gains control over his muscles, he may enjoy some boisterous games. At four or five months he may love to be lifted up above your head or perched on your shoulders. If he's timid—and some babies are—handle him gently until he is more outgoing. Respond to your baby's moods, and let him set the pace of your physical play.

PICKING UP AND PUTTING DOWN A NEWBORN BABY

TALK TO YOUR BABY as you transfer her from one position to another—your voice is familiar and reassuring. Remember that until she is about eight weeks old she cannot control her head or muscles. You need to support her body all the time, so that her head does not flop or her limbs dangle.

PICKING YOUR BABY UP

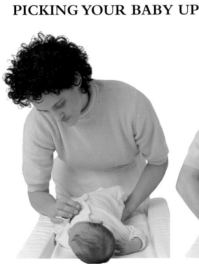

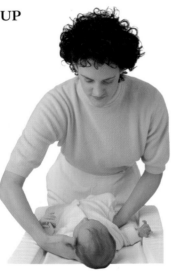

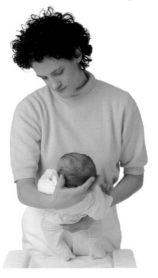

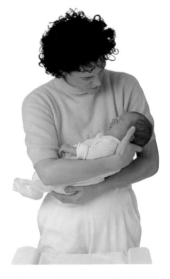

1 When your baby is lying on her back, slide one hand under her lower back and bottom.

2 Slide your other hand under her neck and head, going in from the opposite side.

3 Lift her gently and slowly, so that her body is supported and her head can't loll back.

4 Carefully transfer her head to the crook of your elbow or your shoulder, so it is supported.

PUTTING YOUR BABY DOWN

1 Put one hand underneath her head and neck, then hold her under the bottom with the other. Lower her slowly, gently supporting her until the pad or mattress is taking her weight.

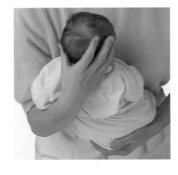

2 Slide your nearest hand out from under her bottom. Use this hand to lift her head a little so you can slide out your other hand, and lower her head down gently. Don't let her head fall back onto the surface, or jerk your arm out quickly.

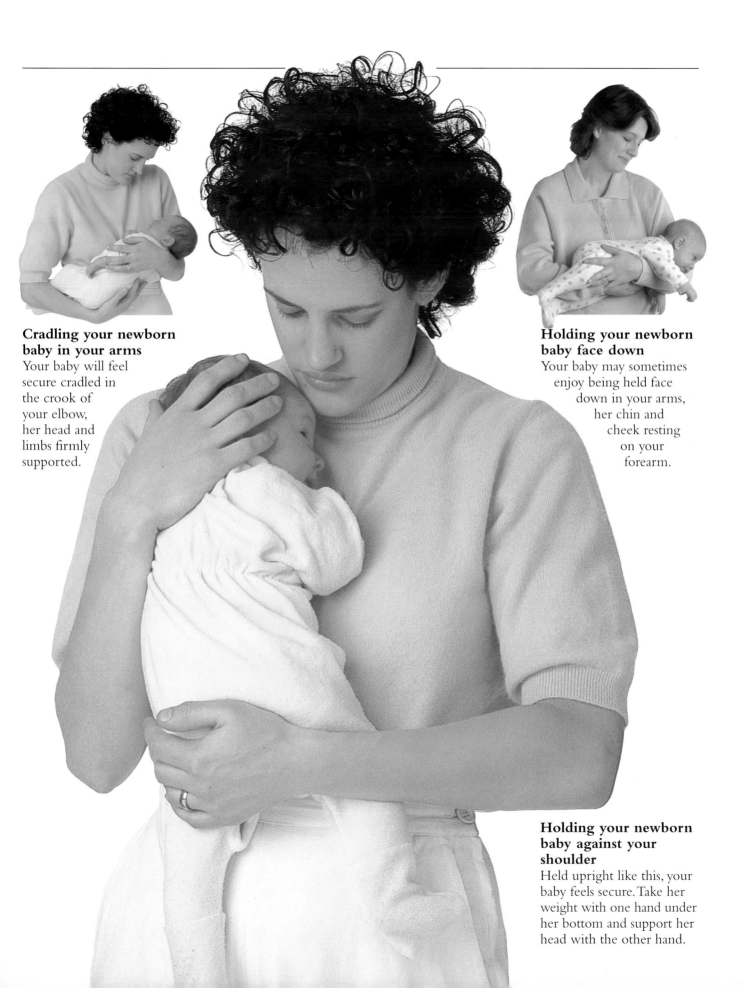

Cradling your newborn baby in your arms
Your baby will feel secure cradled in the crook of your elbow, her head and limbs firmly supported.

Holding your newborn baby face down
Your baby may sometimes enjoy being held face down in your arms, her chin and cheek resting on your forearm.

Holding your newborn baby against your shoulder
Held upright like this, your baby feels secure. Take her weight with one hand under her bottom and support her head with the other hand.

PICKING YOUR BABY UP

1 When asleep in her bassinet or crib, your baby is safest lying on her back or on her side. To pick her up, slide one hand under her neck and head, the other under her bottom.

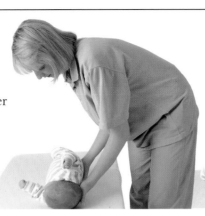

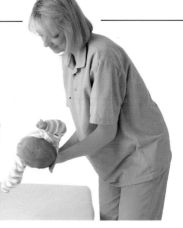

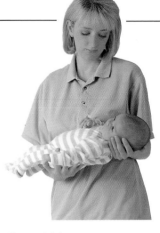

2 Scoop your baby into your arms, making sure her head doesn't flop. Lift her slowly and gently.

3 Hold her against your body, then slide your forearm under her head.

4 Now her head is supported in your elbow, and she feels secure.

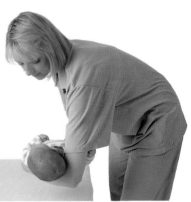

PUTTING YOUR BABY DOWN ON HER BACK OR SIDE

1 When you put your baby down to sleep, lower her to the mattress, keeping her nestled in your arms and her head supported in your elbow.

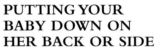

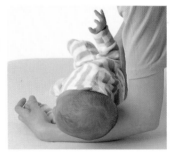

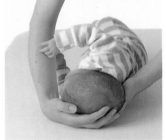

2 Once she is on the mattress, slide out the hand under her bottom.

3 Lift her head so you can slide your arm out and lower her head gently.

PICKING YOUR BABY UP FROM HER FRONT

1 When your baby is lying on her stomach, slide one hand under her chest so your forearm will support her chin when you lift her, and place your other hand under her bottom.

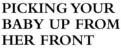

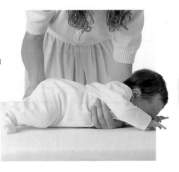

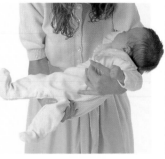

2 Lift her slowly, turning her toward you. Bring her up to your body and slide the arm supporting her head forward, until her head nestles comfortably in the crook of your elbow. Put your other hand under her bottom and legs, so she is cradled and secure.

USING AN INFANT CARRIER

AN INFANT CARRIER is an excellent way of carrying your baby around in the first three months. The contact with your body and the motion as you walk will soothe her, and it leaves your arms free. It's not difficult to put a carrier on when there's nobody to help you; take it off using the same method in reverse.

PUTTING ON AN INFANT CARRIER

1 Slip the carrier straps over your shoulders so that the two metal rings hang down at the front.

2 Attach the padded triangular section by snapping the circular fasteners on the straps into place.

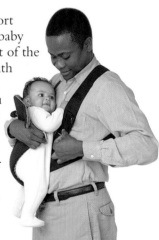

3 Close one side of the carrier by feeding the toggle through the ring and snapping it securely closed.

4 Hold your baby so that she faces you. If she is very young, support her head with your hand. Feed her leg through the hole on the fastened side of the carrier. Keep your arm around her on the open side to ensure that she doesn't fall.

5 Support your baby in the seat of the carrier with one hand while you fasten the toggle and snap under her arm with the other.

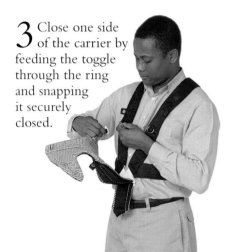

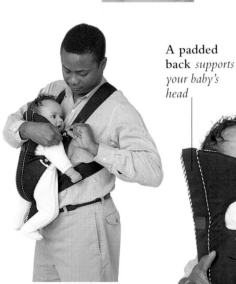

6 Close the top fasteners so that an arm hole is created on each side. The back flap supports a younger baby's head and neck.

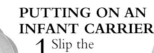

A padded back *supports your baby's head*

WEARING THE CARRIER

After three months, your baby may prefer to face forward. Follow the same sequence, but start with your baby facing forward. With the front flap folded down, she can get a better view of the world around her.

Wide shoulder straps *are the most comfortable*

A machine-washable fabric *is a good idea*

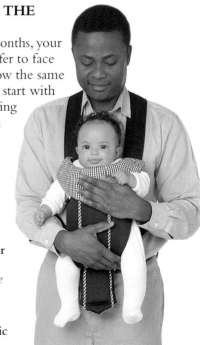

HANDLING AND PHYSICAL PLAY

LET HER FACE FORWARD

Your alert three-month-old has a good view of the world facing forward. Put one hand between her legs, the other around her chest. She doesn't need you to support her head any more.

PLAY BOUNCING GAMES ON YOUR LAP

Your four-month-old baby will love the feeling of being jogged up and down on your knees, in time to a favorite rhyme. Hold his arms in case he jerks backward.

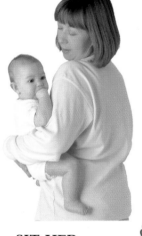

SIT HER ASTRIDE YOUR HIP

Your three-month-old can adjust her own position if she's uncomfortable, and she will cling to you when she needs extra security.

SIT HIM ON YOUR SHOULDER

Sit your six-month-old on your shoulder so he's taller than you are; he will be exhilarated by this new perspective.

EYE-TO-EYE CONTACT

Your baby will love it when you lift her up high. Your face is always the best entertainment of all.

WINDING DOWN

However boisterously you play with your baby, spend a few minutes of gentle, quiet cuddling afterward. Always take your cue from your baby, and forget the roughhousing for today if he's not responding with his usual giggles of pleasure.

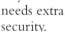

PLAY ROCKING GAMES

Rock her back and forth, going higher and higher if she likes the game. This type of rocking motion is a good way to soothe her, too.

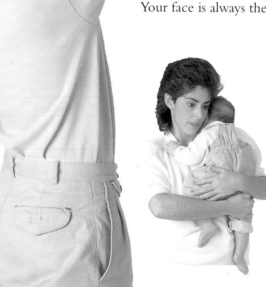

WARNING: Never shake your baby vigorously during any type of play or other handling. It can cause tearing of blood vessels in the brain and permanent damage.

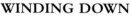

FEEDING YOUR BABY

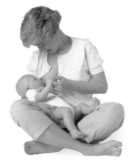

One of the first decisions you and your partner will have to make is whether to breast-feed or bottle-feed your baby. Breast milk meets his needs perfectly and is digested easily, but your baby won't suffer if you decide to bottle-feed. Feeding your baby should be a pleasure, not a challenge, and it will be no pleasure if you breast-feed from a sense of duty, or bottle-feed with a sense of guilt. If instinctively you think you would prefer to bottle-feed, it's a good idea to put the decision off until after your baby is born. There's no substitute for the colostrum that your breasts produce in the first few days (see page 92), and feeding your baby this will provide him with valuable antibodies to help him fight infection in the early months. You can't switch from bottle-feeding to breast-feeding because, without the stimulation of your baby sucking shortly after birth, your breasts will have stopped producing milk. But you can stop breast-feeding and go to bottles. Whichever method you opt for, remember that love, cuddling, and attention are all just as important to your baby as the milk you give him.

BREAST OR BOTTLE

YOU MAY KNOW how you want to feed your baby. If you want to breast-feed, then with information and support you will almost certainly succeed. But even if you're sure bottle-feeding is the method for you, it's worth considering the advantages and disadvantages, and listening to the comments other mothers make. It's a decision that will affect you, your partner, and your baby for months to come.

"I knew that by breast-feeding I was giving him the best possible milk he could have. I could tell he was digesting it easily, and I knew it had exactly the right blend of nutrients."

Breast milk contains substances that help protect your baby from disease until his own immune system has matured. It protects against allergies—which is important if there is a history of allergies in your family. Infant formula can't provide either protection.

"I loved the convenience of breast-feeding my baby: the milk was always there, always sterile, always at the temperature she liked."

"The sheer enjoyment of breast-feeding took me by surprise. It's so intimate, so physically satisfying: her little hand used to come up and stroke my breast, and I could feel her face against my skin. It got better and better, too, as the first year went on."

"The breast was always the best method of soothing my baby when he cried. He wasn't necessarily hungry, he just needed the comfort of sucking."

"The obstetrician told me that the reason I slimmed back to my pre-pregnancy figure so quickly was because I persevered with breast-feeding. So that was an unexpected benefit of listening to her advice."

Breast-feeding is more time-consuming in the early weeks, partly because a breast-fed baby eats more frequently, partly because he likes to suck—in fact sucking is a need and a pleasure quite distinct from the need for food. However, preparing and sterilizing bottles also takes a lot of time and will soon become a chore when you've done it for several months, while nursing becomes less frequent and quicker as your baby gets older.

"I had always been convinced that I couldn't breast-feed—my bust was so small. But I sailed through. I had plenty of milk, and my baby certainly didn't mind my small breasts."

Traveling is easier if you breast-feed: there's no bottle to warm and no danger of storing the prepared formula at too high a temperature.

"The only thing I didn't like about breast-feeding was the nursing at night. I didn't enjoy expressing milk, so the whole burden of those nocturnal sessions fell on me. But it was only for a few weeks of our lives."

"I felt that my decision to bottle-feed was the right one when I saw how much my husband enjoyed feeding our baby: they built a very strong relationship right from the start as a result."

"With a bottle, I could always see how much formula my baby had taken—and that was very reassuring after so many miserable weeks trying to get the hang of breast-feeding."

Exhaustion, illness, or stress which can reduce a breast-milk supply, won't affect the bottle-fed baby's diet.

A bottle-fed baby is more at risk of picking up microorganisms that could cause diarrhea and vomiting.

ESSENTIALS OF FEEDING

DEMAND FEEDING

Feeding on demand simply means giving your baby formula or breast milk whenever he is hungry, not following a timetable.

Hunger is a new sensation for your newborn baby. In the uterus he was being continually nourished. Now he has to go for long periods without food. His digestive system is too immature to cope with large meals at infrequent intervals, so feed him little and often at first.

There is nothing to be gained by keeping your baby hungry once he has cried to be fed—he will only get so distressed that he may refuse to suck. You will have to comfort and calm him until he'll settle down to suck. You're not spoiling your baby by answering his needs. In the early weeks, his empty stomach is the usual reason for waking and crying. As his digestive system matures and his stomach grows, he'll take more at each feeding, and the intervals between feedings will become longer.

How often will he demand food?

Your baby will demand food whenever he needs it, and in the beginning, this will be often. Newborn babies will have no discernible pattern of feeding. By day three or four, feedings will be about every two or three hours, and there may be eight or so a day with a lot of short ones during the evening. At night, you may be feeding your baby two or three times, because few babies under the age of six weeks are able to sleep more than five hours at a stretch without waking with hunger. Breast-fed babies usually need more frequent feedings than bottle-fed babies, because breast milk is more easily and quickly digested than formula.

By three months your baby will probably be settling into a roughly four-hour feeding routine, with five feedings a day, plus one or two at night. If you are bottle-feeding, you will probably be able to establish a four-hour routine more quickly.

SPECIAL CASES

Premature babies A pre-term baby may have a small appetite, but he will need to be fed frequently. He may sleep a lot and may not wake and demand food even though he needs it, so wake your baby every three hours and offer a feeding.

If you managed to express milk for your baby while he was in the hospital intensive care nursery, you will be able to breast-feed once you get him home. It isn't always easy for a baby to adapt to taking milk from a breast. To help him, express a little milk before you start nursing (see page 94) so that the nipple stands out, and rub breast milk over the nipple to give him the taste.

Twins It's perfectly possible to breast-feed twins successfully. Feed them one at a time at first. Then, when you are more confident, you'll find it's easy to feed them both at the same time. Tuck their legs under each of your arms, and their heads can lie in your hands.

GAS AND BURPING

Whether your baby is breast- or bottle-fed, give him the chance to burp up any swallowed air when he pauses for a rest. Gas may be making him feel full. If he doesn't burp after several minutes, give up: he probably doesn't need to bring up any air at that feeding.

Protect your clothes *with a clean cloth diaper*

Your newborn

To help a very young baby bring up gas, put her against your shoulder and rub her back, or lean her forward on your lap, supporting her floppy head under the chin. She's very likely to bring some milk up too, so have a clean cloth diaper or receiving blanket handy.

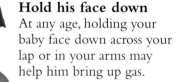

Hold his face down

At any age, holding your baby face down across your lap or in your arms may help him bring up gas.

Rub or pat her back *gently but rhythmically*

Your older baby

By three months, when your baby can sit up for short periods, jiggling him gently on your lap while you rub his back will help him burp up swallowed air.

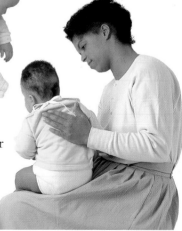

"*Our feeding times were relaxing, calm, and deeply emotional for both of us.*"

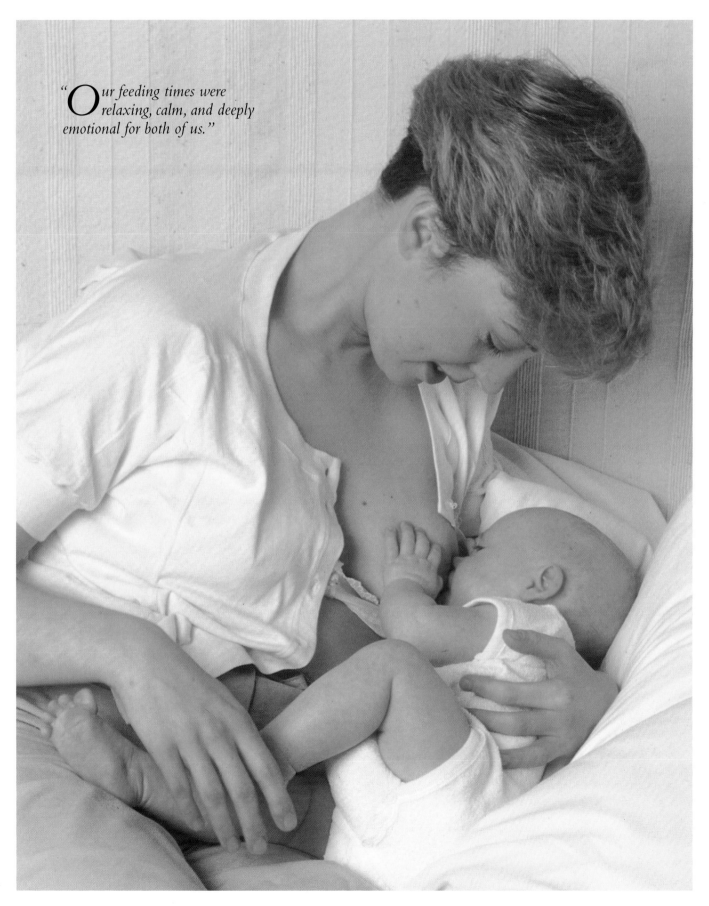

BREAST-FEEDING YOUR BABY

Breast-feeding can be a supremely rewarding aspect of caring for your baby, and you'll be giving her the best nourishment nature can provide, so don't be deterred if you encounter a few problems in the early days. You and your baby have to learn this new skill together, so if at first she doesn't seem to know how to suck, or doesn't suck for very long, be patient with her. She doesn't need a lot of food after birth, and your nipples need time to toughen up and get used to being sucked on. There will be plenty of friends, relatives, and professionals all keen to offer you advice, and it may take some time before you are able to sift out the helpful suggestions and develop a feeling of self-confidence. If you can, talk to someone who has breast-fed successfully and listen to her. It's worth persevering. After the first week or so of possible uncertainty and self-doubt, you can look forward to months of successful and satisfying nursing.

SETTLE YOURSELVES comfortably: you may be there for up to an hour. Take a deep breath and relax your shoulders. The more relaxed you feel to your baby, the easier she will settle down to nurse. Give her plenty of opportunity for skin contact. If you're in private, take your top off: with no clothes in the way, you might find it is easier to get her "latched on"—that is, properly positioned on your breast and sucking efficiently.

FINDING THE NIPPLE

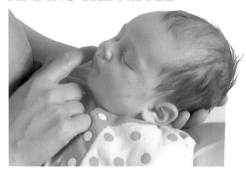

1 Your baby has an instinctive reflex that makes her search for your nipple to find food—this is the "rooting" reflex. Until about her tenth day of life, alert this reflex by touching the cheek nearest to you with your finger or nipple. She will turn toward your breast and search for your nipple.

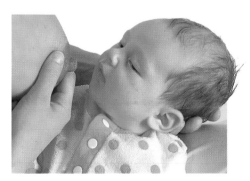

2 If your baby doesn't turn her head instinctively, try gently squeezing just behind your areola until a few drops form on your nipple. Touch her lips with this to encourage her to open her mouth.

GETTING COMFORTABLE

The areola *is the large dark circle around your nipple that your baby "milks" when she nurses*

Nursing your young baby
Sit comfortably in an upright position with your back supported. A low chair without arms is ideal, or sit up in bed with plenty of pillows propping your back. Put a pillow on your lap to bring your baby to the right level, or raise one knee to support her body. To avoid straining your back, position your baby so that she is more on her side than on her back, with her abdomen facing yours. This way you won't have to bend over to get your breast to her.

A pillow *takes the weight of your baby's body*

Make sure your *baby has a hand free to touch and stroke your breast*

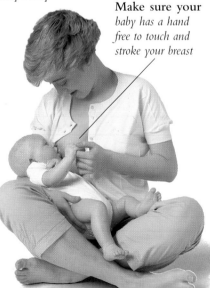

Nursing your older baby
Once you're both adept at breast-feeding, you will find you can nurse in almost any relaxed position. Sitting cross-legged on the bed or floor is excellent, especially if you can lean against pillows or furniture.

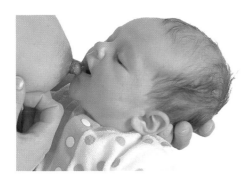

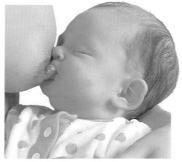

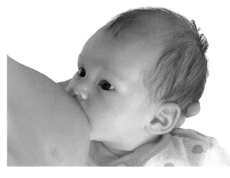

3 Bring her head up close to your breast, so her chin is against it and her tongue is underneath your nipple. Guide your breast in.

1 Once latched on, your baby doesn't just suck, she "milks" the breast with her jaws by pressing on the reservoirs of milk at the base of the areola. Your baby's lips should be curled up and over as much of the areola as possible. If she just sucks on the nipple, you'll get sore and she won't get any milk. If you feel a brief piercing pain, breathe deeply to help you relax.

2 From your viewpoint, your firmly latched-on baby will have her jaws open very wide and her mouth full of your breast. You can tell she is nursing properly when you see her temples and ears moving, indicating that her jaw muscles are working.

THE LET-DOWN REFLEX

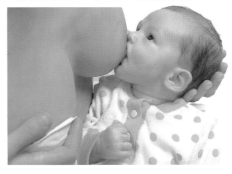

Your baby's sucking action stimulates your breasts to release the milk they have stored. You may feel the warm rush of milk—the let-down reflex—as a tingling sensation soon after your baby has latched on. Not everyone feels it though, so don't be surprised if you don't. If the reflex makes milk leak out of the other breast too, hold a breast pad over your nipple to catch drips.

Talk to your baby
as you feed her: communication is as vital as the milk itself

Hold your baby
with her head higher than the rest of her body

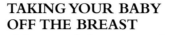

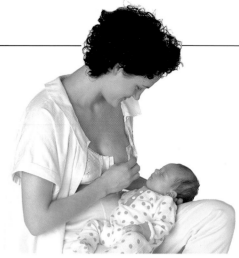

TAKING YOUR BABY OFF THE BREAST

1 Let your baby nurse at the first breast until she drains it—usually seven to ten minutes. Your breast will look smaller, and feel lighter, when all the milk has gone. Your baby will often pause when you are nursing her. She may want to keep sucking though. If after several minutes she doesn't take any milk, remove her from the breast to burp her. Don't pull your nipple away—this will hurt. Slip a finger between her jaws to break the suction.

Use your clean
*little finger to break
your baby's suction*

2 Slip a tissue into your bra on the side your baby has emptied. At the next feeding put her on the other side to begin with, so both breasts get equal stimulation. Sit your baby up to burp her.

OFFER THE OTHER BREAST

1 After a burp or two, offer the other breast. She may be hungry enough to drain this one, too, or she may just suck for comfort—which she needs as much as the milk. Always offer both breasts at each feeding.

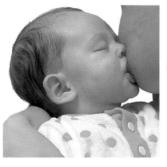

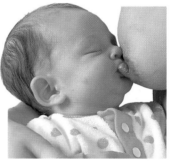

2 When your baby's had enough, she will fall fast asleep in your arms and let your nipple slip from her mouth. Call your pediatrician if she refuses to nurse or her urine and stool output are infrequent.

HOW YOUR BREASTS PRODUCE MILK

In the first days after the birth your breasts produce colostrum, a protein-rich food that supplies your baby with valuable antibodies against infection. Once you begin to produce milk around the fourth day, your baby will naturally stimulate your body into producing plenty.

The key to a good milk supply is feeding your baby when she wants to be fed—and in the early days that means nursing at two- or three-hour intervals. Breast milk production works on a supply and demand system: the more often your baby nurses, and the more she takes, the more your breasts will

produce. Supplementary bottles of formula will undermine this system. If your baby's hunger is satisfied by a bottle, she won't be eager to suck and your breasts won't be stimulated.

Breast milk isn't all the same. At the beginning of the feeding your baby takes what is sometimes called the foremilk, which is watery and thirst-quenching. As she nurses, the fat content of your milk rises, and she soon starts getting the hindmilk, rich in calories. This is why it's important to save prolonged nursing for the second breast offered. This will give her the maximum amount of milk at each feeding.

What you need to do
All you need to do to produce enough milk is to eat a balanced diet with plenty of protein, to drink whenever you're thirsty—have a glass of juice or milk on hand while you nurse—and to rest as much as you can. This is also not the time to diet. Make sure you get the extra calories (and energy) you need from fresh, vitamin-rich foods rather than "empty" carbohydrates. Although breast milk is the best nourishment for your baby, it is very low in vitamin D. If your baby is exclusively breast-fed, she'll require a daily dose (200 IU) of vitamin D.

WHEN YOUR MILK COMES IN

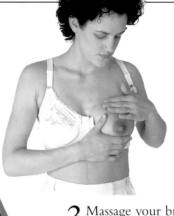

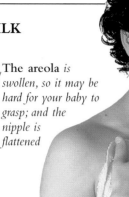

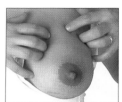

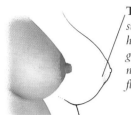

The areola is swollen, so it may be hard for your baby to grasp; and the nipple is flattened

Normal breast   Engorged breast

1 On about the fourth day of breast-feeding your breasts start to produce mature milk, rather than the colostrum that you've fed your baby up to now. You may wake up to find your breasts big, hard, and uncomfortable. This is engorgement, and it may last for 48 hours. Your baby will find it hard to latch on because the nipple isn't sticking out, but is flattened by the swollen areola. The following tips should help her to nurse, lessen the engorgement, and ease your discomfort.

2 Before you try to nurse your baby, soften your breasts by laying warm washcloths or hand towels over them for several minutes, or stand in the shower and run warm water over them.

3 Massage your breasts gently with your hands, and try to express some milk to relieve the swelling and help your baby get the nipple in her mouth (see page 94). Don't worry if you can't get the hang of expressing at this stage. You soon will.

4 When you put your baby to the breast, put your free hand on your ribcage under your breast and push gently upward: this should help the nipple to protrude so your baby can get the areola in her mouth. Her sucking will quickly relieve the engorgement and discomfort.

QUESTION & ANSWERS

"Joe cries a great deal; could it be that he isn't getting enough milk from me?"
When you are breast-feeding, you can't actually see what your baby takes, so it's natural at times to worry that he's not getting enough. But as long as you nurse whenever your baby cries, *and* he is gaining weight normally with occasional spurts, you have no need to worry. After two weeks of age, your baby will gain quickly—about $\frac{1}{2}$ to $1\frac{1}{2}$ ounces a day. Another sign to watch is the number of diapers your baby wets per day. Six to eight is a good indicator that he's getting enough milk.

"Will breast-feeding alter my figure for life?"
Your breasts may be slightly smaller after you've weaned your baby from the breast, because some of the fatty tissue has been replaced by milk glands. Otherwise, you will probably regain your pre-pregnancy figure more quickly if you breast-feed, because the hormones released encourage the uterus to shrink back to normal quickly, and the fat reserves that your body stored during pregnancy are used in the production of breast milk. Your waistline contracts sooner, too.

"Do I have to be as careful about the drugs and medication I take as when I was pregnant?"
What you eat and drink can be passed on to your baby through your milk, so it's vital that you tell your pharmacist or doctor that you are breast-feeding before they suggest any medicines for you. It's sensible to avoid alcohol, nicotine, and caffeine, too. If your baby doesn't sleep well, it may be worth cutting coffee, tea, and other caffeine-containing products, such as soft drinks and chocolate, out of your diet for a few weeks to see if the situation improves.

EXPRESSING MILK BY HAND

THE ABILITY to express your own milk gives you great flexibility. You can freeze the milk (keep it for up to one month), and someone else can give it to your baby when you're out. (See pages 98–107 for bottle-feeding advice.) But expressing by hand can be very difficult for many women. Wash the equipment and your hands. Encourage the flow of milk by having a warm bath, or hold warm washcloths over your breasts. Make yourself comfortable by a high surface, with the bowl in front of you.

■ YOU WILL NEED ■
Large bowl
Clean bottle
Nipple
Plastic funnel

THE FIRST BREAST

Use your *whole hand to massage the breast*

1 Support your breast in one hand and start to massage, working downward from above the breast.

2 Work your way all around the breast, including the underside. Complete at least ten circuits: this helps the flow of milk through the ducts.

3 Stroke downward toward the areola with your fingernails several times. Avoid pressing on the breast tissue.

4 Apply gentle down-ward pressure on the area behind the areola with your thumbs and fingers.

5 Squeeze thumbs and forefingers together, at the same time pressing backward. The milk should spurt out through the nipple. Keep this up for a couple of minutes.

ALTERNATING BREASTS

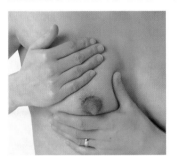

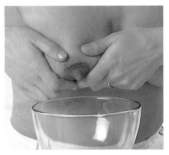

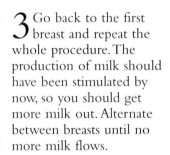

1 Repeat the massaging on the other breast.

2 Squeeze some milk out of the nipple.

3 Go back to the first breast and repeat the whole procedure. The production of milk should have been stimulated by now, so you should get more milk out. Alternate between breasts until no more milk flows.

STORING THE MILK

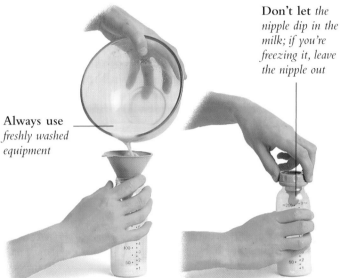

Always use *freshly washed equipment*

Don't let *the nipple dip in the milk; if you're freezing it, leave the nipple out*

1 Pour the milk into a bottle. In the early weeks, you may get 2–3fl oz (60–80ml).

2 Seal the bottle tightly and refrigerate, or cool and freeze. Thaw the bottle under tepid running water, not by using the microwave.

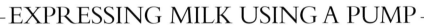

EXPRESSING MILK USING A PUMP

EXPRESSING BY PUMP can be quicker and less tiring than expressing by hand. A wide variety of pumps—manually-operated, battery-powered, or electric; single or double breast—is available for sale or rental. The manual "syringe" type of pump, shown here, is a reasonable and inexpensive choice, but it takes two hands to operate and can be tiring. A high-quality, double breast, electric pump is a faster, more practical option, especially for working mothers.

Funnel

Inner cylinder

Outer cylinder
converts into a baby's bottle

Breast pump

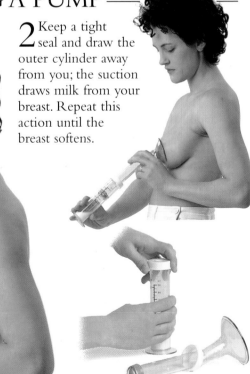

2 Keep a tight seal and draw the outer cylinder away from you; the suction draws milk from your breast. Repeat this action until the breast softens.

1 Wash and dry all the equipment thoroughly, and then wash your hands. Assemble the pump. Soften your breasts using warm washcloths and massage them just as when expressing by hand. Place the funnel of the pump over the areola so that it forms an airtight seal; it needs to press on the milk ducts just as your baby's jaws do.

3 Put the cap on tightly and refrigerate, or freeze until needed.

BOTTLE-FEEDING YOUR BABY

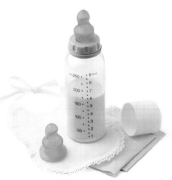

In the last twenty years there has been a dramatic increase in the number of new mothers who are breast-feeding their babies. But if you have decided to bottle-feed, the first rule of thumb is: Don't let anyone make you feel guilty about your choice. It's a good one, and your child is just as likely to thrive as the breast-fed baby. What your infant needs is enough to eat and lots of tender loving care. Cuddling, cooing, and holding your baby in the crook of your arm while you feed him will give him the same kind of security and sense of you that a breast-feeding mother might offer. So don't fall into an insecurity trap. Besides, you'll be able to share the feedings with your mate. There is no other baby in the world quite like yours, and what you bring to him through your choice of feeding is your own particular style of mothering. Someone else's way of doing things is not what he needs. It's you that makes the critical difference in his brand new life, not bottles or breasts. Feeding your baby can be as easy as pouring ready-made formula into a clean bottle and finding a comfortable spot to sit down. With your pediatrician's help, pick a brand of formula, and always follow the directions very precisely when you mix the powder or concentrated liquid kinds.

EQUIPMENT FOR BOTTLE-FEEDING

FOR A FULLY bottle-fed baby you will need 6 to 8 full size 8oz (250ml) bottles. Buy extra nipples and have them ready in a clean jar in case the one you are using is inadequate. Sometimes the holes are either too large or too small. Some bottles have throw-away plastic liners, which reduce the air your baby swallows: the bag collapses as he sucks, so the nipple doesn't flatten and halt the flow.

BOTTLES

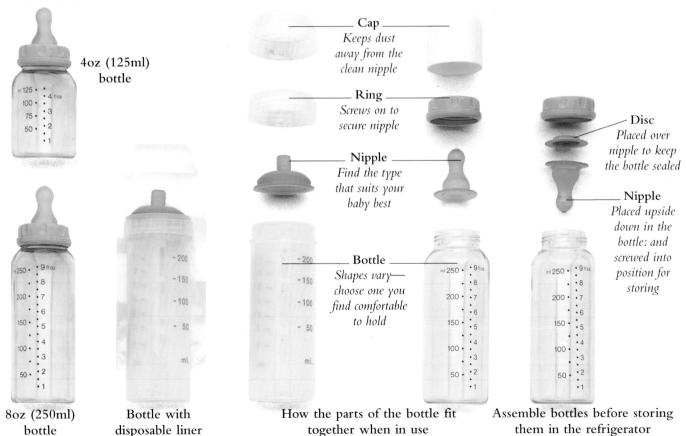

4oz (125ml) bottle

Cap
Keeps dust away from the clean nipple

Ring
Screws on to secure nipple

Nipple
Find the type that suits your baby best

Bottle
Shapes vary— choose one you find comfortable to hold

Disc
Placed over nipple to keep the bottle sealed

Nipple
Placed upside down in the bottle: and screwed into position for storing

8oz (250ml) bottle

Bottle with disposable liner

How the parts of the bottle fit together when in use

Assemble bottles before storing them in the refrigerator

NIPPLES

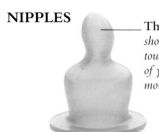

The holes *should point toward the roof of your baby's mouth*

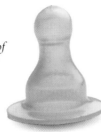

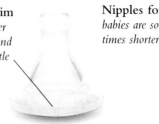

Valve in rim *lets air under the nipple and into the bottle*

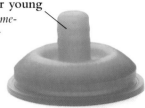

Nipples for young *babies are sometimes shorter*

Natural-shaped nipple
This type is thought to most closely mimic the suction action of breast-feeding. It helps avoid "nipple confusion" in babies who are being both breast- and bottle-fed. It should go into your baby's mouth with the holes up, so formula sprays over the roof of his mouth.

Universal nipple
The standard shape of a nipple gives a sucking action that is not really like sucking from your breast. Nipples are sold with different rates of flow, but check at each feeding: there should be one drop a second. A cross-cut hole gives better flow than a pinhole.

Anti-colic nipple
An anti-colic nipple lets air into the bottle as your baby sucks. This stops the nipple from collapsing, enabling him to get a steady stream without gulping air. Silicone nipples, shown above, last up to a year; latex nipples deteriorate after about one month of heavy use.

Wide-based nipple
This type is not interchangeable among different bottles. As your baby sucks, his lips push against the squashy base and the nipples moves in and out within his mouth, rather than like a human nipple. (Fit the nipple and ring together before assembling the bottle prior to filling.)

OTHER EQUIPMENT

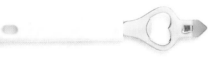

Bottle brush Needed to clean thoroughly inside the bottles. Keep it for this purpose only.

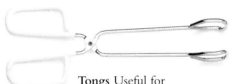

Can opener
For opening cans of formula. Wash well first.

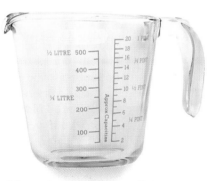

Measuring cup (optional) For mixing powder formula.

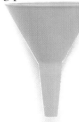

Plastic funnel (optional) Useful for pouring formula into bottles.

Plastic spoon (optional) For stirring formula.

Plastic knife For leveling off scoops of power formula.

STERILIZING BOTTLES

Not all pediatricians agree about the need to sterilize bottles. If you wash them thoroughly using soap and hot water, there may be no need. If you use a dishwasher, the high heat of the drying cycle will kill any potentially dangerous bacteria. However, some doctors do recommend sterilizing, especially for a newborn baby. If this is true for you, you'll need an extra large pot in which to boil your bottles and all your formula-making equipment.

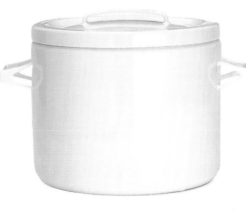

Tongs Useful for gripping hot bottles.

Large pot Choose one big enough to accommodate several bottles.

MAKING UP YOUR BABY'S BOTTLE

IN THE EARLY WEEKS you need to have a supply of bottles ready in the refrigerator so that whenever your baby cries, wanting to be fed, you can respond quickly and easily. Until your baby is a year old, give him an infant formula. Most are modified cow's milk. Your pediatrician will help you choose a brand. You can upset your baby by switching brands, so never do so without professional advice.

Making up formula

Infant formula is most commonly and cheaply available as concentrated liquid or powder that can readily be mixed up as required.

The instructions on the cans tell you the correct amount of liquid or number of scoops to add to each measure of water. It is very important to maintain these proportions exactly. If you add too much formula, the feeding will be dangerously concentrated: your baby may gain too much weight, and his kidneys may be damaged. If you consistently add too little powder, he may gain weight too slowly and could eventually become malnourished.

Mothers used to be advised to dilute formula for a baby suffering from vomiting or diarrhea, but this is no longer the case. If your baby has diarrhea or vomiting, consult your pediatrician, who may advise you to use an oral rehydration solution (see page 179).

Always use fresh, cold tap water to make up your baby's formula, and if boiling is required in your area, boil it only once. Never use:

■ water that has been repeatedly boiled, or left standing in the kettle for more than an hour or two
■ water from a tap with a domestic softener attached—the extra sodium (salt) can damage your baby's kidneys
■ water from a tap with a domestic filter attached—these filters can trap harmful bacteria
■ mineral water—the sodium and minerals may be harmful.

There are two methods of making up your baby's bottle: mixing the formula directly in the bottles, or mixing it in a container or measuring cup first. Use the cup method if you use boottles with disposable liners.

Ready-to-feed formula

Some brands of infant formula are also available ready-mixed in cans and require no extra water. These make a very convenient option.

The formula in the cans has been ultra-heat treated (UHT), so it is already sterile. Store unopened cans in a cool place, and do not use them after the "expiration" date.

Once opened, ready-to-feed formula can be stored in the refrigerator for up to 48 hours, either in a sterile, sealed bottle, or in the can, which must be covered. But unless you can be sure that you won't forget when you put the can in the refrigerator, it's probably safer to pour all the formula into clean, ready-to-use bottles. Throw away any he doesn't drink after each feeding.

How much will my baby want?

Babies' appetites vary from day to day. During the first weeks of life put 4fl oz (125ml) of formula into each of 6 bottles; see how that matches your baby's appetite. As he gains weight, he will often cry for more at the end of a feeding, so gradually increase the amount you put into each bottle. By the time he is six months old you will be making up bottles of 7-8fl oz (200-230ml). As a rough guide, your baby needs about 2$\frac{1}{2}$fl oz of formula per pound (150ml per kg) of body weight every 24 hours. So if a 12lb (5.5kg) baby is on six feedings a day, he may take about 5fl oz (140ml) of formula at each feeding. No baby ever needs more than a quart (1 liter) of formula in a day. If your baby seems to need more, it is worth investigating.

Demand vs. scheduled bottles

It takes weeks and often months for babies to settle into predictable feeding schedules. At first, your baby may be hungry every half hour, then every two, three, or four hours. In years past, mothers were advised to follow strict four-hour feeding schedules, withholding bottles until the appointed hour had arrived. Nowadays, both pediatricians and mothers take a softer approach and believe that babies should take the lead as far as schedules are concerned. By ten weeks, most babies are close to an eating pattern of every three or four hours. If your baby is cranky right after draining a full bottle or within an hour, try burping her or offering some other soothing technique, such as a walk in the stroller or a warm bath.

Should I give anything else?

Most bottle-fed babies don't need anything but formula for the first six months of life. Some doctors recommend vitamin and mineral supplements or additional fluoride, but check first. Too many vitamins can make your baby sick.

The majority of doctors and the American Academy of Pediatrics generally suggest holding off on solid foods until at least four to six months of age. You may be tempted to try some cereal in your baby's diet if he appears not to be satisfied with just formula, but until he can let you know that he wants more or less food, pushing solids can amount to force-feeding, so be patient.

When bottle-fed babies are allergic to formula

Many commercial formulas are modified cow's milk, and some infants have allergic reactions to them. Upset stomachs, diarrhea, irritability, and skin rashes will let you know that something isn't quite right. Call your pediatrician if you suspect an allergy. He or she will be able to recommend formulas that have no cow's milk (soy-based, for instance) as an alternative.

USING CONCENTRATED LIQUID FORMULA

■ YOU WILL NEED ■

Can of concentrated liquid formula

Bottles and nipples

Can opener

1 Boil water in a kettle. Rinse the top of the can by pouring the boiling water over the lid. Shake the formula can well.

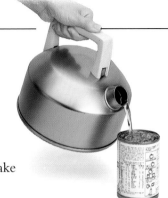

2 Open the can in two places using a clean can opener. Refill the kettle with fresh tap water, boil it, then let it cool for five minutes.

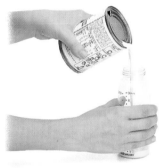

3 Pour the concentrate into a clean bottle until you have half the total feeding amount. Check the amount at eye level.

4 Top off with an equal quantity of cooled boiled water. With the bottle at eye level, make sure you have doubled the amount of concentrate.

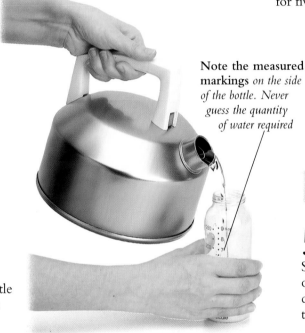

Note the measured markings on the side of the bottle. Never guess the quantity of water required

5 Attach the disc and ring to the bottle. Shake the mixture, leaving out the nipple to avoid coating it in milk. Store in the refrigerator.

USING READY-TO-FEED FORMULA

■ YOU WILL NEED ■

Can of ready-to-feed formula

Bottles and nipples

Can opener

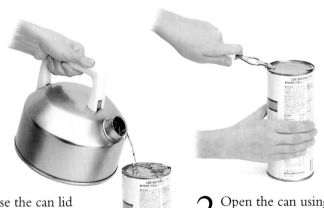

1 Rinse the can lid by pouring boiling water over it. Shake the formula can well to ensure the contents are evenly mixed.

2 Open the can using a clean punch-type opener. Then make a second opening very carefully so the formula does not spill.

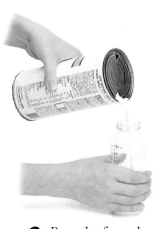

3 Pour the formula into a bottle. Attach the nipple and ring. Shake the bottle, test the temperature, and feed.

MAKING UP POWDERED FORMULA IN BOTTLES

■ YOU WILL NEED ■

Powdered formula
Bottles and nipples
Knife
Paper towels

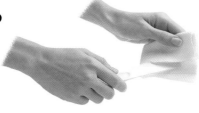

1 Boil water in the kettle to rinse the freshly washed equipment. Pour the boiled water all over the equipment. Drain everything on paper towels. Dry the knife.

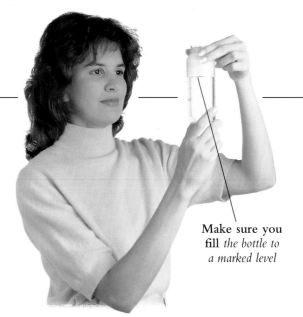

Make sure you **fill** *the bottle to a marked level*

2 Empty the kettle, fill it with fresh, cold tap water, and re-boil. Pour the boiling water into the bottles, filling them to a suitable measure. Check at eye level: the measure must be exact to mix the formula to the right concentration.

3 Open the can of formula and use the special scoop inside. Level each scoop off with the back of a clean knife: *do not* heap the scoop, nor pack the powder down inside it.

4 Drop each scoop of powder into the bottle of water. Add only the number of scoops recommended for that amount of water. The powder will dissolve quickly in the warm water.

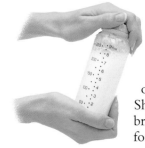

5 Put the disc and ring on the bottle—not the nipple at this stage—and screw on tightly to seal. Shake the bottle briskly to mix the formula thoroughly.

MAKING UP FORMULA USING A CUP

■ YOU WILL NEED ■

Powdered formula or concentrated liquid
Bottles and nipples
Knife
Paper towels
Measuring cup
Spoon
Plastic funnel

1 Make sure your equipment is clean and dry. Boil fresh, cold tap water in the kettle. Fill the cup to an exact full measure. Use the scoop inside the formula can. Level each scoop off with the back of a knife.

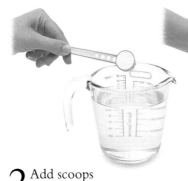

2 Add scoops of powder or the correct amount of concentrated liquid to the cup. Use only the amount recommended for that measure of water, and never any more.

3 Stir the formula well with a spoon until it is thoroughly mixed. The warm water will help dissolve the concentrated liquid.

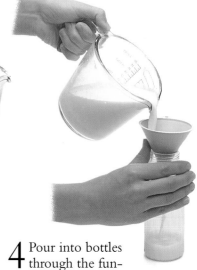

4 Pour into bottles through the funnel. Put the nipple in upside down. Cover with the disc and ring. Make up more formula until the bottles are full.

USING DISPOSABLE LINERS

■ YOU WILL NEED ■
Powdered or concentrated liquid formula
Bottles and nipples
Disposable liners
Knife
Paper towels
Measuring cup
Spoon
Plastic funnel

1 Make up the formula in a measuring cup, a pitcher, or any clean container and follow the manufacturer's directions carefully. If you prefer, open a can of ready-to-use formula (see page 103). Wash your hands. Push the nipple into the ring without touching the tip of it. Tear a pre-sterilized disposable liner off its roll.

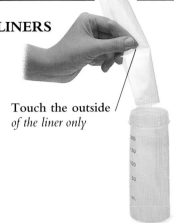

Touch the outside *of the liner only*

2 Fold the liner in half lengthways and place it in the "bottle"—it's not a real bottle, but a plastic sleeve that supports the liner, nipple, and ring.

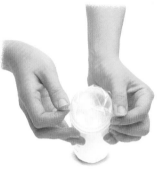

3 Make sure the liner folds well down all round the rim—otherwise milk will spill out.

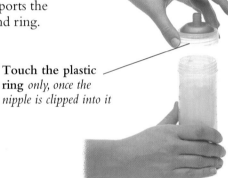

Touch the plastic ring *only, once the nipple is clipped into it*

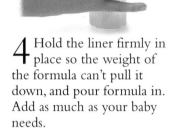

4 Hold the liner firmly in place so the weight of the formula can't pull it down, and pour formula in. Add as much as your baby needs.

5 Screw on the ring with the nipple already secured—this will hold the liner. Pull off the perforated tabs and dispose of them immediately. Put the cap over the nipple of each one and store the bottles in the refrigerator.

STORING THE BOTTLES

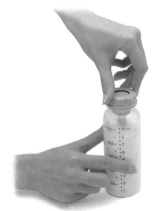

1 To store a batch of feedings, put the nipples in upside down after you've shaken the formula, or insert the nipples later.

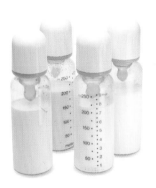

2 Cool the bottles under the cold tap and store in the refrigerator with the caps on. Use stored formula within 24 hours.

STORING OPENED CANS

If you prefer to make up feedings as your baby asks for them, you can store the cans of unused ready-to-feed or concentrate formula in the refrigerator for up to 48 hours. Always cover the can so bacteria cannot enter. It's easy to forget when you opened the can, so use date labels or mark the date on your calendar. Be very strict with yourself about throwing away any formula opened for longer than 48 hours.

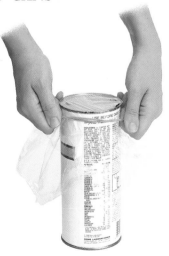

Covering the can
Place plastic wrap over the lid of an opened can and secure with a rubber band.

GIVING YOUR BABY A BOTTLE

FEEDING YOUR BABY is the most important thing you can do for her—but don't make the mistake of thinking that the formula in the bottle is all she needs, or that "anyone" can feed her. Your love, your cuddling, and attention are just as important to your baby as the formula itself. Always hold her close and cuddle her against you, smile and talk to her—just as you would if you were breast-feeding. Never leave your baby alone with her bottle; she may choke.

Right from the beginning, give your baby as much control over feeding as you can. Let her set the pace, pausing to look around, touch the bottle, or stroke your breast if she wants to. Feeding may take as long as a half hour if she's feeling playful. Above all, let her decide when she's had enough.

Make yourself comfortable, put a pillow under your arm, and have a cloth diaper ready to burp her.

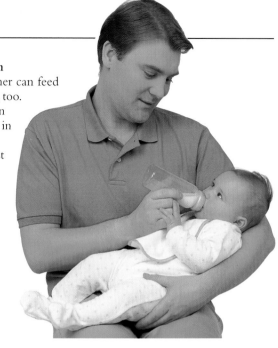

Dad's turn
Your partner can feed your baby, too. Fathers can be critical in a switch from breast to bottle.

FROM BREAST TO BOTTLE

If you decide to switch to bottle-feeding for any reason, remember that the transition from breast to bottle calls for a gradual approach.

Offering one bottle every third day in place of your breast is the best method. Go slowly at first and let your baby set the pace of the transition. Start with a middle-of-the-day nursing. If your baby resists the bottle, don't force the issue. Try again at the same time the following day. If necessary, try a different type of nipple. Or enlist your partner's help and ask him to feed the baby the bottle. Some infants automatically associate breast-feeding with their mothers but will be more daring in their acceptance of a bottle from someone else. Gradually switch other feedings to a bottle, leaving night-time nursings for last.

QUESTION & ANSWER

"My baby never seems to finish her bottle. Is she getting enough?"
A poor appetite could be a sign of illness or of a serious problem that needs medical attention. Check how much formula your baby should be taking for her weight (see page 102), and see if that matches what she drinks. It is important that you have your baby weighed regularly. Your doctor should plot her weight on a growth chart. A baby who is never interested in her bottle or is not gaining weight at a steady rate is always a cause for concern.

GETTING THE BOTTLE READY

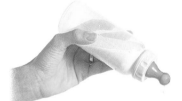

1 Take a bottle from the refrigerator and turn the nipple right side up. Warm in warm water. NEVER use a microwave oven because the formula may get very hot while the bottle still feels cool.

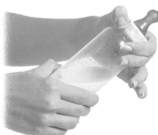

2 Check the flow of formula: it should be one drop a second. Too small a hole will make sucking hard, too large a hole will allow formula to gush out. If the nipple isn't right, swap it for another one and test the flow again.

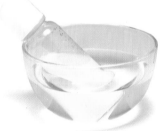

3 Test the temperature by shaking a few drops on the inside of your wrist—it should feel tepid. Cold formula is safe, but your baby may prefer it warm.

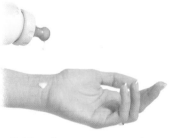

4 Unscrew the ring slightly, leaving it on the bottle, but letting a little air in. This simple step will stop the nipple from collapsing as your baby sucks.

GIVING YOUR BABY HER BOTTLE

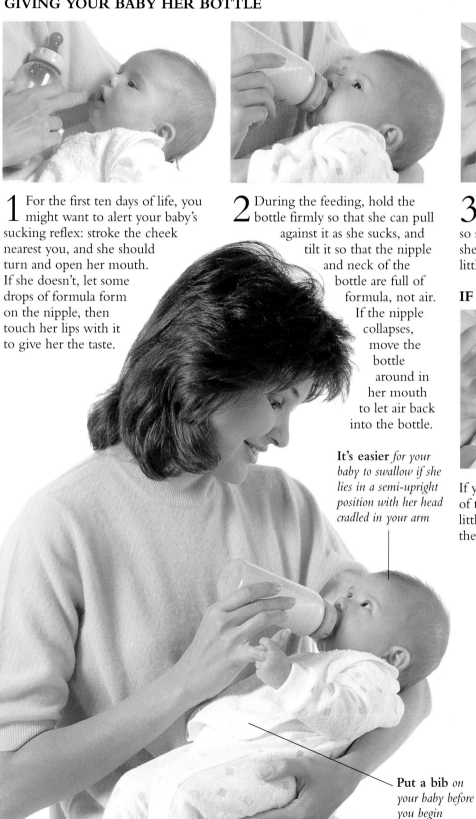

1 For the first ten days of life, you might want to alert your baby's sucking reflex: stroke the cheek nearest you, and she should turn and open her mouth. If she doesn't, let some drops of formula form on the nipple, then touch her lips with it to give her the taste.

2 During the feeding, hold the bottle firmly so that she can pull against it as she sucks, and tilt it so that the nipple and neck of the bottle are full of formula, not air. If the nipple collapses, move the bottle around in her mouth to let air back into the bottle.

It's easier *for your baby to swallow if she lies in a semi-upright position with her head cradled in your arm*

Put a bib *on your baby before you begin*

3 When your baby has finished all the formula, pull the bottle away so she can't swallow too much air. If she wants to suck, offer her your clean little finger or a pacifier.

IF SHE WON'T LET GO

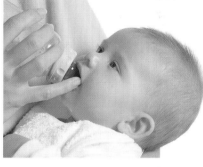

If your baby doesn't want to let go of the empty bottle, slide your clean little finger between her gums and the nipple to release the suction.

SLEEPING DURING A FEEDING

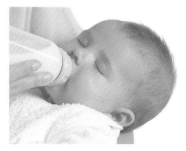

If she dozes off during her feeding, she may have gas, which is making her feel full. Sit her up and burp her for a couple of minutes, and then offer her some more formula.

INTRODUCING SOLID FOOD

Until age four to six months, your baby's food intake should be limited to breast milk or formula, and nothing else—not even juice or water. As she grows closer to six months, however, you may find yourself curious and eager to let her try "real" food. Perhaps she's been watching you from her infant seat while you eat dinner. Or maybe a neighbor has been insisting that she will sleep longer at night if you feed her solids. (Don't believe it! Food isn't the only factor in a sleepless night.)

Check with your doctor before introducing anything into her diet because starting solids too soon can cause problems. But if your baby is between five and six months, your pediatrician will probably agree that she is physically capable of taking her first tastes. Learning to eat is a gradual, enjoyable, and messy process for your baby, and it can be a challenge for you, too. Introduce her to as many new foods as you can to vary her diet and tastes, but let her decide how much she eats.

IS YOUR BABY READY?

WATCH OUT FOR the fascinating signs that your baby might be ready for "real" food. By six months, her sucking reflex is much less intense. She may be trying to bite and chew on anything and everything.

All her drooling means that saliva can help her swallow. And she can move food from the front of her mouth to the back now. All these signs mean you'll soon be needing some new equipment for her.

UTENSILS

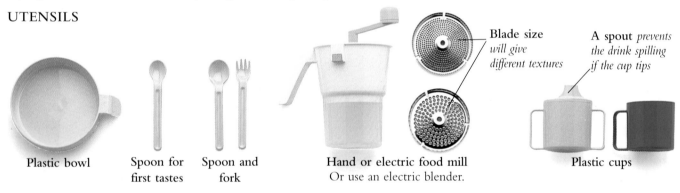

Plastic bowl

Spoon for first tastes

Spoon and fork

Hand or electric food mill
Or use an electric blender.

Blade size *will give different textures*

A spout *prevents the drink spilling if the cup tips*

Plastic cups

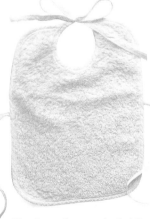

SPILLPROOF BOWL

A plastic bowl with a suction ring on the bottom is difficult for your baby to throw on the floor. This bowl usually has three food compartments as well as a double shell with a stoppered hole, so that you can fill the cavity with hot water to keep food warm for a slow eater.

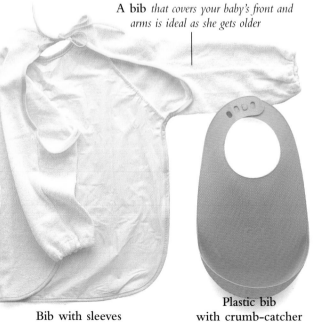

A bib *that covers your baby's front and arms is ideal as she gets older*

Plastic and terrycloth bib
This is the best type in the early months. Plastic backing and ties at the sides insure that your child's clothes are protected.

Bib with sleeves

Plastic bib with crumb-catcher

CHAIRS

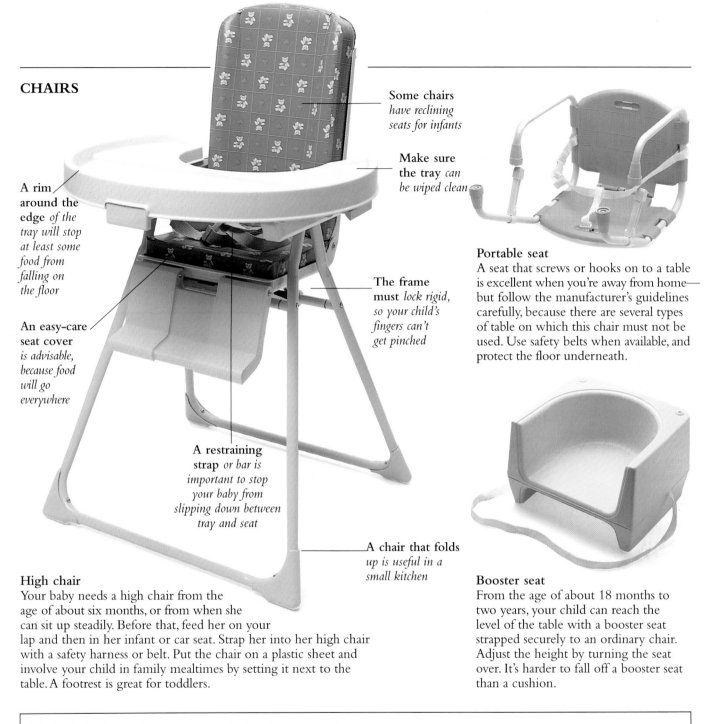

Some chairs have reclining seats for infants

Make sure **the tray** *can be wiped clean*

A rim around the *edge of the tray will stop at least some food from falling on the floor*

An easy-care *seat cover is advisable, because food will go everywhere*

The frame *must lock rigid, so your child's fingers can't get pinched*

A restraining strap *or bar is important to stop your baby from slipping down between tray and seat*

A chair that folds *up is useful in a small kitchen*

Portable seat
A seat that screws or hooks on to a table is excellent when you're away from home—but follow the manufacturer's guidelines carefully, because there are several types of table on which this chair must not be used. Use safety belts when available, and protect the floor underneath.

High chair
Your baby needs a high chair from the age of about six months, or from when she can sit up steadily. Before that, feed her on your lap and then in her infant or car seat. Strap her into her high chair with a safety harness or belt. Put the chair on a plastic sheet and involve your child in family mealtimes by setting it next to the table. A footrest is great for toddlers.

Booster seat
From the age of about 18 months to two years, your child can reach the level of the table with a booster seat strapped securely to an ordinary chair. Adjust the height by turning the seat over. It's harder to fall off a booster seat than a cushion.

WHY WAIT TO FEED YOUR BABY SOLIDS?

Years ago, parents fed their infants puréed or liquefied solids almost from birth. It wasn't unusual for a two-week-old to be sucking pabulum or rice cereal from a spoon. But studies have shown that the digestive tract of a baby that young isn't ready for solid foods. Allergies, indigestion, constipation, and diarrhea are more likely to plague your infant if you start solids too soon. The kidneys and intestines of a young baby are equipped to handle the proportion of fat, protein, and carbohydrates in formula or breast milk, and not much else.

Another reason to hold off on solids is that your baby will be able to let you know when he wants more by leaning forward with an open mouth, or that he has had enough by turning his head away. He can't do this until he has gained head, neck, and upper body control.

Should you balance your baby's diet?
Pediatricians often provide a list of suggested first foods with amounts indicated. But you shouldn't worry if your baby rejects solids at first. At six months, the average infant needs only 800 calories a day, and most of them can come from formula or breast milk. There's no real need to be religious about balancing his diet, but do try a wide variety of foods.

GETTING STARTED ON SOLIDS

PUTTING A LITTLE SPOONFUL of food to the lips of a six-month-old is one of those milestones most parents savor. Your baby's facial expressions alone may amaze you. Whether you choose a small glob of baby cereal, mashed banana, applesauce, or puréed pear, or take this first taste straight from a jar of strained carrots, keep in mind that what you are doing is introducing the idea of solids. Your child is still getting all the nutrition she needs from a bottle, breast, or a combination of both. Try "sandwiching" a first taste into the middle of a regular feeding. She won't be frustrated if she isn't famished, but it might take a while, so be patient. Don't try to speed up the process by placing cereal in your baby's bottle—that could be a choking hazard.

■ YOU WILL NEED ■

Bib
Small plastic bowl
Small spoon
About a tablespoon of applesauce, pear purée, or baby rice cereal
Damp tissue or washcloth

FOLLOW YOUR BABY'S CUES

The American Academy of Pediatrics divides infant feeding into three stages: (1) the nursing period when only formula or human breast milk is given, (2) a transitional period when solids are added, and (3) a modified adult phase during which the bulk of your child's caloric intake comes from the table and less and less from bottle or breast. Most children reach the third stage after their first birthday. Be spontaneous and creative at mealtimes. If your child detests cereal for breakfast and loves sweet potatoes, listen to him. He may not be able to talk, but he's speaking his mind loudly and clearly.

FEED HER FIRST

Sit down with your baby's bowl of food within reach. Put a bib on her, then give her half her usual breast- or bottle-feeding. Let her empty one breast, for instance, or give her half her bottle. Burp her to bring up any gas. She will need her breast milk or formula for several months to come.

"SANDWICHING" HER FIRST TASTES

1 With her still on your lap, scoop a little food onto the spoon—enough to coat the tip. Put the spoon between your baby's lips so that she can suck the food off. Don't try to push the spoon in—she may gag if she feels food at the back of her tongue. She may be surprised at the taste and sensation at first, so be patient and talk to her encouragingly.

2 She may quickly discover that she enjoys this new experience. If she pushes the food out, scrape it up and put the spoon between her lips again. When she's had about a teaspoonful of purée or rice, wipe her mouth and chin and go back to her normal feeding.

IF SHE REFUSES THE SPOON

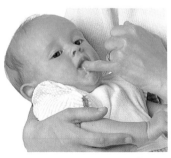

Dip the tip of a clean finger into the food and let your baby suck that. If she still protests, she may not like the taste of that food; try another next time.

YOUR BABY'S NUTRITIONAL NEEDS

HOW YOU BALANCE breast- or bottle-feedings with solid foods will depend very much on your baby's temperament and your lifestyle. Don't rush her away from her bottle or your breast. Take one step at a time, and let her adjust before taking the next. The chart below is just one way you might approach feeding. Some mothers and fathers feel more comfortable having a schedule to rely upon; others prefer a more laissez-faire approach. This schedule begins at the six-month mark, but you and your pediatrician will know the best time to begin. If you are breast-feeding, keep in mind that your body's production of milk must wind down gradually, so don't drop more than one feeding every three or so days.

A STAGE-BY-STAGE GUIDE TO INFANT FEEDING

Stage/Age	What to do	Drinks	Meals and feedings				
			EARLY AM	BREAK-FAST	LUNCH	DINNER	BED-TIME
Weeks 1 and 2 Age 6 months (ages are guidelines only)	Offer small tastes of baby cereal, fruit, or vegetable purée at lunchtime, halfway through the breast- or bottle-feeding. Give the same food for one week to accustom your baby to it.	If you are bottle-feeding, offer your baby occasional tastes of cool water.	■	■	■■■	■	■
Weeks 3 and 4 Age 6½ months	Introduce solid food at breakfast: baby rice cereal or another single grain iron-fortified baby cereal is ideal. Increase the amount of solid food at lunchtime to 3 to 4 teaspoonfuls.	Offer cool water or diluted fruit juice in a cup. Don't worry if she doesn't want any.	■	■■■	■■■	■	■
Weeks 5 and 6 Age 7 months	Introduce solid food at dinner, halfway through the feeding. A week later, offer two courses at lunch: follow a vegetable purée with a fruit one, giving 2 to 3 teaspoonfuls of each.	Continue to introduce a training cup, but don't expect her to be able to drink from it yet—it's just a toy to her.	■■■	■■■■	■■■	■	
Weeks 7 and 8 Age 7½ months	Offer solid food as the first part of lunch, then give breast or bottle. She can have two courses at dinner now, a vegetable and a piece of banana, for example. At breakfast and dinner, continue breast- or bottle-feeding first. She may eat 5 to 6 teaspoonfuls of solid food at each meal now.	You can start to give your baby drinks in her cup, but hold it for her as she drinks from it.	■■■	■■■	■■■■	■	
Weeks 9 and 10 Age 8 months	After lunch solids, offer formula or breast milk from a cup instead of the bottle or your breast. After a few days with no lunchtime bottle, offer solid food as the first part of dinner.	Offer formula in a cup at each meal and cool water or diluted juice at other times.	■■■	■■	■■■	■	
Weeks 11 and 12 Age 8½ months	Offer your baby a drink of formula in a cup instead of a full feeding after her dinner. You may find that she often refuses the bottle or breast after her breakfast solids now.	As before.		■■	■■	■■	■
Week 13 onward Age 9 months	Offer a drink in a cup before breakfast: now your baby is having solids at three meals a day, plus formula to drink. Some doctors suggest cow's milk after the first birthday.	As before. Your baby may be able to manage her own training cup now.		■	■■	■■	■
			Key	■ feeding		■ solid food	

— HOW YOUR BABY LEARNS TO FEED HERSELF —

YOUR BABY WILL WANT to feed herself long before she's able to do so efficiently. However messy this is— be prepared for food to go all over her face and clothes, into her hair, and on the floor—and however long and drawn out it makes mealtimes, encourage her as much as you can. It is her first real step toward independence. Keep a relaxed attitude at meals. If your baby finds them interesting and enjoyable occasions, you are less likely to encounter problems over food and eating in the future.

AT EIGHT MONTHS

Your baby may be making determined efforts to feed herself by this age, but she won't be coordinated enough to get all the food she needs into her mouth. Feed her yourself, but don't stop her from playing with her food. Smearing it over her face may be messy, but it's the first step in learning to feed herself. Have a clean washcloth ready to wipe her when she's finished. Give her plenty of different finger foods, too. They're easy to handle, so she will gain in confidence and dexterity.

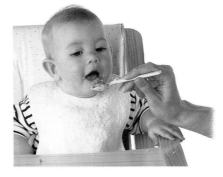

1 She will be hungry at the start of the meal. You may want to hold the bowl and spoon-feed her.

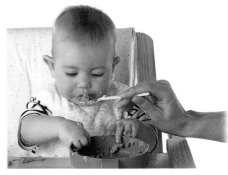

2 Once you've satisfied her initial hunger, let her join in but continue feeding her yourself.

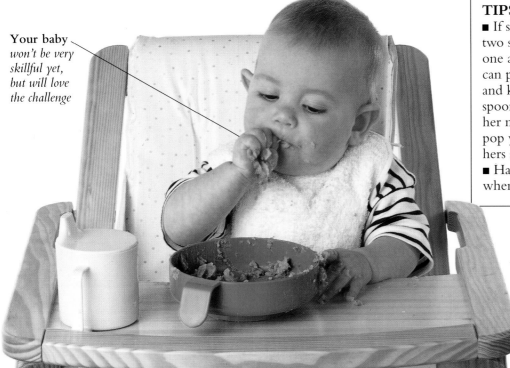

Your baby *won't be very skillful yet, but will love the challenge*

3 Your baby may get so absorbed in the pleasure of dabbling her fingers in her bowl and pushing the food into her mouth that she will lose interest in your feeding her with a spoon. If she's still hungry, she may cry and squirm out of frustration because she can't get the food in quickly enough, so offer some more spoonfuls. Otherwise let her practice her feeding skills. Feeling "I can do it myself" is important to her. She knows when she's had enough.

TIPS TO HELP

■ If she grabs for your spoon, use two spoons at the same meal. Fill one and put it in her bowl so she can pick it up. Fill the other one and keep it ready for when her spoon turns over on the way to her mouth. When this happens, pop your full spoon in, and fill hers so she can try again.
■ Have clean spoons ready for when she drops hers on the floor.

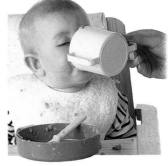

4 Solid food may make her thirsty, so offer formula and tip the cup for her—she won't be able to hold it herself yet. Cow's milk can be introduced after one year.

QUESTIONS & ANSWERS

"How much food should I offer?"
Let your baby decide how much food she wants at each meal. At six months, start with no more than four teaspoons of food in her bowl. Offer more if she eats it all. With cereal, start with about two tablespoons. Some days she will eat voraciously; other days, hardly anything. If she is gaining weight normally, there's no need to worry that she's not getting enough.

"My child will only eat strained fruits and no meats. What can I do?"
Food fads are common and usually don't last more than a couple of weeks. Don't stop offering a variety of foods, but don't worry if he won't eat them. He will not suffer if he's getting vital nutrients from other sources. If you are concerned, ask your pediatrician about diet and supplemental vitamins.

"Should I make him eat things he doesn't seem to like?"
Respect your child's opinions. If he doesn't like something, don't mix it with something he does like because he will only end up disliking both. Try varying the form. For instance, if he doesn't like cooked, cut up, or mashed vegetables, he might eat them raw or in soup. Or, if he always refuses eggs, try egg custard as an alternative to scrambled or hard-boiled eggs.

FIFTEEN MONTHS
Your child will be making a good attempt to feed himself with a spoon or fork with rounded prongs, so cut his food into bite-sized pieces. He may need your help on some days.

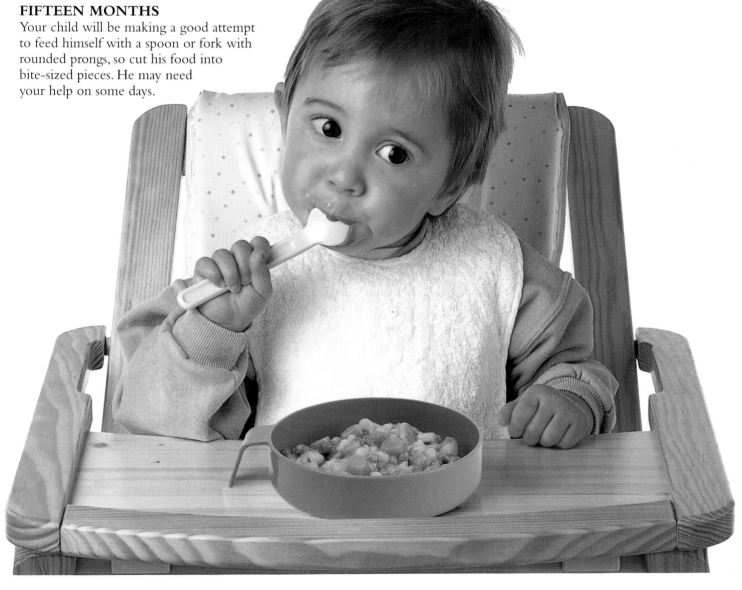

EATING AND YOUR OLDER CHILD

BY THE AGE OF TWO your child will probably be ready to graduate out of his high chair and join you at the table. Mealtimes are important social occasions and learning how to participate as a member of the family is a vital part of your child's social development. What he eats is important too. It's your job to offer enough good food and it's up to him to eat it. Don't force-feed or hover over him worrying about every bite he does or doesn't take. He won't starve, and he knows best how much food he wants.

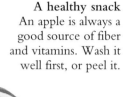

A healthy snack
An apple is always a good source of fiber and vitamins. Wash it well first, or peel it.

Avoiding mealtime problems

The secret to avoiding mealtime problems is to keep your own attitude relaxed and friendly. From the beginning, make your child feel that eating is a pleasurable way to satisfy his hunger. It is always a mistake to battle over eating—you will end up more upset than your child, and he may refuse more vehemently next time. Instead, keep the eating issue in perspective for both of you, for it should be an enjoyable experience:

■ Offer your toddler a varied diet, and let him choose what he wants to eat. He will soon make his likes and dislikes clear.

■ Don't punish him for not eating a particular food, and don't reward him for eating something either. "If you finish your carrots, you can ride your tricycle" will make any child think there must be something terrible about carrots if he has to be rewarded for eating them.

■ Don't spend a great deal of time preparing food especially for him: you will only feel doubly resentful if he doesn't eat it.

■ If he dawdles over his food, don't rush him to finish it. He's bound to be slower than you. If you would expect him to stay at the table while you finish your meal, then you must do the same and wait for him to finish when he's slow.

■ Don't force him to eat more than he wants. Let him decide when he has had enough. He won't starve, and if he's growing normally, you know he's eating enough.

The right diet

Variety is the keynote of a good diet: if you offer many different foods throughout the week, you can be reasonably sure that your child is getting the nutrients he needs. His diet will only be unhealthy if for long periods he eats too much of some kinds of food. For instance, a diet based entirely on crackers, cakes, cookies, highly processed snack foods, or hot dogs and take-out hamburgers is decidedly unhealthy.

Snacks and sweets

Your child will often need a snack to give him energy between meals. Rather than cookies or crackers, offer him healthy, nutritious snacks such as a piece of wholegrain bread, an apple, a carrot, or a banana. If he's not very hungry at the next meal, he won't have missed out nutritionally.

Sweets can be a battleground, but it's not fair or realistic to ban them altogether. Then, your child may learn to covet them even more. But sweets provide few nutrients, and they are very bad for your child's teeth.

Control your child's love of anything sweet by keeping sugary and sweetened foods to a minimum:

■ Provide fruit or unsweetened yogurt for dessert at meals. Cheese is excellent too, because it neutralizes the acid that forms in the mouth and attacks tooth enamel.

■ When you do let your child have sweets, offer them at the end of the meal, not in between meals.

■ Choose sweets that can be eaten quickly, rather than sucked or chewed for a long time.

■ Give pure fruit juices rather than presweetened or carbonated beverages, and provide them only at meals. Offer milk or water at other times.

■ Don't use sweets to reward or punish your child: they will become intensely valuable to him, and thus harder to control.

■ Make brushing with a fluoride toothpaste a routine at least after breakfast and before bed (see pages 144–45).

WAYS TO IMPROVE YOUR FAMILY'S DIET

■ Use vegetable margarine and olive oil instead of butter for spreading and cooking.

■ Keep red meat to a minimum: once or twice a week is enough.

■ Cook chicken or fish at least three times a week.

■ Grill or broil rather than fry.

■ Use fresh rather than processed foods—they will contain more nutrients and less salt and sugar.

■ Buy wholegrain bread and avoid presweetened cereals.

■ Serve vegetables raw as often as possible, or cook them only lightly. Any cooking destroys nutrients, but steaming is best.

CRYING AND YOUR BABY

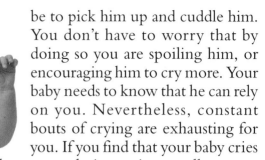

Your baby is bound to cry a great deal throughout his first year. To begin with, it's his only means of communicating his need for food and comfort, but from around three months you will notice a change. Instead of spending much of his waking time crying, he will use that time to learn about the world around him. The crying spells will lessen, and you will become more adept at understanding what he wants. When your baby cries, your instinct will be to pick him up and cuddle him. You don't have to worry that by doing so you are spoiling him, or encouraging him to cry more. Your baby needs to know that he can rely on you. Nevertheless, constant bouts of crying are exhausting for you. If you find that your baby cries so much that you are losing patience, talk to your pediatrician: he may be able to put you in touch with other mothers or voluntary organizations that can help you find ways to cope.

WAYS TO SOOTHE YOUR NEWBORN

THE IMPORTANT THING when your baby cries is to respond quickly, without making a fuss. Letting him cry for a long time will agitate him more. See the next page for other possible causes.

SEVEN WAYS TO SOOTHE YOUR CRYING BABY

Feed her In the first months hunger is the most likely reason for your baby crying, and offering a breast or bottle is the most effective way to soothe her—even if that means frequent feedings day and night.

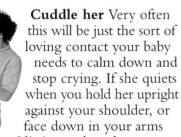

Cuddle her Very often this will be just the sort of loving contact your baby needs to calm down and stop crying. If she quiets when you hold her upright against your shoulder, or face down in your arms (see page 83), it may have been gas that was making her cry. If she has been passed around for relatives and friends to hold, she may just want a few quiet moments of being cuddled by a familiar parent.

Rock her rhythmically Movement often comforts a cranky baby, and may put her to sleep. Rock her in your arms, and if she doesn't quiet down, try rocking faster—perhaps 60 to 70 rocks per minute. Or just jiggle her up and down by shifting from foot to foot, perhaps with your baby in an infant carrier on your chest (see page 85). Or rock with her in a rocking chair, if you have one. Or put her in her stroller or carriage and push her back and forth; if you can take her around the block, the gentle bumping over the pavement will soothe her.

Swaddle him Wrap him up quite firmly in a baby quilt or receiving blanket, tucking the ends under him to make a neat bundle (see page 123). It may comfort him to feel safe and secure. Carry him around in your arms still swaddled up until he seems happier, and put him down to sleep on his back without unwrapping him. If your baby is crying because of something you've had to do to him—perhaps he hates being dressed or washed, for example—swaddling may be the best way to reassure and calm him, and stop the crying.

Pat her Rhythmically patting and rubbing her back or stomach will often calm her down and may help her to bring up gas. The feel of your hand will often comfort her when you first put her down to change her diaper, too.

Give him something to suck Almost all babies are soothed by sucking, and nowadays mothers are often sent home from the hospital with a pacifier for their newborn. Obstetrical nurses have been known to use them, so don't be afraid to try one. You might also offer your cranky baby your own clean little finger. Some newborns suck their own thumbs or fists.

Distract your baby Something to look at may make your baby forget why he was crying, at least for a while. Bright, colorful patterns may fascinate him. He will often gaze intently at postcards, wallpaper, or your clothes. Faces and mirrors are also excellent distractions, and a walk around the house to look at photographs or to peer into a mirror may calm him.

SEVEN REASONS YOUR BABY MIGHT BE CRYING

Often you won't really know why your young baby is crying or why she stops. At times, there may be no reason at all. If you've tried the simple remedies such as feeding, cuddling, and the soothing tactics that usually work (see page 117), all with no success, consider these other possible causes and don't hesitate to call your doctor for advice.

Illness may be making your baby cry, particularly if her crying sounds different from normal. *Always* call your doctor if your baby shows any symptoms that are unusual for her. A blocked nose from a cold may prevent her from feeding or sucking her pacifier or thumb, so she can't comfort herself even though she may not be very ill. Your doctor can prescribe medication to help her breathe easily. (See page 174–175.)

Diaper rash or a sore bottom may make your baby cry. Take her diaper off, clean her thoroughly, and, if possible, don't put a diaper back on for the rest of the day: just lay her on a towel. Take steps to treat the rash (see page 150).

Colic, often called three-month or evening colic, is characterized by a pattern of regular, intense, inconsolable screaming at a particular time each day, usually in the late afternoon or evening. The pattern appears at about three weeks, and can continue until 12 or 14 weeks. The crying spell may last as long as three hours. Always ask for medical advice the first time your baby screams inconsolably. Colic isn't harmful, but you might misdiagnose and miss other, serious symptoms.

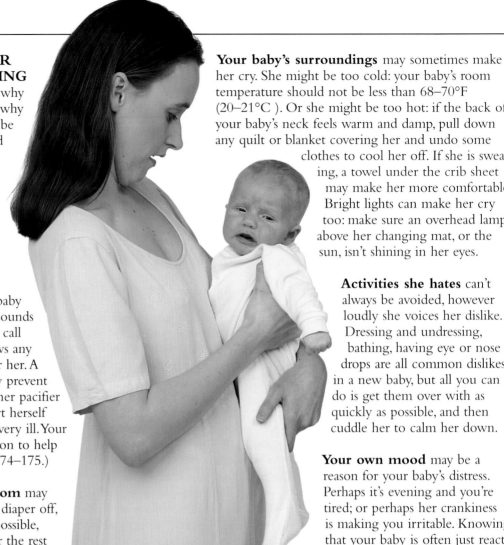

Your baby's surroundings may sometimes make her cry. She might be too cold: your baby's room temperature should not be less than 68–70°F (20–21°C). Or she might be too hot: if the back of your baby's neck feels warm and damp, pull down any quilt or blanket covering her and undo some clothes to cool her off. If she is sweating, a towel under the crib sheet may make her more comfortable. Bright lights can make her cry too: make sure an overhead lamp above her changing mat, or the sun, isn't shining in her eyes.

Activities she hates can't always be avoided, however loudly she voices her dislike. Dressing and undressing, bathing, having eye or nose drops are all common dislikes in a new baby, but all you can do is get them over with as quickly as possible, and then cuddle her to calm her down.

Your own mood may be a reason for your baby's distress. Perhaps it's evening and you're tired; or perhaps her crankiness is making you irritable. Knowing that your baby is often just reacting to your mood may help you to be calmer with her.

Too much fussing can make an upset baby cry all the more. Passing her between you, changing a diaper that doesn't need to be changed, offering to feed her again and again, discussing her crying in anxious voices, may all make her even more agitated, so she cries all the harder. If there's no reason for her crying, don't keep trying to find one: she probably just wants to be held.

COPING WITH COLIC

All you can do if your baby has colic is learn to live with it, in the certain knowledge that she isn't ill or abnormal and that the colic won't last. Don't suffer alone. This will be a difficult three months for you, your partner, and your baby. Try to remember these three points:

■ Do whatever you can to try to soothe your baby. Keeping her in motion, feeding her frequently, rubbing her stomach rhythmically, or just cuddling her, may all soothe her for a short while.

■ Don't resort to medications. You can't cure her colic, so you will be giving your baby large doses of medication for no real purpose.

■ Try to have an occasional evening out. You can leave your partner or a competent, trusted relative to take charge.

YOUR CRYING OLDER BABY

FROM THE AGE of about three months, you may notice a real change in your baby. He's now much more aware of what goes on around him, he's responsive and interested in everything—more of a person altogether. He'll still cry a lot, and will continue to do so for many months to come, but by now you may have a much better idea of why.

SIX REASONS WHY YOUR OLDER BABY MIGHT BE CRYING

Hunger is still an obvious reason for your baby to cry. As his first year progresses and he becomes mobile and moves on to solid food, he will often get tired and cranky between meals—his life is a busy one. A snack and a drink may restore his energy and cheer him up.

Anxiety will be a new reason for crying from the age of seven or eight months, because by then he's discovered his unshakable attachment to you. You are his "safe base"; he'll be happy to explore the world, provided he can keep you in sight. He may cry if you leave him or if he loses sight of you. Be patient with him and let him get used to new people and situations gradually.

Pain, from bumps as he becomes mobile, will be a frequent cause of tears. Often it will be the shock that makes him cry, rather than any injury, so a sympathetic cuddle and a distracting toy will usually help him forget it quickly.

Wanting to get his own way will often be a cause of friction and tears, particularly from the age of two. It's worth asking yourself if you're frustrating him unnecessarily, or perhaps trying to assert your own will; but sometimes he will need to be held back for his safety. If he gets so angry that he throws a tantrum, don't shout at him, or try reasoning with him, or punish him afterward. It's best to ignore the tantrum completely. Wait until the fit of temper has passed and then continue with whatever you were going to do (see also page 170).

Frustration, as your baby tries to do things that are beyond his capabilities, will be a more and more common reason for crying. You can't avoid this although you can make life easier for him. For example, put his toys where he can reach them. Distraction is the best cure: introduce a new game or toy and his tears may soon be forgotten. Or help him if he's struggling, but don't take over completely.

Overtiredness will show itself in whininess, irritability, and finally tears. By the end of his first year your child's life is so full of new experiences that he can run out of energy before he's run out of enthusiasm. He needs you to help him relax enough to get the sleep he needs. A quiet time sitting on your lap listening to a story may work, and a calming, enjoyable bedtime routine (see pages 124–25) that you all stick to every evening will help, too.

QUESTION & ANSWER

"Every new tooth my toddler cuts is preceded by days of crying. What can I do to help him?"
The first teeth shouldn't cause any trouble, but the back teeth, cut during the second year, can be painful. Your child will probably drool a lot and have a red cheek for a couple of days. There are ways you can help him:

- Rub his gums with your little finger.
- If you use a gel- or water-filled teething ring, put it in the refrigerator to cool it. Don't put it in the freezer: frozen ones can cause frostbite.
- Check for sharp edges on his smaller toys.
- Avoid giving repeated doses of medications or teething gels.

SLEEP AND YOUR BABY

Your newborn baby will sleep as much as she needs to. The only trouble is that she may not always sleep when you would like her to. Broken nights and lack of sleep for you will be a fact of life for many weeks until she settles into a routine that coincides more closely with yours. At around nine months, new problems might develop. She may be very reluctant to let you say good night and leave her, or she may settle into a pattern of night waking. Careful handling at bedtime from around the middle of your baby's first year can help to avoid problems later. A relaxing and loving bedtime routine that takes place in exactly the same way *every* night will give her the sense of security she needs. Until at least the age of two and a half, and probably much longer, some daytime sleep will be essential. Your toddler's life is an active, exciting one, and she will need a reviving nap during the morning or afternoon to prevent her from becoming overtired and irritable.

EQUIPMENT FOR SLEEP

WHAT YOU BUY for your baby to sleep in will be a significant investment, so shop around and ask friends what worked for them. If you buy a secondhand crib, make sure any paint is lead-free and that decorative trim cannot be picked off. You will need plenty of machine-washable bedding. Until your baby is a year, tuck the bottom end of the top sheet and blankets well under the end of the mattress, so that the top ends come only halfway up the crib. Put your baby to sleep lying halfway down the crib, with her feet near the end. It may look strange, but in this position she is unlikely to slip down beneath the bedclothes and overheat or suffocate.

Crib Your baby will be sleeping in this from at least three months to around age three, so it's worth investing in a sturdy, well-made one. Safety is paramount: choose a crib that conforms to Consumer Products Safety Codes.

WHAT TO SLEEP IN

Convertible carriage (see page 156) For your young baby, a carriage that will eventually convert into a stroller is a good investment. A bassinet or a cradle that rocks is a good alternative.

Infant seat
For the first few months a seat with carrying handles is very useful. The base is adjustable so that when your baby is awake she can sit up and even rock.

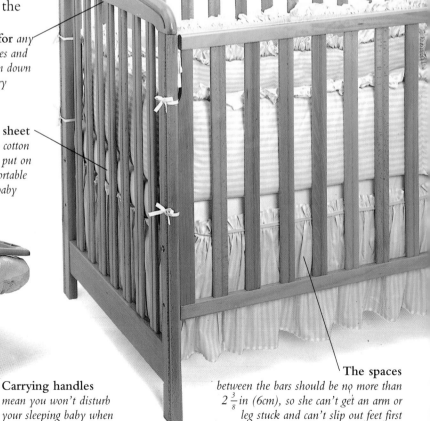

Watch for *any sharp edges and sand them down if necessary*

A fitted sheet *in 100% cotton is easy to put on and comfortable for your baby*

Carrying handles *mean you won't disturb your sleeping baby when you have to transport her*

The spaces *between the bars should be no more than $2\frac{3}{8}$ in (6cm), so she can't get an arm or leg stuck and can't slip out feet first*

YOUR BABY'S BEDDING

Mattress Choose a foam type with a fabric cover and air holes at the head end. Vinyl over the rest of the mattress protects it from leaky diaper damage.

Valance or dust ruffle

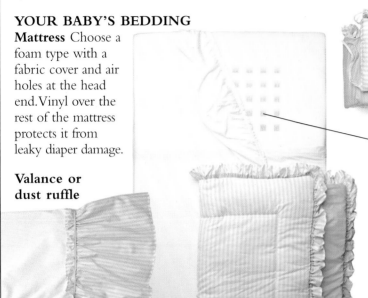

Air holes are for added safety

Crib bumper This will cushion and guard against drafts. Make sure any ties are no longer than 6in (15cm). Long ties can become dangerous and should be removed altogether when a baby begins to stand.

Fitted sheet and comforter A firm crib mattress covered by a fitted sheet is the safest bedding. A crib-sized quilt or comforter will be warm and light. Choose a machine-washable product that has a non-allergenic, man-made filling. Alternatively, a sheet plus layers of blankets is enough for your baby if you keep his room at the recommended temperature.

TOYS FOR THE CRIB

Mobile Hang a colorful mobile above the crib. Remove it before she can reach it

Teddy bear

YOUR BABY'S ROOM

■ Keep the room warm: 68–70°F (20–21°C) is the ideal temperature.
■ Install a dimmer switch or night-light, so you can check on your baby while she's asleep without disturbing her.
■ You may need a smoke alarm installed in your baby's room, unless you live in a small apartment and already have one in the hallway.
■ Never tie a toy or pacifier to a string, as it could entangle her.

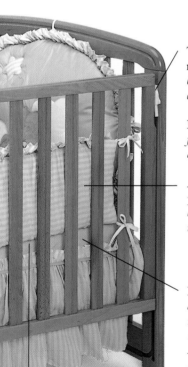

The dropside mechanism should be one that your baby can't release by herself

Do NOT use pillows *for your baby until she's at least two years old*

A crib bumper protects your baby's head if she bumps it against the bars; it also keeps drafts out

If the crib doesn't come complete with a mattress, follow the instructions on what size to buy. It must fit snugly so your baby can't get her face trapped

The mattress base should be fixed securely to the bed frame. The mattress should be at least 2ft (60cm) from the top edge of the crib, so your baby cannot climb out. You should be able to lower the base

SLEEPTIME SAFETY

■ Put your baby to sleep on her back. Doctors believe this is the safest position.
■ **Never** let your baby sleep on soft surfaces, such as pillows, until at least age two years: they could smother her.
■ Remove any plastic packaging from the mattress and don't use a plastic sheet.
■ Don't let your baby get too hot or too cold.
■ Don't smoke, and keep your baby in a smoke-free atmosphere.

CRIB DEATH A few babies die unexpectedly each year in their cribs. There is no explanation for crib death, or sudden infant death syndrome (SIDS), but doctors have suggested safety precautions (see left) that help to minimize the risk.

If you think your baby is unwell, consult your doctor immediately.

DAYTIME AND NIGHTTIME SLEEP

IN THE EARLY DAYS your baby will sleep in short bursts randomly throughout the day and night. The chart below shows how her sleep pattern might develop. As the months pass, her longest period of sleep coincides more and more with the hours of night, and her wakeful times become longer. However, babies vary. Don't worry if your baby takes longer than you expected (or hoped) to sleep through the night.

Emphasizing day and night

Right from the newborn stage, make a clear distinction between how you treat daytime and nighttime sleep, to help your baby learn which time is for play and which for sleep. During the day put her to sleep in a carriage, cradle, or bassinet. If you're using a crib already, save it for nighttime only. A carriage or stroller can go outside in a shady spot, *always* covered with an insect net and with the brakes on. Indoors, make sure pets can't get into the room where your baby is, but there is no need to keep the house especially quiet for her. When your baby cries, pick her up and make the most of her waking time: help her to associate daylight hours with play and wakefulness.

At night, swaddle your baby firmly so her jerking limbs won't wake her, and put her to sleep in her crib if you're already using one. Keep the light dim. When she wakes and cries for a feeding, pick her up and feed her quietly, talking as little as possible and only changing her diaper if she's very wet or messy. She will gradually learn that nighttime feedings are business only, not social times, and her sleep pattern will become more like yours as the weeks go by.

Your toddler's naps

From the age of about six months, bedtime will become a more and more important ritual in your baby's day, and she needs to be tired and ready for bed if she is to sleep through the night. She needs some daytime sleep to give her energy for her active life, and will go on needing it throughout toddlerhood, but don't let her nap for too long. Allow two hours for each nap (she may wake earlier); then wake her. She may be grumpy and confused if she was deeply asleep, so give her plenty of time before introducing the next activity.

QUESTION & ANSWER

"My ten-month-old wakes up at 6 am, and won't go to sleep again. Is there anything we can do?"

Early-morning waking probably just means your baby has had enough sleep. Put a few toys in his crib each night to occupy him for a while when he wakes. When he tires of his toys and calls for you, changing his diaper and offering some new toys in his crib may gain you an extra hour's sleep.

If early waking is a regular pattern, you could try adjusting his sleep times throughout the day so he has a later bedtime. Put thick curtains up in his bedroom so the sun won't wake him.

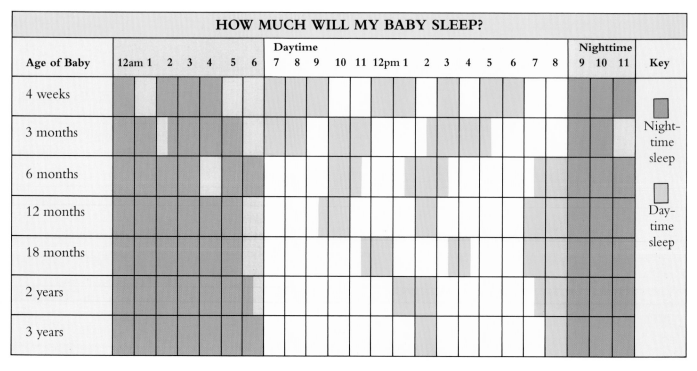

HOW MUCH WILL MY BABY SLEEP?

SWADDLING YOUR NEWBORN BABY

YOUR BABY will probably drift off to sleep much better in his first three months if you wrap him up snugly in a blanket. Although swaddling isn't necessary, especially in a warm room, it does make your baby feel safe and secure, and stops his limbs from jerking and twitching as he drops off to sleep. Fold your baby's blanket in half diagonally. If he's crying, don't upset him by putting him down to swaddle him; wrap him up on your lap. Discontinue swaddling after your baby is three months old.

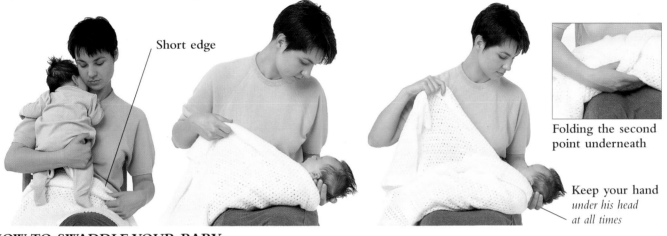

Short edge

Folding the second point underneath

Keep your hand *under his head at all times*

HOW TO SWADDLE YOUR BABY

1 Hold your baby against your shoulder while you arrange the blanket over your lap, the long edge of the triangle along one thigh, the point hanging down on the other side.

2 Supporting his head, lay your baby across your knees, his neck just level with the edge of the blanket. Bring the far corner up, pulling it taut.

3 Tuck the corner under his botom, smoothing it out. Bring the other corner up, again pulling it taut, and take it over to tuck under him. Fold the point beyond his feet loosely under his bottom.

PUTTING HIM DOWN TO SLEEP

Once your baby is swaddled and has calmed down, he's ready to be put into his cradle or crib for sleep. Doctors believe that the safest sleeping position is lying on his back—there is no evidence to suggest that babies tend to vomit and then choke in this position. Babies who sleep on their tummies run an increased risk of crib death (see page 121).

If you do put him down on his side, make sure you pull his elbow well forward so he can't roll onto his front. After the age of three months, when you stop swaddling him, your baby will roll into whatever position suits him best, however you put him down.

Always *put your baby down to sleep on his back*

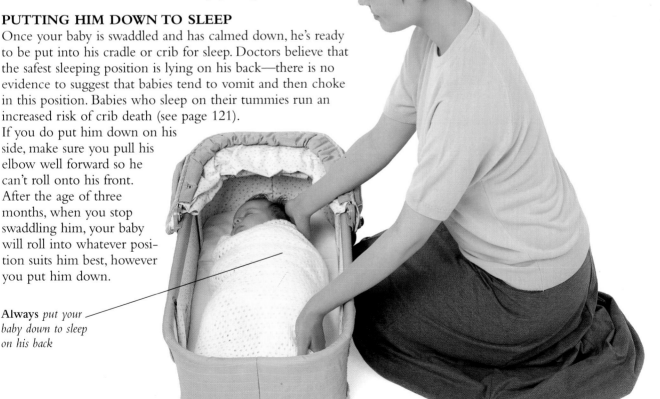

SETTLING DOWN TO SLEEP

THE FEELING of a full stomach will often be enough to send your baby contentedly off to sleep, but there will also be many times when she needs you to help her relax. Be confident, calm, and gentle when you're soothing her for sleep. Tickles, giggles, and jerky movements won't help: she needs a quiet period in your arms to make her feel safe, secure, and relaxed.

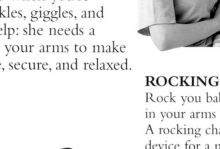

SOOTHING CONTACT

Rubbing your baby's stomach rhythmically may soothe her enough to put her to sleep. Don't alter the rhythm or you will disturb her and don't stop until her eyelids have closed.

ROCKING

Rock you baby back and forth in your arms to lull her to sleep. A rocking chair is a wonderful device for a new mother. You may have to rock for some time, but it's still a good method to get her to sleep.

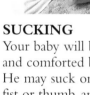

SUCKING

Your baby will be soothed and comforted by sucking. He may suck on his own fist or thumb, and on occasion, your own little finger will do nicely as well. Pacifiers are also soothing, but they can cause dependence; prolonged use can result in dental problems.

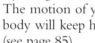

Ensure adequate *support for his head*

AN INFANT CARRIER

If your baby wakes every time you put him down, try using an infant carrier. The motion of your body will keep him asleep (see page 85).

YOUR OLDER BABY'S BEDTIME ROUTINE

FROM ABOUT six months, your baby will settle down to sleep much more happily if the whole process takes place in exactly the same way every evening—babies love routine and rituals. From now on, her sleep patterns will be easily upset by a change in surroundings or routine, so try to keep to her routine even if you're away from home. Make getting ready for bed as much fun as you can, so it's a pleasurable, but undemanding, part of your baby's day. It's never too early to start reading to your baby, and bed-time is an ideal opportunity.

WHAT TIME IS BEDTIME?

It's up to you and your partner to choose a time that fits in well with your own routine—and one that you can stick to more or less every day. Make sure it's late enough so that you're both home, and not so late that the routine takes up all your evening. Any time between 6 pm and 8 pm would be suitable.

THE BEDTIME ROUTINE

1 Start the routine in the same way every evening. A bath is ideal because it's both fun and relaxing. If she doesn't like being bathed, twenty minutes spent playing a gentle game together might help her unwind.

2 If your baby still has a bedtime feeding, give it to her in her room so she understands this to be a friendly, familiar place, not somewhere she is banished to at night while family life continues elsewhere.

3 Put your baby into her crib with her favorite teddy or soft toys and her security blanket if she has one.

4 Now perhaps your partner could take over, so you're both involved in the bedtime routine. This last half hour or so needs to be always the same, and as enjoyable as possible for your baby, to mark it clearly as the end of the day.

RHYTHMIC MOVEMENTS

Pushing her back and forth in her carriage will often soothe her to sleep, although she may keep trying to look at you. When she does drop off, don't lift her out to put her in her cot, even if it's nighttime.

A CAR RIDE

If you get desperate, try putting your baby in his car seat and going for a drive around the block: the motion will probably put him to sleep automatically. When you get home again, leave him undisturbed in his seat and carry both indoors. Cover him with a blanket to keep him warm.

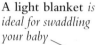
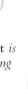
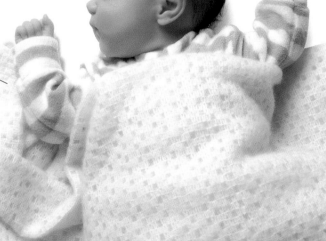

A light blanket is ideal for swaddling your baby

SWADDLING

Not all babies like to sleep with their arms tucked in. Don't worry if you wrap your baby securely (but not tightly) and he works his arms loose. He won't get cold and it won't matter if you leave his arms free when swaddling him.

OTHER METHODS

Lullabies, as you rock your baby back and forth, are an age-old method of soothing her to sleep. Your baby won't mind if you can't sing in tune.

Taped music sometimes helps. Gentle music playing softly in her room may help your baby to drop off to sleep.

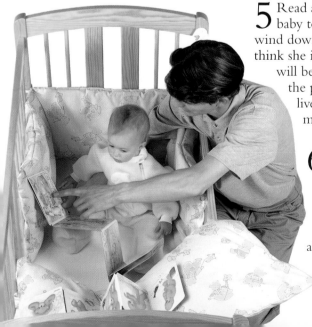

5 Read a favorite story with your baby to relax her and help her wind down. Don't give up if you think she isn't paying attention: she will be tired and won't respond to the pictures with her usual lively interest, but that doesn't mean she isn't listening.

6 Position your baby's favorite toy or security blanket next to her and kiss her good night. Turn the light down, or switch a night-light on. Don't leave abruptly: spend a moment or two puttering around the room before you go out.

QUESTION & ANSWER

"Is it a good idea to take my baby into bed with me?"
The American Academy of Pediatrics specifically cautions parents about sleeping with their baby. There is little evidence to support bed sharing, and it is not encouraged. A healthy baby should be put to sleep on his back in his own crib. Soft bedding, such as pillows or comforters, should not be placed beneath the baby; it may increase the risk of crib death, or sudden infant death syndrome.

OVERCOMING SLEEPING PROBLEMS

■ NIGHT FEEDINGS ■	■ NIGHT WAKING ■	■ UNSETTLED BEDTIME ■
By the time your baby is six months old, she can go until morning without food; but she may well settle into a pattern of waking to be fed. If you want to wean her off these nighttime feedings, start by reducing the feedings gradually, then stop them but go in to see her and offer reassurance for as long as she cries.	The tactics below provide a way of reassuring your older baby when she wakes at night that all is well and you have not abandoned her, while conveying the message that she is only going to get the minimum of attention from you during these hours. If she is not sleeping through within a week, ask your pediatrician's advice.	From the age of about nine months, establish a method of handling bedtime, then stick to it. If your baby gets into a pattern of not settling when you put her to bed, a week of resolutely following the tactics below may break it. She will soon get the message that you *will* always come to her if she cries, but you *won't* pick her up again.

NIGHT FEEDINGS

At her bedtime feeding, try not to let your baby fall asleep with the breast or bottle in her mouth: she needs to learn to fall asleep on her own, not rely on sucking to relax her. As soon as her eyelids droop, take her off the bottle or breast. Tuck her in the crib.

↓

For a few nights, feed her when she wakes, but reduce the amount. Put her back in her crib, asleep or not, kiss her, and *leave*.

↓

If you are breast-feeding, your partner will have to take over at this point because your baby will smell your milk and want to be nursed. If she continues to cry, wait five minutes, then go back in to give her a pat and rub her back to reassure her. Then go back to bed, even if she's still crying.

↓

Continue to go back every five minutes. Pick her up only if she is beside herself with crying; when her sobs subside put her back in her crib and leave her for a few minutes more. You may have a couple of hours of this, but persevere.

↓

For the next few nights, stop offering the feeding; instead, adopt the tactics for night waking for as long as it takes to teach your baby to sleep through the night.

NIGHT WAKING

If your baby whimpers at night, wait a few minutes to see if she goes back to sleep again.

↓

If she cries loudly, go in to make sure that nothing is wrong. Soothe her and calm her down: rubbing her back may be enough, but try not to pick her up and cuddle her. When the crying has subsided into sniffles, tuck her in so she is snug and warm, and kiss her good night. Then go back to bed yourself.

↓

If the crying continues, or increases in intensity again, call out reassuringly from your own bed if you are near enough to be heard, but wait five minutes before going in to her.

↓

When you do go back, just reassure her by patting and rubbing her back—don't pick her up unless she's really upset—then tuck her in and leave her.

↓

Continue going back in this way at five-minute intervals for as long as it takes her to fall back to sleep. After half an hour, increase the intervals between visits to 10 minutes, but never let her cry for more than 15. A week of gentle firmness on your part should be enough to establish a more sociable sleeping pattern.

UNSETTLED BEDTIME

Keep to a bedtime routine, making it fun for your baby but relaxing and loving as well. If she cries when you leave her after tucking her in for the night, go back and give her a reassuring kiss, but *don't* pick her up, and *don't* stay more than a moment or two.

↓

If she cries again, call out to her reassuringly, but wait five minutes before going in again.

↓

When you do go in, make sure that nothing's wrong, such as a wet diaper or something chafing. Pat her back to soothe her, kiss her good night again, and tuck her in. Be cheerful but firm, and then *go*. Don't hesitate—your baby's will is stronger than yours at this point, and you'll be only too easily persuaded to stay.

↓

If she keeps on crying, continue going in for a brief look at five-minute intervals. After half an hour, start to increase the intervals between visits, but never let your baby cry for longer than a quarter of an hour.

↓

Eventually she will realize that the brief reward of you coming in at intervals isn't worth all the effort that she's putting in, and she will drop off to sleep.

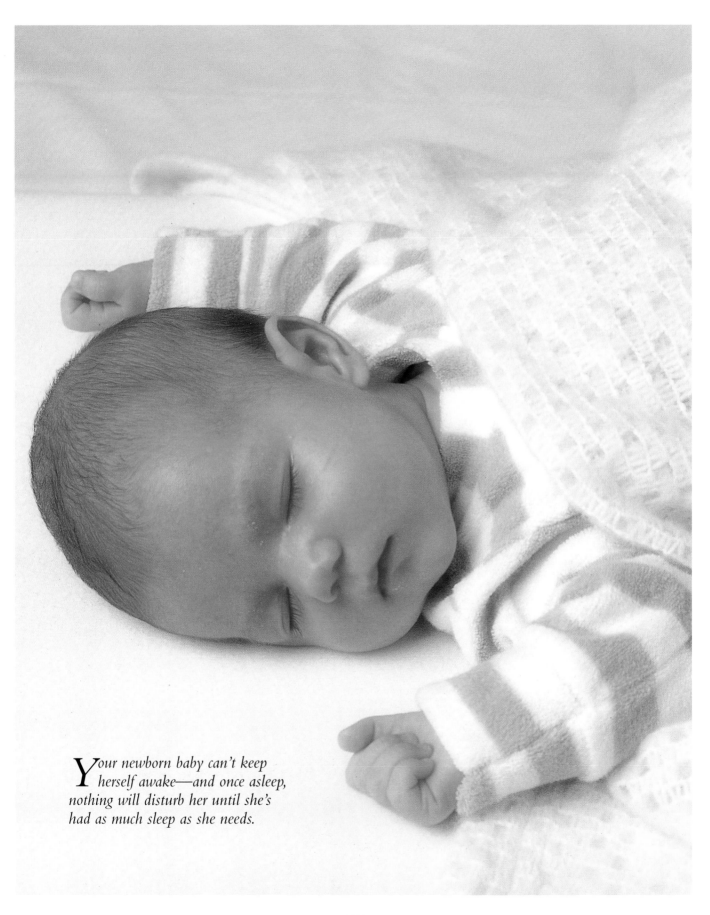

Your newborn baby can't keep herself awake—and once asleep, nothing will disturb her until she's had as much sleep as she needs.

CLOTHES AND DRESSING

In the early weeks you will be dressing and undressing your baby frequently; he may need clean clothes as often as he needs a clean diaper, so you will want to have plenty of newborn sizes on hand. Ask friends and relatives for hand-me-downs. When your child turns into a toddler, start looking for clothes that are as comfortable and unrestricting as possible, but be reassured that you may not need as many outfits then. Don't invest in an extensive "dress-up" wardrobe unless you have very special occasions in mind; fancy clothes are often outgrown long before they are outworn. It's much better to buy a few things at a time and replace them when they become too small. Choose carefully: easy-to-manage openings and pants with elastic waistlines, for example, will help him as he learns to dress and undress himself. Above all, buy clothes that are easy to care for and machine washable. Staying neat and clean is not number one on a child's list of priorities. In fact, neither of you should need to worry about his clothes.

BUYING CLOTHES FOR YOUR BABY

CLOTHES FOR A YOUNG BABY should be easy to put on, machine washable, and if possible made from natural fibers, which allow your baby to regulate his own temperature as well as he can. Don't use harsh detergents or fabric conditioners to wash baby clothes, because they may irritate his skin. The basic item of clothing now and throughout the first six months is the all-in-one stretchsuit.

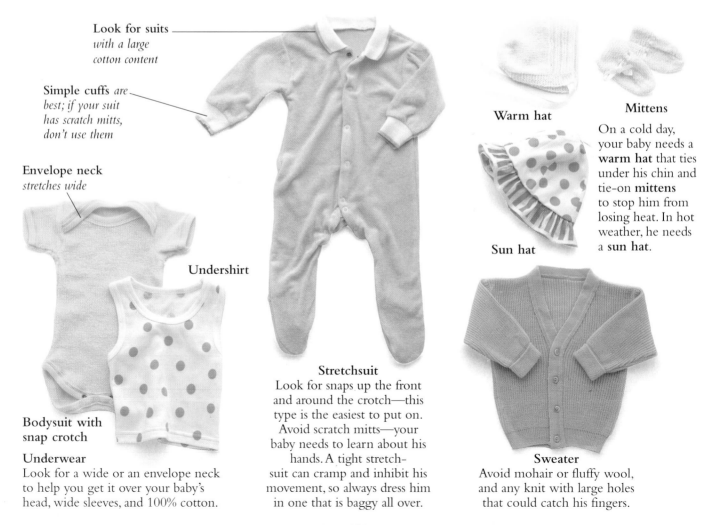

Look for suits *with a large cotton content*

Simple cuffs *are best; if your suit has scratch mitts, don't use them*

Envelope neck *stretches wide*

Undershirt

Bodysuit with snap crotch

Underwear
Look for a wide or an envelope neck to help you get it over your baby's head, wide sleeves, and 100% cotton.

Stretchsuit
Look for snaps up the front and around the crotch—this type is the easiest to put on. Avoid scratch mitts—your baby needs to learn about his hands. A tight stretch-suit can cramp and inhibit his movement, so always dress him in one that is baggy all over.

Warm hat

Sun hat

Mittens
On a cold day, your baby needs a **warm hat** that ties under his chin and tie-on **mittens** to stop him from losing heat. In hot weather, he needs a **sun hat**.

Sweater
Avoid mohair or fluffy wool, and any knit with large holes that could catch his fingers.

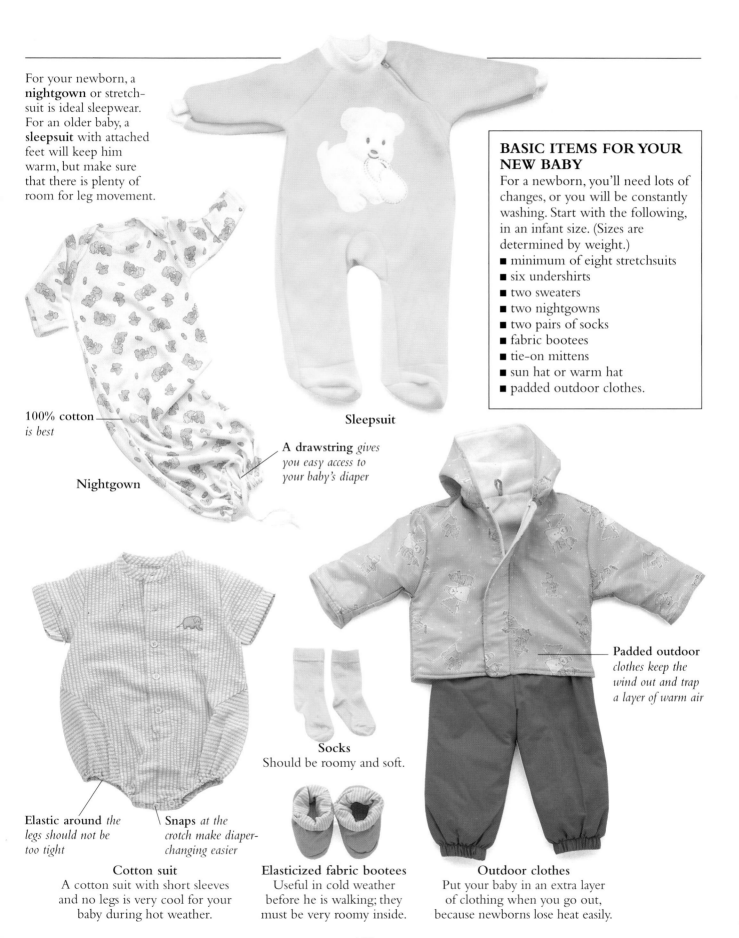

For your newborn, a **nightgown** or stretch-suit is ideal sleepwear. For an older baby, a **sleepsuit** with attached feet will keep him warm, but make sure that there is plenty of room for leg movement.

BASIC ITEMS FOR YOUR NEW BABY
For a newborn, you'll need lots of changes, or you will be constantly washing. Start with the following, in an infant size. (Sizes are determined by weight.)
- minimum of eight stretchsuits
- six undershirts
- two sweaters
- two nightgowns
- two pairs of socks
- fabric bootees
- tie-on mittens
- sun hat or warm hat
- padded outdoor clothes.

Sleepsuit

100% cotton is best

Nightgown

A drawstring *gives you easy access to your baby's diaper*

Padded outdoor *clothes keep the wind out and trap a layer of warm air*

Socks
Should be roomy and soft.

Elastic around the legs should not be too tight

Snaps at the crotch make diaper-changing easier

Cotton suit
A cotton suit with short sleeves and no legs is very cool for your baby during hot weather.

Elasticized fabric bootees
Useful in cold weather before he is walking; they must be very roomy inside.

Outdoor clothes
Put your baby in an extra layer of clothing when you go out, because newborns lose heat easily.

HOW TO DRESS YOUR BABY

DRESSING and undressing your baby is a lovely opportunity to let him learn about his own body by stroking and caressing his soft skin. He may hate being dressed, but you can make it pleasurable with lots of nuzzling, cuddles, kisses and talk; be especially gentle, too. Gather the clothes you need and undo all the snaps. Lay your baby on a changing mat.

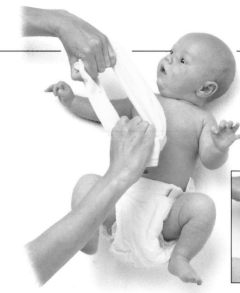

PUTTING ON UNDERWEAR

1 Hold the shirt or bodysuit with the front facing you and gather it into your hands. Put the back edge at his head.

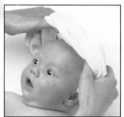

Position the back edge at the top of his head

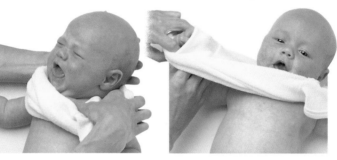

2 With one swift, gentle movement bring the front edge of the shirt down to your baby's chin. Hold all the fabric gathered together and stretch it as wide as you can, so that none of it drags on his face and upsets him.

3 Gently lift your baby's head and upper body and pull the back of the shirt down so it is around his neck and lying behind his shoulders. Lower him to the pad without jolting or letting his head flop.

4 If your baby's shirt has sleeves, put the fingers of one hand down through the first sleeve and stretch it wide, then with the other hand guide his fist into your fingers.

5 Hold your baby's hand with your first hand, and ease the sleeve over his arm with the other. Pull the shirt down below his arm. Do the same with the other sleeve, pulling the fabric, not your baby.

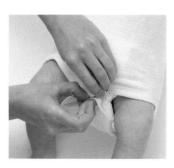

6 Pull the shirt over his stomach. If it's a one-piece bodysuit, lift his lower body by his ankles and pull the back down. Close the snaps at the crotch.

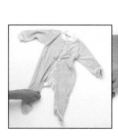

Lay the stretchsuit out flat

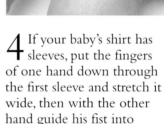

PUTTING ON A STRETCHSUIT

1 Pick your baby up while you lay the clean stretchsuit out flat on the changing pad, the front facing up and all the snaps undone. Lay your baby on top of it, his neck in line with the stretchsuit's.

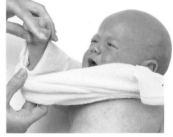

A shirt *underneath the stretchsuit is essential in anything but the hottest weather*

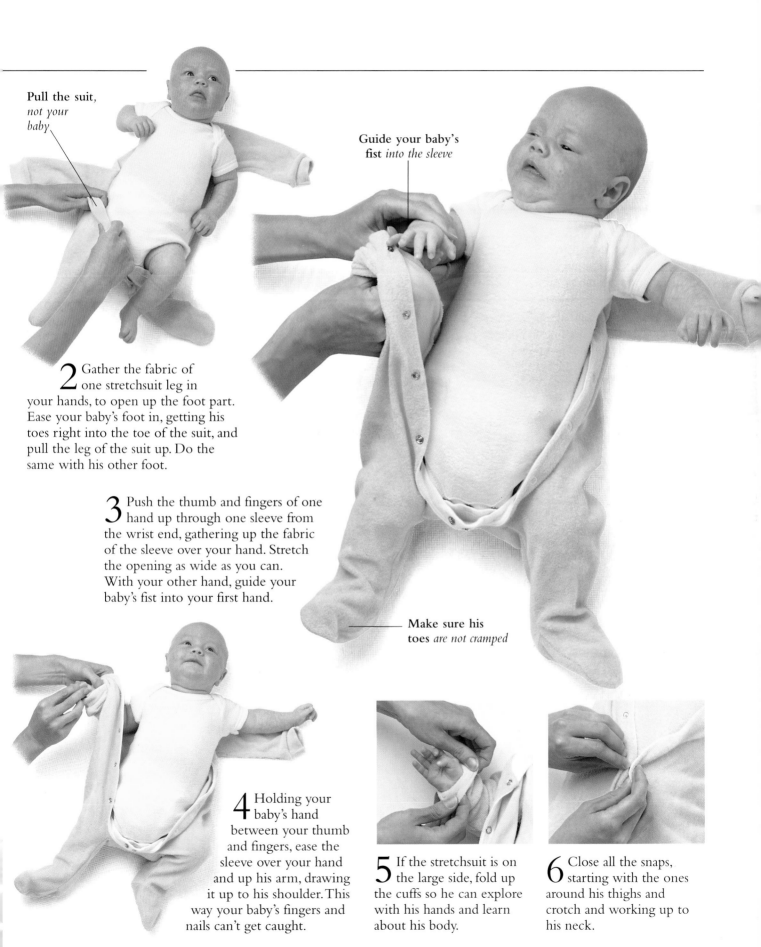

Pull the suit, *not your baby*

Guide your baby's fist *into the sleeve*

2 Gather the fabric of one stretchsuit leg in your hands, to open up the foot part. Ease your baby's foot in, getting his toes right into the toe of the suit, and pull the leg of the suit up. Do the same with his other foot.

3 Push the thumb and fingers of one hand up through one sleeve from the wrist end, gathering up the fabric of the sleeve over your hand. Stretch the opening as wide as you can. With your other hand, guide your baby's fist into your first hand.

Make sure his toes *are not cramped*

4 Holding your baby's hand between your thumb and fingers, ease the sleeve over your hand and up his arm, drawing it up to his shoulder. This way your baby's fingers and nails can't get caught.

5 If the stretchsuit is on the large side, fold up the cuffs so he can explore with his hands and learn about his body.

6 Close all the snaps, starting with the ones around his thighs and crotch and working up to his neck.

BATHING AND WASHING YOUR BABY

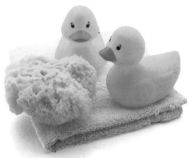

One day you will look back at your baby's baths as some of the most luxurious moments of parenting. But at first, that's not always the case. You may be nervous, and newborn babies don't always enjoy the sensation of being naked or being in water. Many babies cry that first month. Talk to your pediatrician about when to introduce a full bathtub, but be assured that little babies don't really need daily bathing. In fact, until the belly button is completely healed, you'll probably be advised to stick to sponge bathing. Change diapers often and keep bottoms free of wet or soiled diapers. Get into a habit of washing his face, hands, and diaper area with a soft baby washcloth at the same time every day. This will help inch you both toward a more predictable schedule. Coo, cuddle, and reassure your baby if he is unhappy. He knows your voice already, and soon you will both enjoy those bathing experiences.

EQUIPMENT FOR BATHING AND WASHING

THERE ARE plenty of products available designed to make bathtime easier for you, but you can keep costs down by just buying the things you genuinely need. Some mothers even use the kitchen sink at first. It's the right height and with a bath towel on the bottom for soft cushioning, you'll be all set. Don't use adult shampoos, soaps, or creams. They contain too many additives and chemicals to be safe for a baby.

EQUIPMENT FOR BATHING

Baby bathtub
Until your baby is ready to go into an adult bathtub (some time between three and six months), a babytub may make bathtime easy for you. Place it at a convenient height on a tabletop, or put it on a towel on the floor and kneel beside it. If you put it on a changing table, make sure it's secure.

Tissues

Cotton balls

Baby wipes

Baby washcloth

You may want to position such essentials near the bathing area and within easy reach.

A rubber bath mat *stops your baby slipping down*

Waterproof apron
A cotton fabric with waterproof backing will feel softer to your baby than plastic.

Rubber bath mat
Once your baby moves into the big bathtub, a suctioned rubber bath mat is a must to stop him from sliding on the bottom of the tub. The small size will also fit into a baby bathtub to give you more confidence.

BABY TOILETRIES

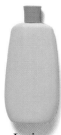

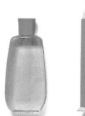
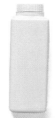
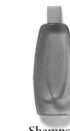
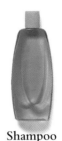

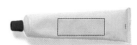
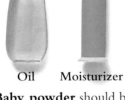

Bath liquid   Lotion   Oil   Moisturizer   Powder   Shampoo   Soap   Cotton swabs   Fluoride toothpaste

Baby bath liquid is an excellent alternative to both soap and shampoo.
Diaper lotion is useful for cleaning your baby's diaper area, particularly if his skin is very dry.
Baby moisturizer can be used instead of baby oil.

Baby powder should be used sparingly, if at all; it can cake in the creases of the skin and cause irritation if you use too much. Don't put any powder on an area where you will be putting diaper cream.
Baby shampoo may be needed once a week.

Baby soap is very mild; avoid pure soap because it is too alkaline. Choose moisturizing soaps rather than those with dyes and perfumes. Remember that a soapy baby will be very slippery, so hold him firmly.
Cotton swabs are useful for cleaning between your baby's fingers and toes, but never push them into his ears, nose, eyes, or bottom.
Toothpaste can be an adult brand or a lower fluoride baby toothpaste. Try not to let your child eat toothpaste, especially the adult type—if he does, stop using it until he's old enough *not* to eat it (see page 144).

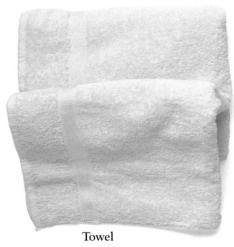

Towel

Keep a large, very soft towel for your baby's use only. Some baby bath towels have a corner piece that makes a hood.

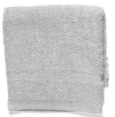

Natural sponge

Baby washcloth

Keep a new washcloth or sponge for you baby's use, and put the washcloth in the washing machine regularly. Don't let an older baby suck on the sponge.

HAIR, NAILS, AND TEETH

A hairbrush should have soft bristles and be small enough for your child to brush his own hair from about eighteen months. Choose a small comb with rounded teeth, and make sure there are no sharp points or edges. Use the baby comb and brush daily. It will help prevent cradle cap—and your baby will probably like having his scalp massaged.
Baby nail scissors have rounded ends

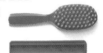

Baby hairbrush and comb

Nail scissors

Toothbrush

and short blades, so there's no danger of accidentally jabbing your baby.
Your child's **toothbrush** must have a small head so it can reach into the corners of his mouth, and soft, rounded bristles. Let your baby play with a baby-size brush, but use a child-size brush to clean his teeth for him. Change his brush regularly, and check with your dentist that it is cleaning adequately.

TIPS FOR WASHING YOUR YOUNG BABY

- Until your baby's navel has healed, rely on sponge baths. When you do start using a tub or sink, keep the water level to 2in (5cm).
- Only clean the parts you can see—do not try to poke inside the baby's nose or ears. Just wipe away any visible mucus or wax with damp cotton balls. Otherwise you may push the dirt back up into the nose or ear.
- With a baby girl, you can gently spread the outer vaginal lips and wipe near the anus. Remember, though, that the natural flow of mucus washes bacteria out.
- With an uncircumcised baby boy, never push back his foreskin to clean under it: you may hurt him, or damage the foreskin.
- Always wipe from front to back when you are cleaning a baby girl's diaper area. This prevents germs from spreading into the vagina and causing infection.
- When wiping your baby's eyes and ears, use a fresh cotton ball for each one, or you may spread minor infections.
- Always clean your baby's bottom last, and use a moistened washcloth, tissue dipped in baby oil, or a diaper wipe, whichever you prefer.

SPONGE BATHING A YOUNG BABY

SPONGE BATHING simply means cleaning only the parts of your baby that really need attention—her hands, face, neck, and diaper area. You don't even need a "sponge." A baby washcloth or cotton balls will do. Sponge bathe as part of your routine. It's an excellent alternative to a bath during the first six weeks, when neither of you will feel very sure about bathing in a bathtub. Make sure the room is warm. Wash your hands. Lay your baby on her changing table or on a pad on the floor and un-dress her down to her under-wear and diaper. Sponge bathe her in this position or on your lap.

■ **YOU WILL NEED** ■
Warm tap water
Cotton balls
Tissues
Washcloth
Warm towel
Diaper-changing equipment
Clean clothes

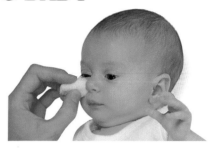

1 Wipe each eye from the nose outward with a cotton ball dipped in water. Use a fresh ball for each wipe, and for each eye. Dry gently with a tissue or soft cloth.

Wipe away *dirt and fluff behind her ears*

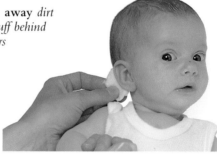

5 Uncurl her fingers *gently to wipe her hands*

2 With a fresh moist tissue, cotton ball, or washcloth, wipe each ear. Don't try to wipe inside: just go over and behind it. Dry with the towel.

CLEANING YOUR BABY'S NAVEL

The shriveled up stump of your baby's umbilical cord will probably remain until he is about 10–14 days old. Until it drops off, you must clean it every day. Your pediatrician or the nurse in the hospital can show you how. Careful cleaning prevents infection and helps keep the cord dry. Use a cotton swab dipped in rubbing alcohol and then squeezed to clean the base of the stump where it meets the skin. Also, keep the diaper folded down below the cord to keep urine from soaking it.

Once the stump has dropped off, you will need to clean the navel area every day as part of your routine until it is fully healed.

Consult your pediatrician or midwife as soon as possible if the navel looks red, swollen, inflamed, or starts to ooze fluid, although a small amount of bleeding is normal.

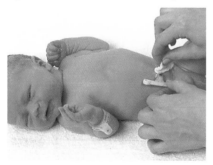

Moisten a cotton ball or swab with rubbing alcohol, and carefully wipe in the skin creases around the navel. He may cry as the alcohol feels cold to his skin. Let the alcohol dry on the cord, and fold the diaper down to expose the cord. This will help the cord to dry out and fall off sooner.

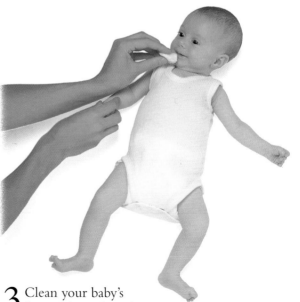

3 Clean your baby's face of formula and drool by wiping around her mouth and nose. Then, go over her cheeks and forehead. Dry with the towel.

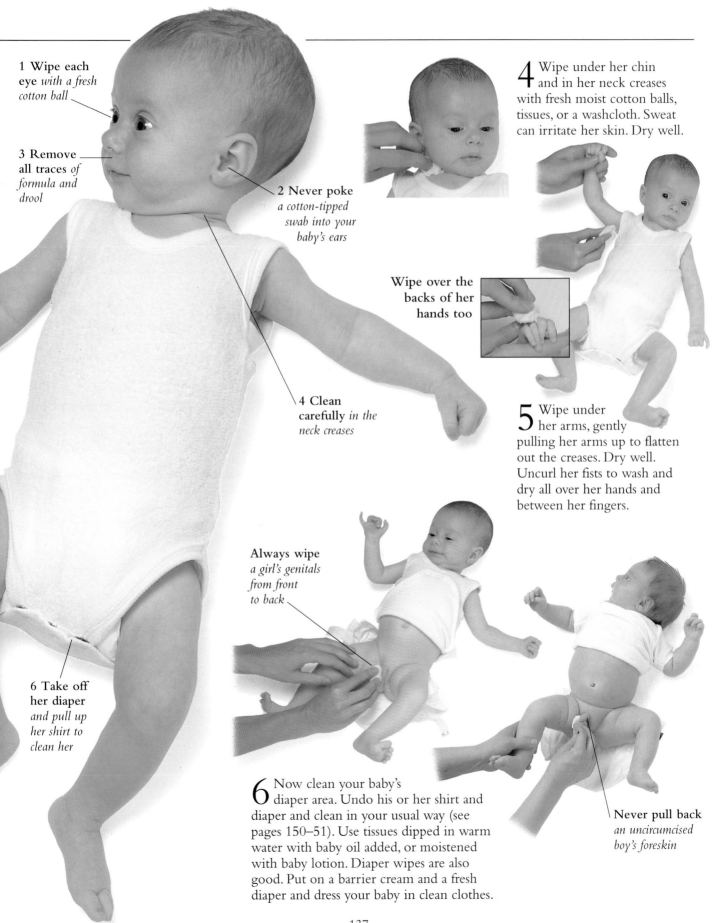

1 Wipe each eye *with a fresh cotton ball*

3 Remove all traces *of formula and drool*

2 Never poke *a cotton-tipped swab into your baby's ears*

4 Clean carefully *in the neck creases*

6 Take off her diaper *and pull up her shirt to clean her*

4 Wipe under her chin and in her neck creases with fresh moist cotton balls, tissues, or a washcloth. Sweat can irritate her skin. Dry well.

Wipe over the backs of her hands too

5 Wipe under her arms, gently pulling her arms up to flatten out the creases. Dry well. Uncurl her fists to wash and dry all over her hands and between her fingers.

Always wipe *a girl's genitals from front to back*

6 Now clean your baby's diaper area. Undo his or her shirt and diaper and clean in your usual way (see pages 150–51). Use tissues dipped in warm water with baby oil added, or moistened with baby lotion. Diaper wipes are also good. Put on a barrier cream and a fresh diaper and dress your baby in clean clothes.

Never pull back *an uncircumcised boy's foreskin*

BATHING YOUR NEW BABY

MOST BABIES eventually love getting a bath, but in the early days you and your baby will probably both have mixed feelings. A new baby often dislikes the feeling of being "unwrapped," and you may feel nervous holding the small, slippery body. In the first weeks you can just sponge bathe your baby to keep her clean. Practice with a full bath once a week, including a hair/scalp wash. Make sure the room is warm. Kneel, sit, or stand to bathe your baby, but don't strain or your back will start to ache.

■ YOU WILL NEED ■
Baby bathtub
Changing mat
Two baby bath towels
Waterproof apron
Cotton balls
Baby soap
Diaper changing equipment
Baby powder (optional)
Clean clothes

■ WARNING ■
■ **NEVER** leave your baby unattended in a bath. It only takes seconds for an infant to drown.

GETTING READY FOR THE BATH

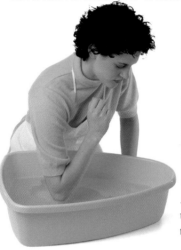

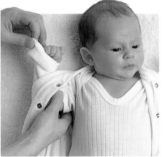

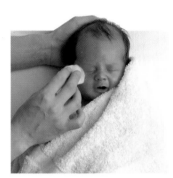

1 Put in cold water, add hot, and mix. Test with your elbow. The water should feel just warm and be 2in (5cm) deep.

2 Lay the bath towel on the changing mat and undress your baby down to her diaper.

3 Wrap her up snugly in a bath towel and wipe her face with moistened cotton balls.

QUESTION & ANSWER

"My four-week-old baby has ugly crusty patches on his scalp. What can I do?"

This is a harmless form of dandruff called cradle cap. Shampoo the area and then gently stimulate the scalp using a fine-toothed comb to help clear away the dead skin cells clogging the pores. Rinse with clear water. Repeat for several days until the condition clears.

RINSING YOUR BABY'S HAIR

1 Cradle her head in one hand, her back along your forearm, and tuck her legs under your elbow. Gently pour water over her head with a cupped hand. Don't splash her face and do keep smiling and chatting.

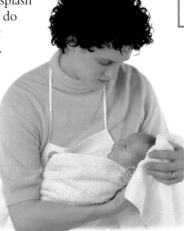

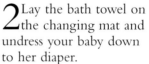

Avoid splashing *water over her face*

2 Bring your baby back to your lap to pat her head dry gently with the second towel.

SOAPING HER

1 Lay your baby on her mat and unwrap the towel. Moisten the soap and make a lather in your hands. Then rub your hands all over her upper body. Rinse your hands.

2 Take off her diaper and clean her bottom (see pages 150–51). Then, make your hands soapy again and run them over your baby's bottom and legs.

PUTTING YOUR BABY IN THE BATHTUB

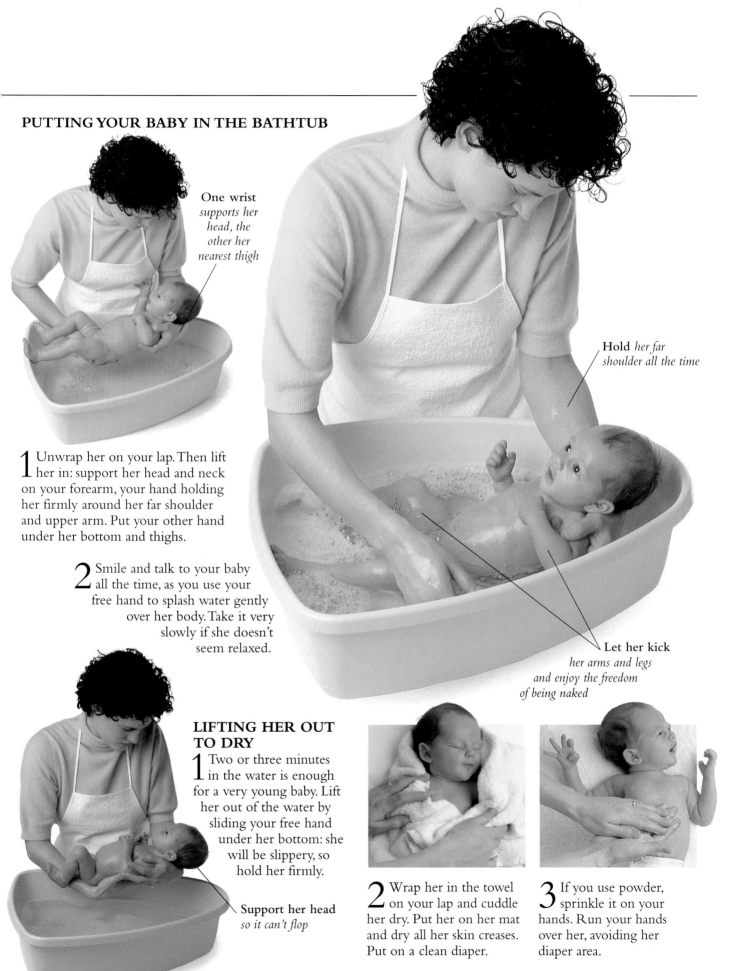

One wrist *supports her head, the other her nearest thigh*

Hold *her far shoulder all the time*

1 Unwrap her on your lap. Then lift her in: support her head and neck on your forearm, your hand holding her firmly around her far shoulder and upper arm. Put your other hand under her bottom and thighs.

2 Smile and talk to your baby all the time, as you use your free hand to splash water gently over her body. Take it very slowly if she doesn't seem relaxed.

Let her kick *her arms and legs and enjoy the freedom of being naked*

LIFTING HER OUT TO DRY

1 Two or three minutes in the water is enough for a very young baby. Lift her out of the water by sliding your free hand under her bottom: she will be slippery, so hold her firmly.

Support her head *so it can't flop*

2 Wrap her in the towel on your lap and cuddle her dry. Put her on her mat and dry all her skin creases. Put on a clean diaper.

3 If you use powder, sprinkle it on your hands. Run your hands over her, avoiding her diaper area.

139

BATHING IN THE BIG TUB

YOUR BABY will probably be ready to graduate to the exciting territory of the big tub at the age of three or four months—and some babies are happy in it even earlier. If your baby hasn't yet learned to enjoy bathtime, don't rush the change—give him a few more weeks of being bathed in his own tub, until he really is too big for it, or is more confident.

To bathe your three-month-old, arrange everything you will need beside the tub. Make sure the room is warm. Put the rubber mat on the bottom of the tub and run in cold water, then hot, so that the water is just warm. Put your baby on his changing mat to wash his face, eyes, and ears before you put him in the tub. Take the diaper off and clean his bottom last.

■   **YOU WILL NEED**   ■
Rubber bath mat
Waterproof apron
Baby soap and baby shampoo (shampoo not needed every time)
Large soft towel
Baby's own sponge or washcloth
Equipment for washing your baby's face
Diaper-changing essentials
Pouring and other toys for an older baby
Toothbrush for an older child
Clean clothes

WASHING YOUR BABY

1 Lay your baby in the tub on a rubber mat. Keep his head and shoulders supported on your arm, his ears clear of the water.

Always kneel *beside the tub so that you can hold your baby securely*

Bathtime *is a time to talk to and enjoy your baby*

The water *should not be deep: 2in (5cm) is enough*

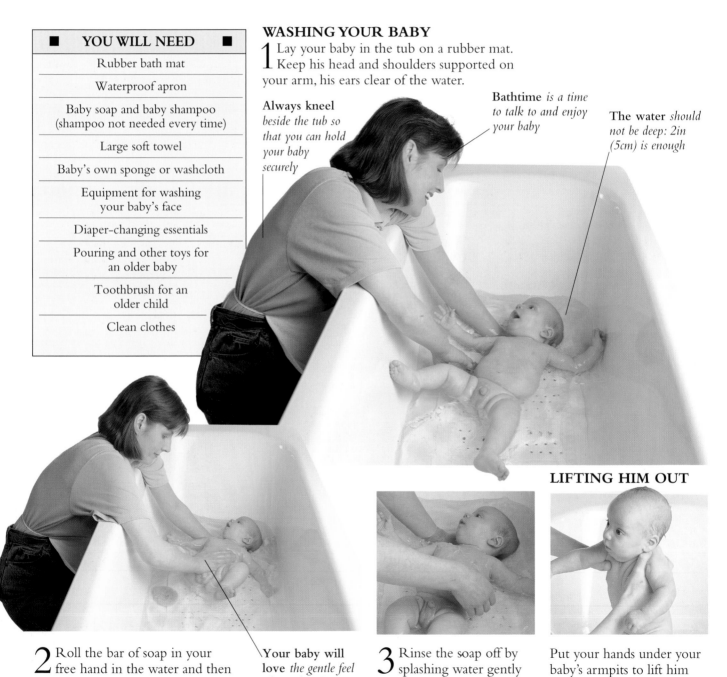

LIFTING HIM OUT

2 Roll the bar of soap in your free hand in the water and then run your hand over his body. There's no need to scrub him—he's unlikely to be that dirty!

Your baby will love *the gentle feel of your hand*

3 Rinse the soap off by splashing water gently over him, talking to him and reassuring him all the time that bathtime is fun time.

Put your hands under your baby's armpits to lift him out. He will be slippery. Wrap him in his towel and cuddle him dry.

WASHING YOUR BABY'S HAIR

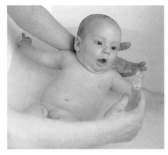
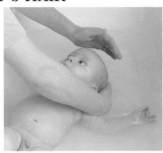
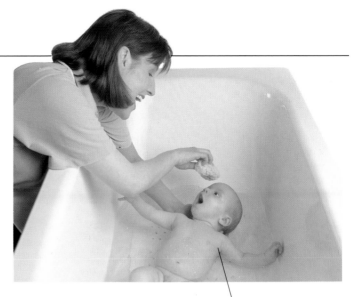

1 Wash his hair about once a week. Wet it first. If using shampoo, slide your supporting hand forward and pour a small amount into the palm.

2 Support your baby's head with your free hand and rub shampoo over his hair. Don't worry about hurting the fontanelle, the soft spot on his head.

3 Swap hands again and wipe most of the suds off with a wet, well squeezed out sponge or washcloth.

Take your cue *from him—he might enjoy a teasing game*

■ BATHTIME SAFETY ■

Always follow these few rules:
- **Never leave a baby or small child alone in the tub, or move out of easy reach, even for a second.** It takes no time for a child to slip and drown, even in very shallow water.
- **Never** let your child pull himself to standing in the tub even if he can stand steadily, and even though you have a rubber mat in the bathtub.
- Even when your baby can sit steadily, keep a hand ready to support him if he slips.
- A rubber suction mat in the bottom of the tub is essential.
- Never add extra hot water while your child is in the water. If any adjustment is necessary, mix hot and cold water in a pitcher so it's just warm, then pour it in.
- Make sure your water heater thermostat isn't set higher than 120°F (49°C).
- If the faucet gets hot when you run it, tie a washcloth around it so your child can't be burned.
- If you bathe with your baby, make the water cooler than you usually have it.

MAKING BATHTIME FUN

Once your baby can sit steadily, bathtime becomes a wonderful playtime— not just a way of getting him clean. Gather together bath toys: things that pour, like plastic beakers and funnels, clean sandcastle buckets with holes, even plastic colanders—all will fascinate him. Floating toys like boats or ducks are ideal too. About once a week use a pouring toy to wash his hair, but don't let the water run down his face—he will probably hate it.

Always supervise bathtime, *and never leave your child alone in the bathtub, not even for a minute. Let another person answer the phone.*

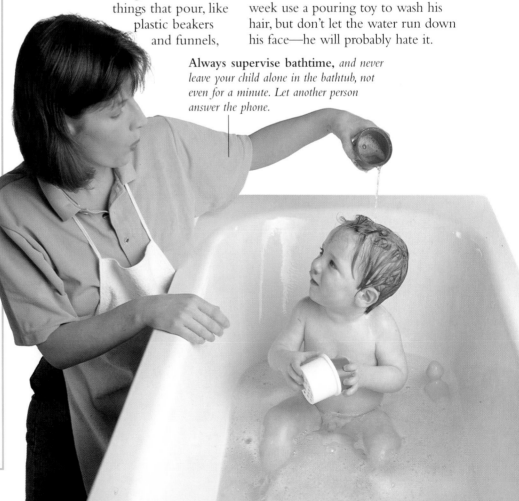

BABIES WHO HATE WATER AND WASHING

BABIES WHO HATE BATHING

Some newborns are frightened by bathtime—and often a baby or toddler may suddenly fight it. Give up baths altogether for a while. Light sponge bathing will keep a small baby clean, though a mobile baby may need a thorough sponge bath on your lap (see below). After two or three weeks, try having a bath with him to help him overcome his fear.

Playing with water

Sit your baby beside a bowl of water on the kitchen floor and let him splash and play. Pouring cups and floating toys can often persuade a child that water can be fun.

BABIES WHO HATE WASHING

Even if your child hates having his hands washed, it's important to do so before and after every meal. Make it more fun by washing his hands between your own wet and soapy ones.

BABIES WHO HATE HAIR WASHING

Babies and young children often particularly dislike having their hair washed, even if they love bath-time. Around two-and-a-half to three years is often the most difficult time. If your child doesn't like hair washing, abandon it for a couple of weeks. Help him to be more reasonable about his dislike; for example, go out together in the rain and show him how pleasurable rain-drops feel on his face.

Reintroduce hairwashing at bathtime gradually. It may help to give him a washcloth to hold over his eyes and face. Often it's the feel of water on the face that children hate most. If your child will wear one, you could try putting a plastic "halo" around his hairline to keep the water off his face.

Sponging her hair

You can keep your child's hair clean by sponging out any bits of food and dirt with a damp washcloth or sponge.

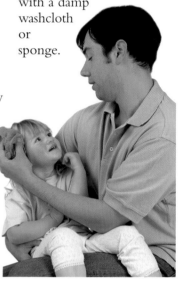

SPONGE BATHING YOUR OLDER BABY

IF YOUR BABY doesn't like water, there's no need to bathe him: Once he can hold his head up, a daily sponge bath on your lap is enough. First, lay your baby on his mat and wipe his eyes, face, and ears with a clean washcloth or cotton balls. Sit him on your lap with everything you need within reach.

■ YOU WILL NEED ■
A sink filled with warm water
Baby soap
Waterproof apron that covers your upper body
Your baby's own sponge or washcloth
Warm towel
Diaper-changing equipment

TOP HALF

1 Take off the top half of your baby's clothing. Wet the sponge, squeeze it out well, then rub a little soap and wash his neck.

Wear an apron *that covers your upper body*

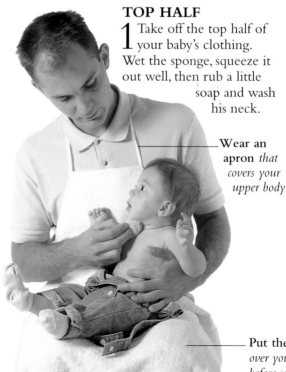

2 Wet and soap the sponge again, squeezing it out so it doesn't dribble. Then, wash all over his chest and stomach. Rinse the soap off as before. Dry him well with the towel.

Put the towel *over your lap before you begin*

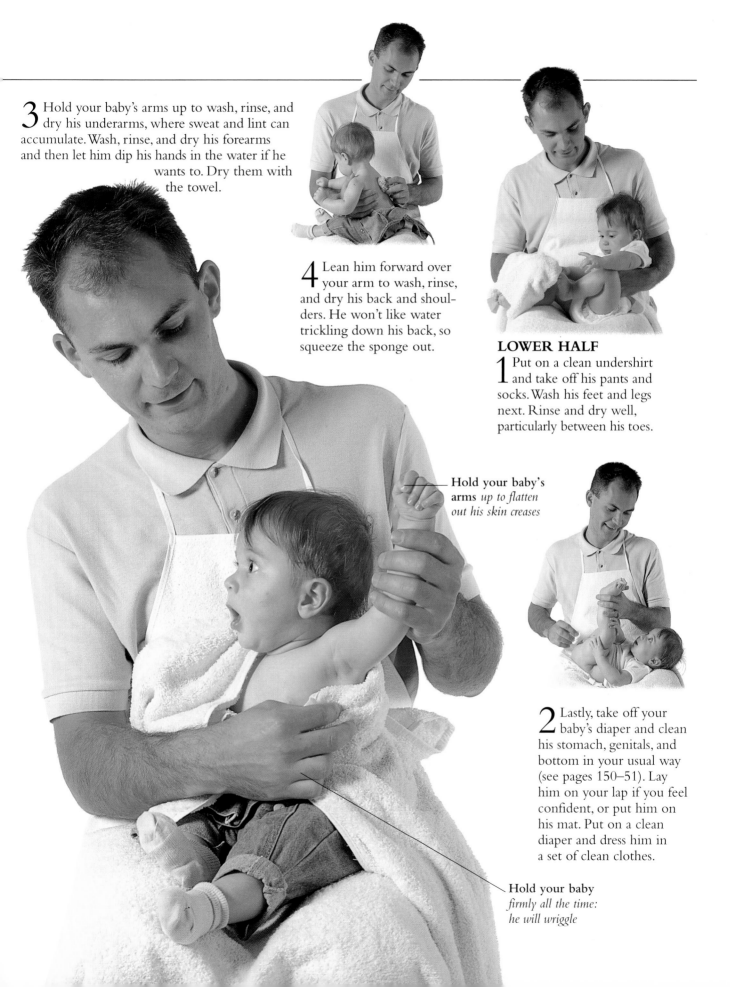

3 Hold your baby's arms up to wash, rinse, and dry his underarms, where sweat and lint can accumulate. Wash, rinse, and dry his forearms and then let him dip his hands in the water if he wants to. Dry them with the towel.

4 Lean him forward over your arm to wash, rinse, and dry his back and shoulders. He won't like water trickling down his back, so squeeze the sponge out.

LOWER HALF

1 Put on a clean undershirt and take off his pants and socks. Wash his feet and legs next. Rinse and dry well, particularly between his toes.

Hold your baby's **arms** *up to flatten out his skin creases*

2 Lastly, take off your baby's diaper and clean his stomach, genitals, and bottom in your usual way (see pages 150–51). Lay him on your lap if you feel confident, or put him on his mat. Put on a clean diaper and dress him in a set of clean clothes.

Hold your baby *firmly all the time: he will wriggle*

CARING FOR YOUR CHILD'S TEETH

IT'S NEVER TOO EARLY to start cleaning you child's teeth. Once your baby has two or more, wipe his teeth and gums each evening with a damp handkerchief (see below). Twelve months is a good age to introduce him to a child's toothbrush. Clean his teeth for him after breakfast and at bedtime, but let him play with a brush himself at bathtime too. Taking care of the first, or "milk," teeth helps to ensure that when the permanent teeth come in around age six, they will be correctly positioned and in healthy gums—and you will be establishing good, lifelong habits in your child.

At any age, the more of a game teeth cleaning seems, the more your child will be encouraged to cooperate. Playing dentist, cleaning your own teeth with him, and spitting out messily will all help.

CLEANING YOUR BABY'S TEETH

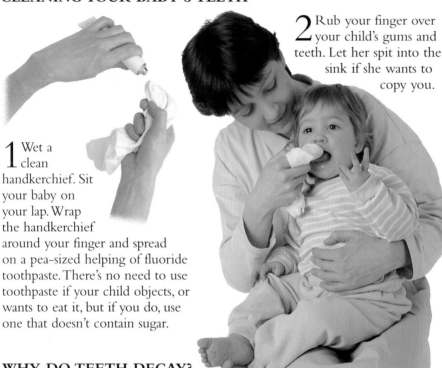

1 Wet a clean handkerchief. Sit your baby on your lap. Wrap the handkerchief around your finger and spread on a pea-sized helping of fluoride toothpaste. There's no need to use toothpaste if your child objects, or wants to eat it, but if you do, use one that doesn't contain sugar.

2 Rub your finger over your child's gums and teeth. Let her spit into the sink if she wants to copy you.

WHY DO TEETH DECAY?
Teeth decay because bacteria in the mouth react with sugar to form acid, which eats through the hard enamel covering teeth. Candy and sugary foods increase the risk of tooth decay, particularly if they're eaten between meals, because the teeth are bathed in sugar most of the time. So try to confine candy to mealtimes, brush your child's teeth afterward, and give him snacks that don't contain a lot of sugar (see page 116).

The biggest contributor to decay of the primary teeth is prolonged bottle-feeding. Babies should be weaned to a cup between 12–15 months of age, and babies more than 18 months old should learn other ways of falling asleep and not continue to rely on sucking.

Fluoride
Children's teeth can be protected with fluoride, a chemical that hardens tooth enamel and even heals small breaches in it. Twice-daily brushing with a fluoride toothpaste will help protect your child's teeth from decay, particularly if you let the paste linger in his mouth. Ask your pediatrician about giving your child a fluoride supplement (drops or tablets) if your local water supply isn't fluoridated.

Too much fluoride?
You needn't worry if your child swallows a little toothpaste as you brush his teeth, but he might love the taste that he wants to eat it from the tube. Don't let him. If he's getting fluoride from water or supplements, the extra in the toothpaste might be excessive.

VISITING THE DENTIST
From the time your child has a complete set of first teeth (at about age two and a half) you should arrange regular dental checkups every six months. Your dentist will have treatments available to prevent tooth decay, and he will be able to advise you about fluoride supplements. If there are any cavities, it's important that they are spotted promptly. Get your child used to the idea of going to the dentist before he has any treatment. If he seems frightened, sit him on your lap, and show him what the equipment does.

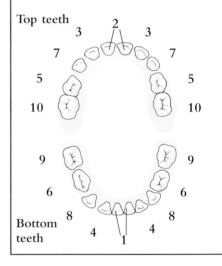

HOW THE TEETH COME IN
Your baby might cut his first tooth at any time during the first year, and he will be teething into his third year. Babies' teeth usually appear in the same order.

Top teeth

Bottom teeth

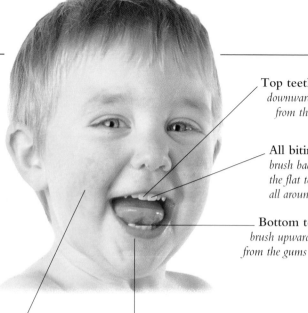

CLEANING YOUR CHILD'S TEETH

From the age of 18 months, start cleaning your child's teeth for him with a wet toothbrush and a pea-sized helping of fluoride toothpaste. Brush them for him for as long as he will let you. He will probably want to brush them himself from the age of about two. Always supervise—he needs to brush correctly. Teach him by standing behind him in front of a mirror and, holding his hand, showing him the correct movements.

Top teeth: *brush downward, away from the gums*

All biting surfaces: *brush back and forth along the flat tops of the teeth, all around the mouth*

Bottom teeth: *brush upward, away from the gums*

Get the brush *right to the back of your child's mouth*

Brush the gums *with a circular motion, both on the outsides and on the inside by the tongue*

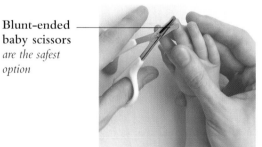

Making a game of teeth cleaning
Play games at bathtime to encourage your child to copy you. Clean his teeth properly afterward.

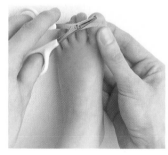

Cleaning your child's teeth
Stand your child on a step at the sink, with you behind her and to one side. Hold her head back so you can see into her mouth as you brush. Let her rinse and spit out—that's most of the fun.

CUTTING NAILS

YOUR NEWBORN BABY

Keep your baby's fingernails short so that there's no chance of his scratching himself. Kept short, fingernails are also easier to keep clean. Trim the nails with small, blunt-ended baby scissors or a soft emery board. Follow the natural curve of the fingertip, making sure not to cut the nails uncomfortably short.

Remember that a baby's nails may grow so quickly that you may have to trim them twice a week.

If your baby wriggles and won't keep still when you cut his fingernails, try cutting them while he is asleep.

CUTTING FINGERNAILS   CUTTING TOENAILS

Blunt-ended baby scissors *are the safest option*

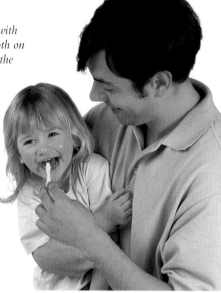

Sit your baby on your lap, facing forward. Hold one finger at a time and cut her nails with baby scissors, following the shape of her fingertips and checking for sharp points.

Lay a young baby on a mat; sit an older baby on your lap. Hold her foot firmly as she will kick. Cut the nails straight across, otherwise the side edges might grow into the skin.

DIAPERS AND DIAPER CHANGING

The first few weeks of your newborn's life will probably seem like a constant round of diaper changing. Because your baby's bladder is small, she wets often, so at the very least you need to change her after a feeding, after she wakes, before she goes to bed, and in the early weeks often after night feedings too. In fact, change her whenever her diaper is wet or soiled, because a dirty diaper makes it more likely that she will get diaper rash. Changing her isn't always your first priority. When she wakes in the morning she will be hungry, so try to give her half her feeding before you stop to change her. Diaper changing need not be a chore: it's a time for games and cuddles and an important way to show your baby that you love her. Make it easy on yourself by keeping a full set of everything you need in one place. If you live in a two-story house, put a duplicate set downstairs for the first weeks. As the months go by, you'll notice that her diaper needs changing less and less often. By around the age of two and a half, your child may start to recognize the feeling of a full bladder and may be ready for potty training.

THE CONTENTS OF YOUR BABY'S DIAPER

All these are common sights on a baby's diaper:

■ **greenish-black, sticky tar (first two or three days only):** this is meconium, which fills the bowels before birth and must be pased before digestion begins
■ **greenish-brown or bright green semifluid stools, full of curds (first week only):** "changing stools" show that your baby is adapting to feeding through her digestive system
■ **orange-yellow, mustard-like stools, watery with bits of milk curd in them, often very copious:** the settled stools of a breast-fed baby
■ **pale brown, solid, formed, and smelly stools:** the settled stools of a bottle-fed baby
■ **green or green-streaked stools:** quite normal, but small green stools over several days may be a sign of under-feeding
■ **changes in stool color, consistency, and odor** are a normal result of adding solid foods to your baby's diet. Cereals may also cause constipation (see page 213).

Consult your doctor if:
■ the stools are very watery and smelly, or your baby is vomiting and not eating. (Diarrhea is life-threatening in a young baby; see page 179.)
■ you see blood on the diaper
■ anything at all worries you.

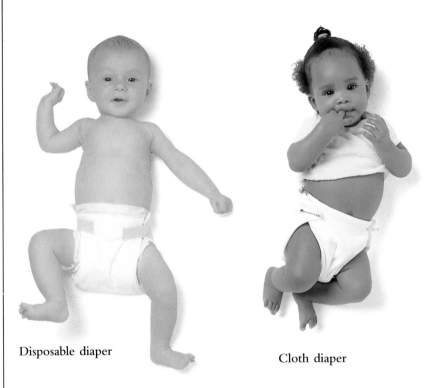

Disposable diaper

Cloth diaper

TYPES OF DIAPER

Your baby won't mind whether you use disposable or cloth diapers, provided the diaper is comfortable and she's not left in a wet or dirty one. Disposables tend to fit snugly. Cloth diapers are bulkier, and the clothes you buy your baby may need to be a few sizes larger to accommodate the diaper. Using a diaper service, especially in the newborn stage, is a good idea. Many are as cost-effective as disposables.

A mat with a raised edge *won't stop your baby from rolling off*

CHANGING YOUR BABY'S DIAPER

Since you will be changing your baby's diaper frequently, make your changing area a pleasant place for both of you: a mobile above your baby's head, a teddy bear nearby, bright decals on the walls or furniture alongside will all amuse your baby—

and encourage her to lie still for you. A changing mat is cheap and very convenient, and your baby will be safe if you put the mat on a reasonably clean and dry floor. A specially designed changing table may be useful for storing clean diapers and

toiletries, but your baby can fall off unless she is buckled on with a restraining belt, and she will soon outgrow it. If you do buy one or use a countertop, chest of drawers, or your bed to change the baby, never turn your back, not even for a second.

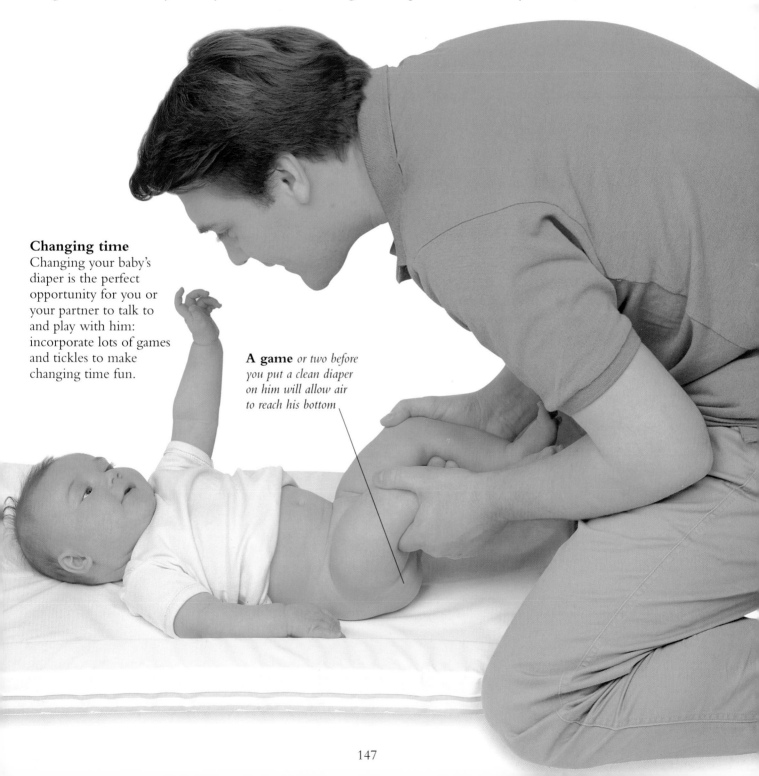

Changing time
Changing your baby's diaper is the perfect opportunity for you or your partner to talk to and play with him: incorporate lots of games and tickles to make changing time fun.

A game *or two before you put a clean diaper on him will allow air to reach his bottom*

EQUIPMENT FOR CHANGING YOUR BABY'S DIAPER

SUCH AN EXTENSIVE ARRAY OF EQUIPMENT need not seem daunting: the cotton balls, washcloths, and baby wipes, for example, are alternatives. The cotton balls or washcloths can be moistened with water or diaper lotion. You may be able to flush used tissues, diaper liners, and wipes down the toilet, but put disposable diapers into a pail lined with a plastic bag. Drop dirty cloth diapers into a special pail, too, so you can launder them separately or send them out, if you have a regular diaper laundering service.

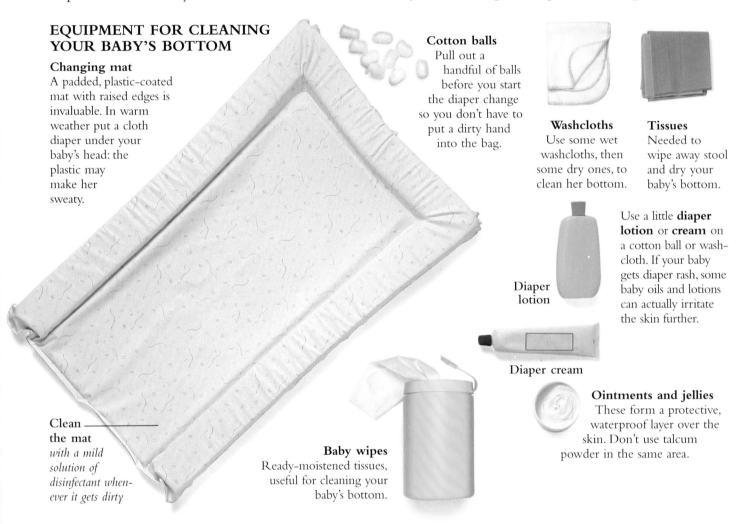

EQUIPMENT FOR CLEANING YOUR BABY'S BOTTOM

Changing mat
A padded, plastic-coated mat with raised edges is invaluable. In warm weather put a cloth diaper under your baby's head: the plastic may make her sweaty.

Clean the mat *with a mild solution of disinfectant whenever it gets dirty*

Cotton balls
Pull out a handful of balls before you start the diaper change so you don't have to put a dirty hand into the bag.

Washcloths
Use some wet washcloths, then some dry ones, to clean her bottom.

Tissues
Needed to wipe away stool and dry your baby's bottom.

Diaper lotion

Use a little **diaper lotion** or **cream** on a cotton ball or washcloth. If your baby gets diaper rash, some baby oils and lotions can actually irritate the skin further.

Diaper cream

Ointments and jellies
These form a protective, waterproof layer over the skin. Don't use talcum powder in the same area.

Baby wipes
Ready-moistened tissues, useful for cleaning your baby's bottom.

WHAT KIND OF DIAPERS SHOULD YOU USE?

You really have three choices when it comes to diapering your baby: use disposables, hire a diaper service, or buy and wash your own cloth diapers. Cotton cloth diapers that you'll be washing at home really are the cheapest option, but don't forget to consider your time and labor when it comes to cost. You'll also be buying more laundry soap and using more water to run all of the diapers through the washing machine rinse cycle several times to help rid the diaper of soap. When economists compare the costs of diaper services with disposable diapers, they are almost even. A good service provides up to 90 diapers per week, picks up dirty ones and returns a properly washed and dried supply. You still need to purchase waterproof pants and diaper pins, however. Disposables, which are the most extensively used, are clearly the most convenient. Initially at least, you may want to use both cloth and disposable diapers. Having some cloth handy for emergencies is always a good idea. You'll need up to 70 disposables weekly so plan shopping trips ahead; big boxes take up grocery cart space.

DISPOSABLE DIAPERS

Disposable diapers are absorbent paper pads and plastic pants all in one. When you're happy with a brand, buy in large quantities: in the first weeks you may be changing your baby 10 or 12 times a day, so 70 diapers will only be one week's supply. A diaper that is too small might be uncomfortable, so buy the next size up if it looks tight. "Ultra" brands are slim and very absorbent; those labeled "standard" are cheaper and bulkier, but you will have to change your baby more often.

You will also need:
Plastic bag or pail with a liner inside: drop the used diaper into this, and then when the bag is full, seal it and put it with your garbage. Disposable diapers are guaranteed to stop up your toilet.
A dozen cloth diapers: for general mopping up around your baby.

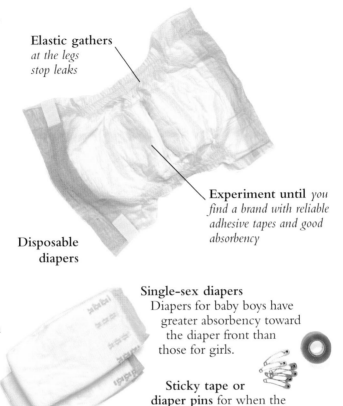

Elastic gathers *at the legs stop leaks*

Experiment until *you find a brand with reliable adhesive tapes and good absorbency*

Disposable diapers

Single-sex diapers
Diapers for baby boys have greater absorbency toward the diaper front than those for girls.

Sticky tape or diaper pins for when the tapes won't stick, or you need to reseal the diaper.

DISPOSING OF THE DIAPERS

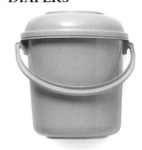

Diaper pail Place the used disposable diapers in a pail with a plastic liner inside.

Recycling disposables
Several disposable diaper manufacturers have joined forces to solve the growing problem of trash. Used plastic-covered, disposable diapers are being converted into pulp for wallboard and plastic that can be molded into park benches.

CLOTH DIAPERS AND WATERPROOF PANTS

When you use **cotton cloth diapers** you will need a pair of waterproof pants over the top. Unless you hire a service that provides diapers and launders them weekly, you will have the extra work of washing the diapers. Buy the best quality **100% cotton cloth diapers** you can find. You need 24 to begin with. They are bulkier than disposables, so the smallest sizes of baby clothes may not fit her for long.

Always buy *100% cotton cloth diapers*

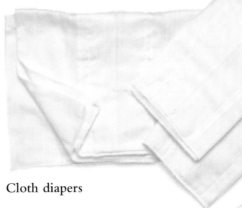

Cloth diapers

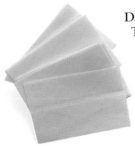

Diaper liners
These are sometimes used inside a cloth diaper to allow moisture to seep through to the diaper but not back again. The disposable type can be flushed down the toilet with your baby's messes.

Safety diaper pins The hood locks the pin shut. As you take each pin off, attach it to your clothing, and discard any that become blunt.

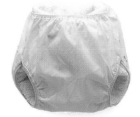

Pull-on pants
These do prevent leaks, but can also promote diaper rash.

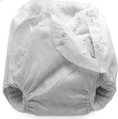

Snap-on pants
When you leave the bottom snaps undone, air circulates inside.

CLEANING A GIRL

CLEAN your baby's bottom thoroughly at every diaper change; otherwise she will soon get red and sore. Wash your hands first. Put your baby on a mat or changing table and undo her clothing and diaper. If she's wearing a cloth diaper, use a clean corner to wipe off most of any mess. With a disposable, wipe off the worst of the mess with tissues and push them down into the diaper. Lift your baby's legs and fold the diaper down under her.

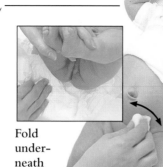

Fold underneath

1 Wipe away stool with tissues. Then using a moist baby washcloth, clean all over her stomach up to her navel.

2 With a fresh washcloth, clean inside all the creases at the tops of her legs, wiping downward and away from her body.

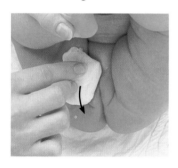

3 Lift her legs with a finger between her ankles and clean her genitals next. Always wipe from front to back to prevent germs from the anus entering the vagina. If necessary, gently spread the outer vaginal lips to clean near the anus; otherwise, do not try to clean inside the vaginal lips.

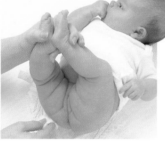

4 With a fresh washcloth or baby wipe clean her anus, then her buttocks and thighs, working inward toward the anus. When she's clean, remove the disposable diaper, seal the tapes over the front, and drop in the pail. Wipe your hands.

Dry the skin creases well

5 Dry her diaper area with tissues, and then let her kick for a while without a diaper so that her bottom is open to the air.

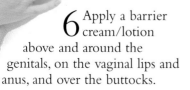

6 Apply a barrier cream/lotion above and around the genitals, on the vaginal lips and anus, and over the buttocks.

DIAPER RASH

All babies get a red or sore bottom from time to time. Consult your doctor if the rash won't clear up.

To avoid diaper rash:
■ change your baby's diaper frequently
■ clean and dry her bottom and skin creases thoroughly
■ let your baby go without a diaper for short periods
■ use a diaper rash cream
■ if using cloth diapers, buy breathable diaper pants or wraps, because they allow air to circulate

■ wash and rinse cloth diapers thoroughly.

At the first signs of redness:
■ use a healing diaper rash cream
■ change diapers more frequently
■ let your baby go without a diaper for as much of the day as possible
■ if using cloth diapers, try an absorbent type of liner
■ stop using waterproof pants: they make a rash worse because they help keep urine close to the skin. If you don't like the leaks, switch to disposables for a while.

CLEANING A BOY

YOUR BABY BOY'S urine may go everywhere, so you need to clean his bottom very thoroughly at every diaper change to guard against diaper rash. Wash your hands. Put your baby on a mat or changing table and undo his clothing and diaper. If he's wearing a cloth diaper, wipe off the worst of any mess with a clean corner. With a disposable, undo the tapes, and pause. He may wet then.

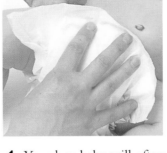

1 Your boy baby will often urinate just as you take his diaper off, so pause for a couple of seconds with the diaper held over his penis.

2 Open the diaper out. Wipe off the mess with tissues and drop them into the diaper, then fold it down under him. Moisten cotton balls with water, or use a washcloth or diaper wipe to clean him. Wipe his stomach up to his navel.

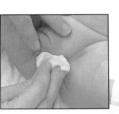

Clean carefully under his testicles

3 With fresh cotton balls or a diaper wipe clean thoroughly in the creases at the tops of his legs and at the base of his genitals, wiping away from his body. Hold his testicles out of the way while you wipe underneath them.

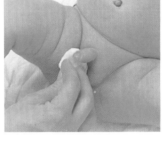

4 With fresh cotton balls or diaper wipes clean your baby's testicles, including under his penis. There may be traces of urine or feces here. Hold his penis out of the way if necessary, but take care not to drag the skin.

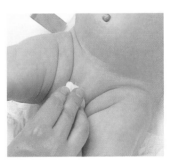

5 Clean his penis, wiping away from the body: do not pull the foreskin of an uncircumcised boy back to clean underneath.

Put a barrier cream or lotion *over his stomach for protection*

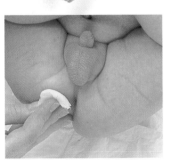

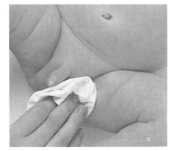

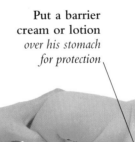

6 Lift your baby's legs to clean his anus and buttocks, keeping a finger between his ankles. Wipe over the backs of his thighs too. When he's clean, remove the diaper.

7 Wipe your hands, and dry his bottom with tissues. Let him kick for a while if he has a rash, but keep tissues close at hand just in case he urinates.

8 Apply a barrier cream generously above the penis (but not on it), around the testicles and anus, and over the buttocks.

PUTTING ON A DISPOSABLE DIAPER

IF YOU WANT a disposable diaper to stay on your baby, there are two things to keep in mind: choose the right size for her weight and always wipe your own hands before you open the tabs. When they get greasy, they don't stick.

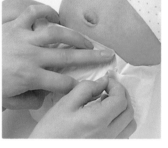

1 Open out the diaper with the tapes at the top. Lift your baby by her ankles with one finger between them and slide the diaper under her, until the top edge lines up with her waist.

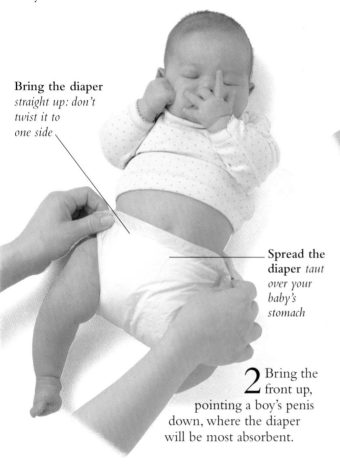

Bring the diaper *straight up: don't twist it to one side*

Spread the diaper *taut over your baby's stomach*

2 Bring the front up, pointing a boy's penis down, where the diaper will be most absorbent.

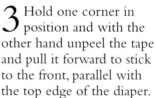

3 Hold one corner in position and with the other hand unpeel the tape and pull it forward to stick to the front, parallel with the top edge of the diaper.

4 Do the same with the other side, making sure the diaper is snug around your baby's legs, and not twisted around to one side.

QUESTION & ANSWER

"How can I make my 15-month-old son lie still while I change his diaper? He wriggles so much I can't clean him properly or get the diaper on."
No self-respecting toddler will lie quietly while you change him— but you must still get his bottom clean. First of all, make sure to use disposable diapers. They go on very quickly, with no awkward pins to worry about. Remember to make changing time fun, with tickling games and some interesting toys for him to hold. If he's very dirty, it will be easiest to clean him by standing him in the bathtub on a non-slip mat and, if possible, hose his bottom down with warm water from a shower attachment. Dry him well.

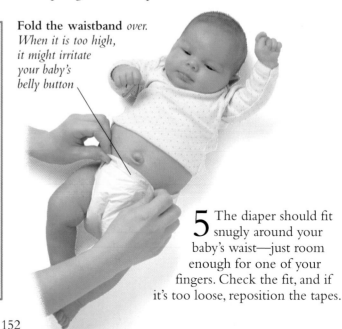

Fold the waistband *over. When it is too high, it might irritate your baby's belly button*

5 The diaper should fit snugly around your baby's waist—just room enough for one of your fingers. Check the fit, and if it's too loose, reposition the tapes.

PUTTING ON A CLOTH DIAPER

YOU WILL QUICKLY get to know the best way to put on your baby's diapers. Be creative, and experiment with the folding until you get the maximum absorbency right where it's needed.

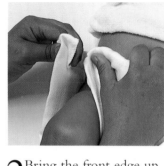

1 Lift up her lower body by the ankles and slide the folded diaper under her.

Make sure a protective cream *is applied all over your baby's bottom*

2 Bring the front edge up over her stomach. Draw one front corner of the diaper over to meet the back corner over her hip.

FOLDING A CLOTH DIAPER

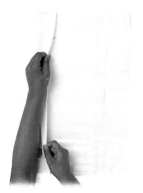

1 Lay the diaper and liner out flat. Fold the side edges in: make the folds shallow for a large baby, deep for a smaller one.

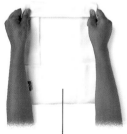

Extra padding *at the front is better for a baby boy*

2 Fold in each end to give most padding wherever your baby seems to get wettest.

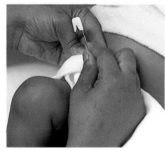

3 Keeping the fingers of one hand between the diaper pin and her body, pin the back edge of the diaper on to the front corner. **Make sure the hood locks the pin shut.**

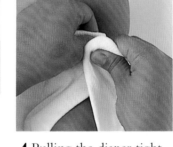

4 Pulling the diaper tight over her body, pin the second corner in the same way as the first

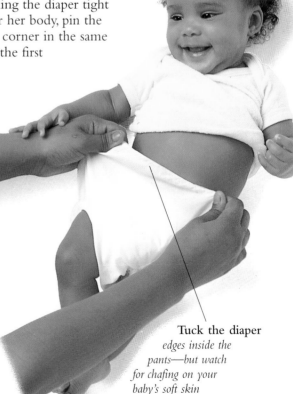

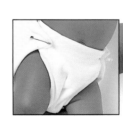

The diaper should *fit tightly at first: it will loosen.*

5 Put waterproof pants over your baby's diaper, holding the leg hole wide as you ease them up over her foot and knee. Then pull them over the diaper, lifting her at the ankles to pull them up at the back. Tuck the cloth edges up into the pants to keep the wetness in.

Tuck the diaper *edges inside the pants—but watch for chafing on your baby's soft skin*

GIVING UP DIAPERS

Becoming toilet-trained is a big step in your toddler's life. You can't force him to use a potty chair any more than you can force him to walk. It's all part of his natural development, and it may take a day, a week, a month, or half a year. Just wait until he's ready and then provide encouragement as you help him understand what's happening. Until your child turns two, he is probably physically incapable of recognizing the signs of a full bladder or bowel or of using his muscles to control them. And if he's one of those children who finds no discomfort in wearing a dirty, wet diaper, there's no reward for him to become potty-trained. Be patient and nonjudgmental when he has an accident. Bowel control usually comes first, during the second year, followed by daytime bladder control. Staying dry at night is last. Most, but certainly not all, children are potty-trained by three years of age.

Training pants
Extra padding and sometimes a waterproof backing make these more absorbent than ordinary underpants.

TIPS TO HELP

Remember, too much pressure from you can be confusing, as your child struggles to understand and do what you want.
■ Choose a time for potty-training when your child's life is relatively free of new situations, *and* when you can approach it with a relaxed attitude, infinite patience, and sense of humor.
■ When he's successful, don't be too wildly enthusiastic—you want him to accomplish this big step for himself and not just to please you.
■ When he has an accident, be sympathetic, nor angry or irritated about it.

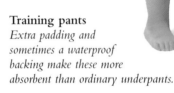

Your child and his potty chair
Let him play with it and on it. He will soon understand what it's for.

ACHIEVING DAYTIME CONTROL

1
Wait until your child is ready
Your child may be ready to use the potty chair if he:
■ is two and a half (some boys may not be ready to do so until age three)
■ recognizes that he's done something in his diaper, perhaps by pointing and shouting, or by telling you that it's wet
■ is often dry after a nap

2
Introduce the potty chair
Show him a potty chair and tell him what it's for. Put it in the bathroom for a few days or even months so he gets used to it. Show him how to sit on it, with or without his diaper on at first.

3
Set aside a suitable time
The ideal arrangement for potty-training is to start in the summer when your child can wear training pants while playing outside in the yard. Accidents won't be as disastrous in the grass and you won't have to worry about outer clothing. Set up his potty where he can see it outside. You might try letting him play in a pail of water or a little wading pool. Don't start when your routines are upset for any reason or when you are away from home.

4
Buy or borrow a pile of training pants
Make sure that you keep a stack of clean training pants in the bathroom so when he has an accident, he can quickly discard one pair for another. Buy or borrow a dozen. Don't put him in overalls with complicated straps, difficult zippers, or buttons, Time is of the essence when he's got to go.

5

Help him to use the potty chair
Be encouraging about sitting on the potty chair, but don't pressure him. Buy him pants he can pull down by himself but help him to sit down on the chair, tucking a boy's penis in. If he's managed to *tell* you he needs it, thank him.

If your child jumps up immediately
Suggest that he sit a little longer and make it easier by distracting him with a toy or a book. If nothing happens, let him get up and keep on playing.

When he does go in the potty
When he does use the potty chair successfully, praise him and tell him what a good boy he is. Wipe off any drips of urine with toilet paper or clean his bottom quickly (wipe a girl from front to back). Hold the potty steady as he stands up. Let him pull up his own pants. Don't show disgust at the potty contents, just flush it away, wipe the pot clean, rinse it, and wash your hands.

6

When your child has an accident, don't scold him
You can't expect him to be able to use the potty every time at this stage. When he wets or dirties his pants, don't scold him. Clean him up and be sympathetic. Have a supply of clean training pants handy in the bathroom.

7

Take the diaper off during naps
Once your child is using the potty chair fairly reliably during the daytime, *and* his diaper has been dry after a nap for about a week, you can take his diaper off—he may even ask you to remove it. Suggest that he sit on the potty chair after he wakes from his nap. Napping without diapers will help him stay dry at night.

8

When you go out
Until your child is fairly reliable, put a diaper on him when you go out, but talk to him about it. Try to make sure, without forcing him, that he uses his potty chair beforehand. For car trips, a diaper might be essential unless you will be able to stop easily. Take a potty chair along, spare clothes, and an old towel in case of accidents.

9

Suggest using the toilet
After a few weeks or months of using the potty chair during the day, suggest that he might try using the toilet. Clip a child's seat on it to give him confidence that he won't fall in, and put a step in front so he can climb up. Help him the first few times, until he gets the hang of it. If he just wants to urinate, lift the seat and lid and show him how to aim his penis. Otherwise encourage him to pull his pants down and climb up to sit on the seat; do the same for a girl. Stay nearby until he's finished, wipe his bottom, and help him down. Many children aren't able to wipe their own bottoms until at least four. He will probably want to flush the toilet afterward— that's part of the fun. Then wash his and your hands.

Potty chair
This chair converts into a seat that sits on an adult toilet with two steps up.

ACHIEVING NIGHTTIME CONTROL

1

Wait until your child is already dry at night
If you have taken a dry diaper off your child in the morning for at least a week, he can start going without one at night.

2

Don't force the issue of staying dry at night
Your child will stay dry at night when his bladder is mature enough and you aren't pressuring him. If you make a toddler nervous or anxious about something he has no control over—urinating when he is asleep—achieving nighttime control will only take longer. If you both feel more comfortable wearing the diaper at night, keep it on. If he wants to wear his training pants, let him.

3

If he wets the bed
If your child starts to wet his bed, do not scold, punish, or blame him. Has he suffered some upheaval in his life? There are numerous explanations for why some children never wet their beds and others are unable to stay dry. Because bed-wetting seems to run in families, doctors have looked for physical causes. Is he a deep sleeper, unable to wake when the urge to use the bathroom might be extreme? The size of the bladder is also linked to bed-wetting. Whatever you do, be patient and keep in mind that your child isn't unusual. Put a night-light in his room alongside the potty chair. Try waking him to use the toilet at 10 or 11 pm. Limit beverages in the early evening and totally avoid caffeine-containing drinks to help prevent night-time accidents.

TAKING YOUR BABY OUT

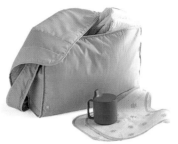

Some form of carriage or stroller and a car seat are essential pieces of equipment for your new baby. Other useful items are an infant carrier (see page 85) or a backpack if your baby is older. A diaper bag with detachable changing mat is convenient for parents on the go: pack it with disposable diapers, changing equipment, spare clothes, plastic bags for used diapers, and whatever feeding equipment you need (but see page 101 for how to transport formula safely). It's a good idea to take a container of diluted juice or water and a bottle or training cup, and don't forget her favorite toy or security blanket. Your older baby will get enormous enjoyment from your adventures. Whether you're going to the zoo to show her the animals, to the park, or a friend's house, there's always something to see. Everything is fascinating to her—traffic jams, store windows, other people—so try to look at the world through her eyes, answer her questions, and don't dismiss her when she points excitedly at something that seems trivial or mundane to you.

WHAT KIND OF CARRIAGE?

WHILE IT MAY NOT be quite as difficult as buying a car, deciding on what kind of carriage to purchase for your baby can be almost as troublesome. These checklists should help you sort out the pros and cons of baby carriages and strollers. Before you go shopping, however, consider how many months of the year you'll be using your purchase, how old your baby is, and where you'll be walking. You don't want to succumb to a sale on an old-fashioned baby carriage if you'll be able to use it for only a month, for instance.

CARRIAGE
Use from birth
☑ Gives your young baby good protection in bad weather.
☑ Gives your baby a comfortable ride.
☑ Can be used up to about one year.
☒ Can't easily be used on public transportation.
☒ Needs ample storage space at home.

CONVERTIBLE CARRIAGE-STROLLER
Use from birth as a carriage
Use from three months as a stroller
☑ Your young baby can ride facing you.
☑ When your baby is older you can convert to the stroller position so she can ride looking forward and see around her.
☑ As a carriage, it gives your young baby good protection in bad weather.
☑ Your young baby can sleep in the carriage day and night.
☑ Your young baby can be snug under a baby blanket or comforter.
☑ As a stroller, the rigid seatback gives good support.
☑ In either position the carriage is light, and easy to maneuver.
☑ It can be easily stored when folded flat.
☒ It can be awkward to take on public transportation.

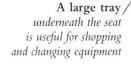

As a carriage
To your newborn baby, the carriage position gives all-round protection and comfort so she can catch her daytime naps in it.

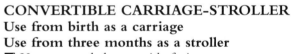

A large tray
underneath the seat is useful for shopping and changing equipment

As a stroller

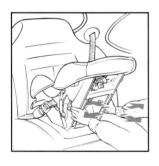

UMBRELLA-STYLE FOLDING STROLLER

✔ Folds up neatly so it's good on public transportation and if storage space is limited.
✔ The cheapest option; also the lightest.
✘ Soft seatback offers poor support, so not suitable for babies under six months.
✘ Some models don't feature shopping pockets or trays.

YOUR WALKING CHILD

A harness is an ideal way to keep your child from wandering off, and gives her more freedom than holding her hand. Take the stroller with you too.

■ CARRIAGE AND STROLLER SAFETY ■

■ Check that a stroller is firmly locked into position before you put your baby in.
■ In a stroller, always strap your child in with the seat belts or stroller harness.
■ In a carriage, fit and always use a harness when you baby starts to sit up.
■ Put the brake on as soon as you stop.
■ Never let your child pull herself up or stand in the carriage; she may tip it over.
■ Never hang heavy shopping bags on the handles: you may tip the stroller over.
■ Never let your child play with a folded stroller.

SAFETY IN THE CAR

EVERY CHILD must be securely strapped into an approved safety seat when traveling in a car. The seat must suit your child's age, size, and weight. The safest place in a car for all children under 12 years of age, including babies, is a rear seat, especially the middle one. Until your baby is at least one year old *and* weighs more than 20 pounds, she should ride in an infant safety seat positioned so that she faces backward (i.e., toward the rear of the car). A deploying airbag can seriously injure a child. Never allow children under 12 years of age to ride in a seat protected by an airbag.

WHAT SEAT FOR WHAT WEIGHT?

Birth to 20lb (9kg): Tub-shaped infant seats are specifically constructed to hold your baby in a semi-reclining position. They are designed to face the rear of the car whether in the back seat or front, but must **never** be installed in a front seat that has an airbag.

Birth to 40lb (18kg): Convertible seats can be used either rear-facing, for infants who are under one year of age and weigh 20lb (9kg) or less, or forward-facing, for babies who are over one year of age and weigh more than 20lb (9kg).

20–40lb (9–18kg): Combination seats are for toddlers who have outgrown infant seats and are old and heavy enough to ride facing forward. This type of seat can later be converted into a belt-positioning booster.

30–80lb (13.5–36kg): Booster seats enable lap and shoulder belts to be positioned properly on children who have outgrown toddler seats.

IN-CAR ENTERTAINMENT

Make car trips fun by:
■ bringing along children's cassettes of songs or stories;
■ singing songs or reciting nursery rhymes;
■ packing a bag full of books, toy, and games;
■ having portion-sized snacks and drinks handy;
■ stopping frequently.

■ TRAVELING TIPS ■

Don't fool yourself into thinking that a baby is safe in an adult's arms when you are in a car. You should **always**:

■ Select a child safety seat that fits your child and your car and use it correctly and every time.
■ Use only child safety seats that meet Department of Transportation requirements.
■ Have children under 12, including infants, ride in the back seat and out of reach of an airbag.
■ Face infants toward the **rear**.
■ Follow carefully the manufacturer's directions for securing the safety seat either with the car's seat belt or with the newer, more convenient built-in attachment system called LATCH (Lower Anchors and Tethers for Children).
■ Use the correct harness slots for your child and fasten the harness snugly over her shoulders.

GROWING AND LEARNING

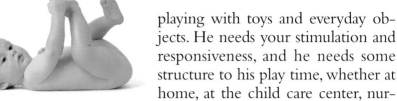

Watching your child grow and learn is a fascinating experience. Physically and emotionally, being a parent is the hardest work you may ever do, but every stage brings something new and rewarding from your baby. At first it's rolling over, using his hands, and then sitting, crawling, walking. The next thing you know he'll be talking to you. Throughout these preschool years, play is critical. Everything your child knows about the way things behave, colors and shapes, cause and effect, he learns through playing with toys and everyday objects. He needs your stimulation and responsiveness, and he needs some structure to his play time, whether at home, at the child care center, nursery school, or with the babysitter. If you are working away from home and burdened by chores, try to approach them, as well as your baby, like a wonderful game. When you turn on a "let's play" mentality, getting him dressed, unpacking groceries, setting the table can become happy times together. That's what your baby needs from you.

THE FIRST SIX MONTHS

DURING THESE MONTHS you will see your baby develop into a real personality. He'll become someone who is able to reward you with enchanting smiles and gurgles. Although there are toys aimed at this age group, he needs—and loves—people most of all. When he's wakeful, take the time to talk, smile, and respond to the facial expressions. Stimulate him with things to look at, sounds to hear, and textures to explore. You don't really need expensive toys. Position old postcards and photographs near him. Try a child's nonglass mirror so he can smile at himself. Put a rattle in his hand and take him on a tour around your home.

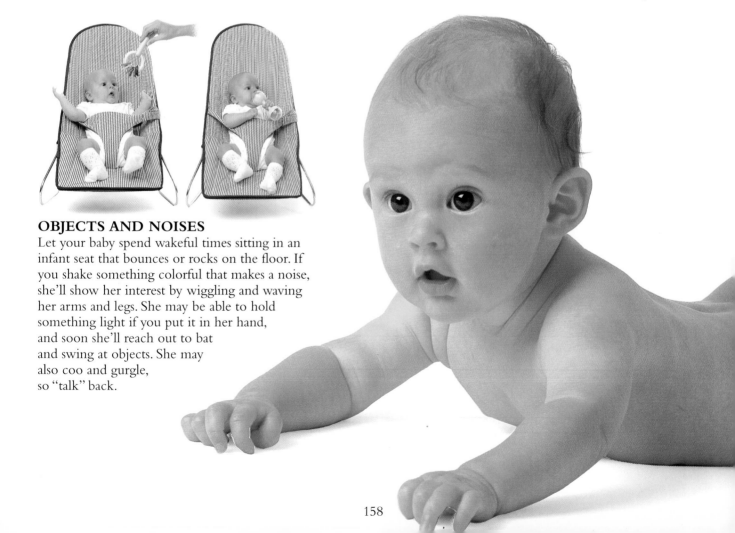

OBJECTS AND NOISES
Let your baby spend wakeful times sitting in an infant seat that bounces or rocks on the floor. If you shake something colorful that makes a noise, she'll show her interest by wiggling and waving her arms and legs. She may be able to hold something light if you put it in her hand, and soon she'll reach out to bat and swing at objects. She may also coo and gurgle, so "talk" back.

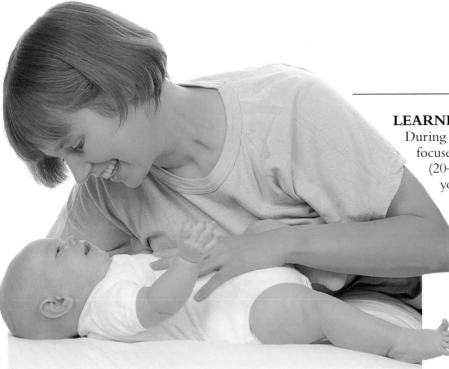

LEARNING ABOUT EACH OTHER

During the first few months of life, your baby focuses best on objects that are 8–12in (20–30cm) away. Keep this in mind when you talk to her by exaggerating your expressions and smile. It's this kind of contact that helps your baby become a person and shows her what a loving relationship is all about.

ROLLING OVER

Sometime during these six months, your baby will learn to roll over, from front to back first, then from back to front. It will give him a great sense of achievement: at last he's beginning to make his body move for him. Remember that even before he's learned to roll he can fall, so never leave him unattended on a high surface, not even the center of a bed.

SITTING

As your baby gains more control over his body, help him learn to sit by surrounding him with pillows. They will let him balance and protect him if he falls over.

USING HER BODY

Give your baby the chance to explore what she can do with her limbs and body. Lying on her stomach, she will push up on her arms and kick her legs out behind her; she may even balance on her stomach. She will probably enjoy your massaging her gently with baby oil too.

PREMATURE BABIES

Your premature baby will probably reach all his developmental milestones later than other babies. Remember that in reality he has two "birthdays": one is the day he was born, but the more important one for the first few months is the date on which he was *expected* to be born. If you take those missing weeks in the womb into account, you may find that his progress is not slow at all. Your pediatrician will be monitoring him each month, and he should catch up with other children born at the same time by the age of two.

THE SECOND SIX MONTHS

YOUR BABY will cram a great deal into these months. He will sit up unsupported, and he may crawl, stand, and even walk by his first birthday. It won't be steady progress, and not every child goes through each stage. Some children never crawl, for example, but this doesn't hinder walking development. This is the age when he learns to explore every new thing by putting it in his mouth—so finger foods are ideal. From now until around age two, make sure he can't grab anything sharp or toxic, or small enough to swallow.

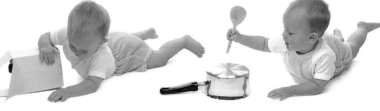

EXPLORING BOXES

Don't be surprised if your baby finds the boxes her toys arrive in just as fascinating as the toys. Be sure to remove any staples.

MAKING NOISES

A wooden spoon and a saucepan make a perfect drum—your baby will love banging away and listening to the noise.

SITTING UP

Your baby will lean forward and spread her legs out wide and straight when she first learns to balance sitting up. (Put a pillow behind her until she's really steady.) Now she has both hands free to explore. A board book is easy to handle, and even more fun if you look at it with her and point out the action, objects, and characters. Start a lifelong reading habit now by reading to your baby often.

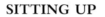

CRAWLING

Moving around on all fours is a great achievement. She may not use each leg in the same way: a lop-sided shuffle with one knee and the other foot is quite normal.

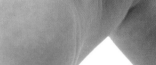

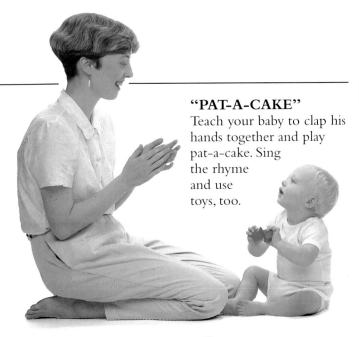

"PAT-A-CAKE"
Teach your baby to clap his hands together and play pat-a-cake. Sing the rhyme and use toys, too.

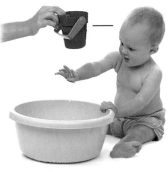

WATER PLAY
Fill a plastic kitchen bucket or tub half full and let your baby splash, scoop, pour, and feel the wonder of water.

BOXES AND OBJECTS
Offer your baby a box of small plastic toys, blocks, or shapes. She may play this "fill and dump" game over and over again.

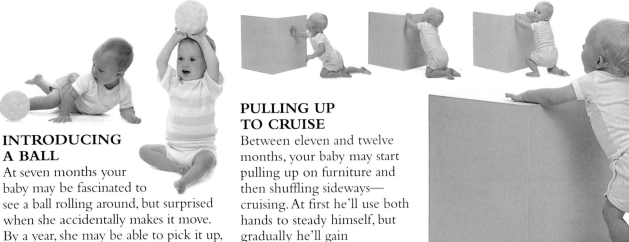

INTRODUCING A BALL
At seven months your baby may be fascinated to see a ball rolling around, but surprised when she accidentally makes it move. By a year, she may be able to pick it up, throw it, and roll it—she's learned how a ball behaves.

PULLING UP TO CRUISE
Between eleven and twelve months, your baby may start pulling up on furniture and then shuffling sideways—cruising. At first he'll use both hands to steady himself, but gradually he'll gain coordination. When he falls, kiss the "Boo-Boo" and make light of the tears.

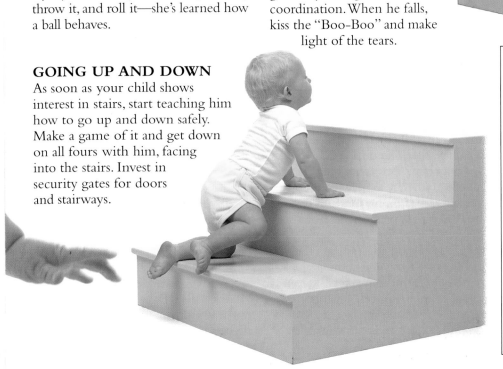

GOING UP AND DOWN
As soon as your child shows interest in stairs, start teaching him how to go up and down safely. Make a game of it and get down on all fours with him, facing into the stairs. Invest in security gates for doors and stairways.

PLAYPENS AND BABY WALKERS
Though it has fallen out of favor, a **playpen** can be one of the safest spots for an active baby when you have to temporarily leave him alone. It can serve as a great storage spot for toys, too. The key to a successful playpen is not overusing it.
A **baby walker** is a chair on wheels that your baby can propel using his feet. Many doctors agree that they should be taken off of the market; they are a major cause of injuries, encourage tight heel cords and toe walking, and promote gait problems in premature babies. Instead, consider a wagon or kiddie push car.

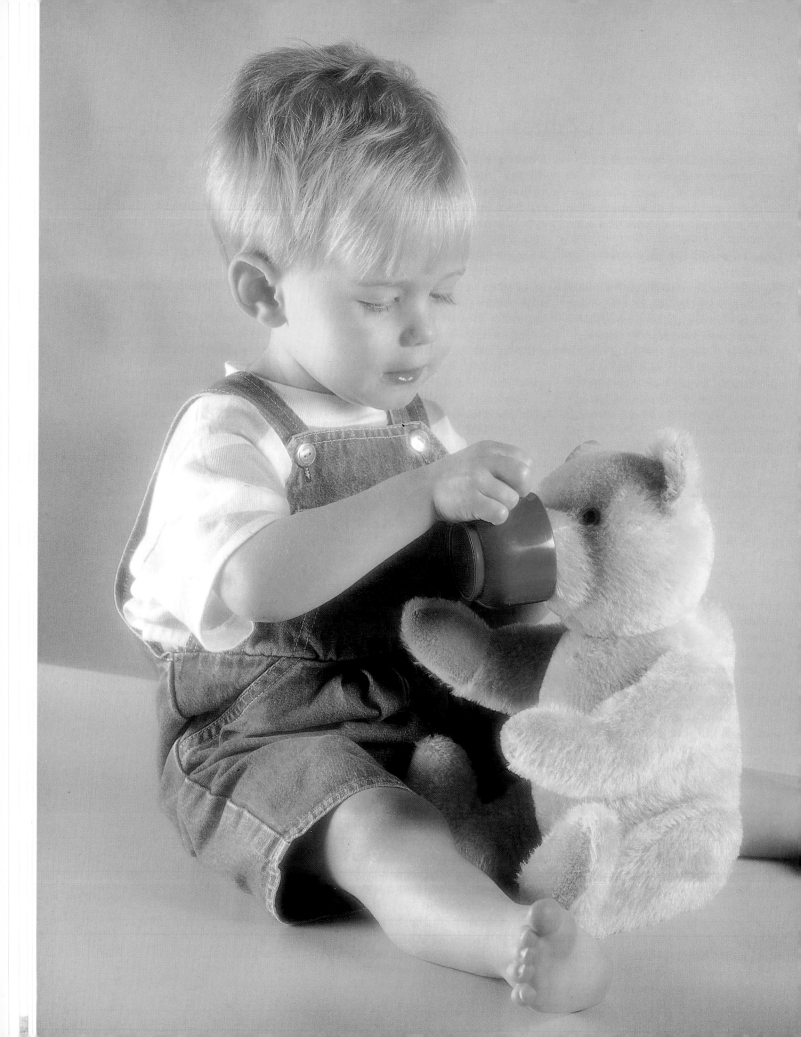

3

HEALTH CARE

■ ■ ■ ■ ■ ■

*Everything you need to know to recognize
and treat common childhood
illnesses, plus a guide to first aid.*

THE FIRST THREE MONTHS

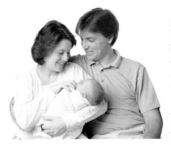

It is always difficult to be sure whether or not a baby is truly sick, especially if you are a first-time parent. Everything about your infant is new in those early months, including the way he'll let you know when he isn't feeling well. But babies can become seriously ill quickly and any infection may be dangerous so don't take chances: be cautious and call you doctor immediately if you think your baby might be sick. If you notice anything about his behavior that frightens you, look at the symptoms listed on these two pages. These are the most common health risks for babies under three months olds. The guide will direct you to the relevant section on pages 176–79, but is not intended as a definite medical diagnosis—only a doctor can offer you that. If you can't find your baby's symptoms here, look at the guide on pages 180–81, which covers illnesses for babies and children of all ages. Babies are born with a natural immunity to many infections, since antibodies (which destroy germs) are passed to them from their mother's blood. This immunity lasts for about two months following birth for a full term infant. Nevertheless, take precautions—keep your baby away from anyone who has a cough or cold and don't take him into crowded public places. Breast-fed babies also receive antibodies from their mother's milk. This immunity lasts for about six months, so before this age your baby is very unlikely to catch any of the infectious illnesses that are common in childhood.

PREMATURE BABIES
Babies who were very small at birth, or who were born a month or more before their due date, are very vulnerable to infections during their first weeks.

Jaundice
This is a yellowing of the eyes and skin caused by a buildup in the blood of a chemical called bilirubin. The condition, known as hyperbilirubinemia, is common during the first two weeks after birth, and usually clears up on its own in a few days. Light-exposure therapy is used to treat persistent cases (see page 70). Call your doctor if you notice your baby's skin and eyes turning increasingly yellow. It's especially important to seek medical attention if your baby was born prematurely, if there's a family history of jaundice, or if you also notice a decrease in appetite and urine output.

■ EMERGENCY SIGNS ■
Call for emergency help immediately if your baby:
▲ brings up green vomit
▲ has a temperature over 102.2°F (39°C) for more than half an hour (Call your doctor for a fever that is between 100.4°F and 102.2°F.)
▲ vomits AND cries uncontrollably as if in great pain
▲ is breathing very noisily or rapidly but is not congested

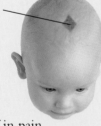

Fontanelle

▲ has a taut, bulging fontanelle when he isn't crying
▲ screams as if in pain and turns pale when he screams
▲ has BMs containing blood and mucus, which resemble red currant jelly.

Loss of appetite
If your baby does not want to feed, but seems generally healthy and contented, there is no need to worry. If he refuses two feedings in succession, or does not demand a feeding for eight hours, **call your doctor now.**

■ CALL THE DOCTOR ■
Don't wait to call your doctor if your baby seems unwell or:
▲ cries more than usual, or doesn't cry in her usual way over a period of about an hour
▲ seems abnormally quiet, drowsy, or listless, or is difficult to arouse
▲ refuses two successive feedings, or does not demand a feeding for eight hours
▲ produces less urine than usual
▲ seems particularly irritable or restless.

Crying
If none of your usual soothing methods calms your baby after an hour or so, or if his crying sounds unusual, **call your doctor now.** If your baby cries inconsolably for two or three hours at about the same time each day, but shows no other signs of illness, he might have colic (see page 118). This may continue for several weeks, but there is no treatment for it.

Slow weight gain
If you baby does not seem to be gaining weight at the normal rate (see charts on pages 246–49), consult your pediatrician. Occasionally an underlying illness can make a baby grow more slowly than normal.

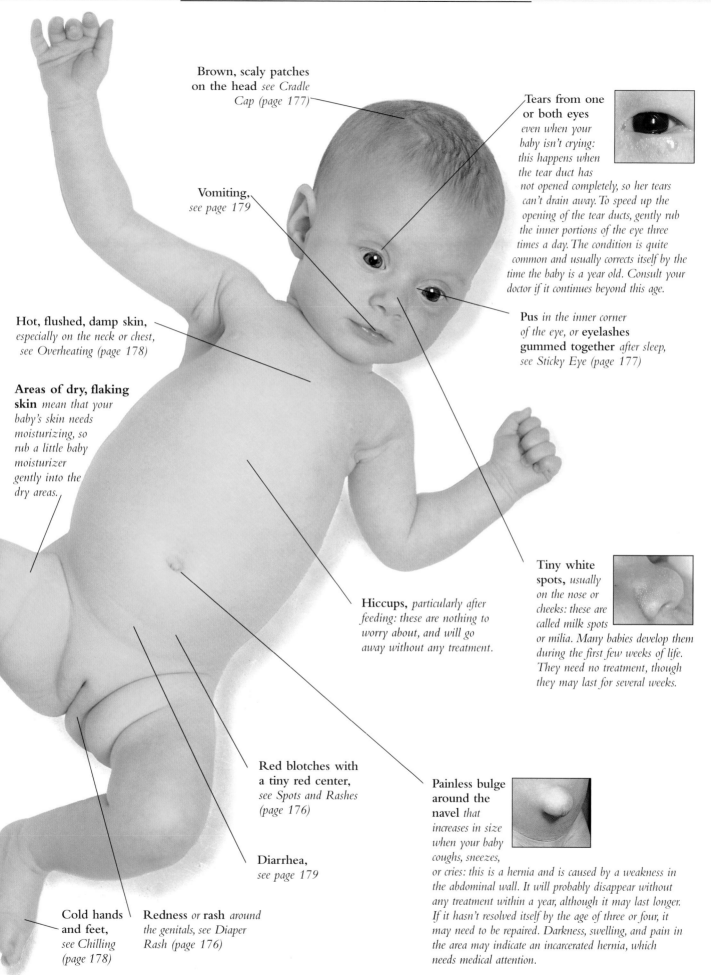

Brown, scaly patches on the head *see Cradle Cap (page 177)*

Tears from one or both eyes *even when your baby isn't crying: this happens when the tear duct has not opened completely, so her tears can't drain away. To speed up the opening of the tear ducts, gently rub the inner portions of the eye three times a day. The condition is quite common and usually corrects itself by the time the baby is a year old. Consult your doctor if it continues beyond this age.*

Vomiting, *see page 179*

Pus *in the inner corner of the eye, or* eyelashes gummed together *after sleep, see Sticky Eye (page 177)*

Hot, flushed, damp skin, *especially on the neck or chest, see Overheating (page 178)*

Areas of dry, flaking skin *mean that your baby's skin needs moisturizing, so rub a little baby moisturizer gently into the dry areas.*

Tiny white spots, *usually on the nose or cheeks: these are called milk spots or milia. Many babies develop them during the first few weeks of life. They need no treatment, though they may last for several weeks.*

Hiccups, *particularly after feeding: these are nothing to worry about, and will go away without any treatment.*

Red blotches with a tiny red center, *see Spots and Rashes (page 176)*

Painless bulge around the navel *that increases in size when your baby coughs, sneezes, or cries: this is a hernia and is caused by a weakness in the abdominal wall. It will probably disappear without any treatment within a year, although it may last longer. If it hasn't resolved itself by the age of three or four, it may need to be repaired. Darkness, swelling, and pain in the area may indicate an incarcerated hernia, which needs medical attention.*

Diarrhea, *see page 179*

Cold hands and feet, *see Chilling (page 178)*

Redness *or* rash *around the genitals, see Diaper Rash (page 176)*

SPOTS AND RASHES

What are they?
Many newborn babies go through what might be called a spotty stage, so don't worry if your baby develops a few spots—they don't mean that he is sick; it's just that his skin is delicate. One of the most common rashes is *erythema toxicum*; it usually appears during the first week of life.

What can I do?
If your baby has *erythema toxicum* (see symptoms box), the spots will disappear on their own within about two or three days, so don't put any lotions or creams on them. Don't alter your baby's feedings—the spots are not due to formula disagreeing with him.

■ SYMPTOMS ■

▲ Red blotches which can be 1–2in (2.5–5cm) in width, each with a tiny red center, and which come and go on different parts of the baby's body, and last only a few hours.

■ CALL THE DOCTOR ■

Call your doctor now if the spots are flat and dark red or purplish (a petechial rash—a sign of bleeding under the skin). Consult your doctor as soon as possible if:
▲ a spot has developed a pus-filled center
▲ you think a spot has become infected.

DIAPER RASH

What is it?
Diaper rash is an inflammation of the skin on a baby's bottom. It may occur if your baby has been left in a dirty diaper for too long. Constant contact of the baby's skin to a wet diaper results in skin irritation, swelling, and skin breakdown. It can also be due to an allergy to laundry detergent or fabric conditioner. A similar-looking rash may be caused by yeast which causes thrush in the mouth (see page 206), and can travel through the intestines and cause a rash from its presence in feces and skin.

■ SYMPTOMS ■

▲ Red, spotty, sore-looking skin in the diaper area
▲ smell of ammonia from your baby's diaper.

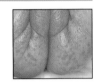

What can I do?
1 Buy a diaper rash cream (from a drugstore) and apply it when you change her diaper, to protect, soothe, and heal the skin.

2 Change your baby's diaper frequently, and clean and dry her bottom thoroughly at each change (see pages 150–51). Use an extra-absorbent type of liner inside cloth diapers, or switch to disposable diapers.

3 Whenever possible, let your baby lie on a diaper with her bottom exposed to the air. Don't use waterproof pants over cloth diapers until the rash subsides.

Spread the cream *evenly all over your baby's diaper area*

4 Don't use harsh detergents or fabric conditioner to wash cloth diapers because they can trigger an allergy. Rinse her diapers thoroughly.

5 Look for white patches inside your baby's mouth. If you see any, she may have thrush (see page 206).

■ CALL THE DOCTOR ■

Consult your doctor as soon as possible if:
▲ the rash lasts several days or becomes worse
▲ you think your baby has thrush and it is painful.

What the doctor might do
The doctor may prescribe an antibiotic cream if the rash has become infected, or an antifungal cream if your baby has thrush.

CRADLE CAP

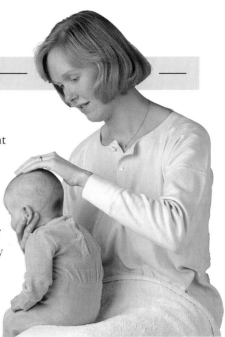

What is it?
Yellowish to brown, crusty patches on a baby's head are known as cradle cap. Sometimes it may spread to the baby's face, body, or diaper area, producing a red scaly rash. Although it looks as if it might be irritating, cradle cap doesn't seem to distress the baby.

SYMPTOMS
▲ Yellowish to brown, scaly patches on the scalp.

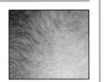

CALL THE DOCTOR
Consult your doctor as soon as possible if the rash spreads and:
▲ seems to irritate the baby
▲ looks infected or begins to ooze
▲ does not clear up after five days.

What can I do?
1 Cradle cap is best managed by frequent shampooing. Rub the scales on your baby's head with a small amount of baby oil to soften them. Then wash his hair—most of the scales should simply wash away.

2 If the rash spreads, keep the affected areas clean and dry.

What the doctor might do
If the condition persists, or if the rash looks infected or starts to ooze, your doctor may prescribe a cream to be rubbed gently on the area.

STICKY EYE

What is it?
This common mild eye irritation may be the result of poorly functioning tear ducts. If your baby has any of the following symptoms after she is two days old, she may have conjunctivitis (see page 202) or a blocked tear duct.

SYMPTOMS
▲ Eyelashes gummed together after sleep
▲ pus in the inner corner of the eye.

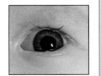

CALL THE DOCTOR
Call your doctor now if your baby has a bad discharge of yellow pus or is very irritable.
Consult your doctor as soon as possible if:
▲ your baby develops symptoms of sticky eye after the first two days of life
▲ sticky eye does not clear up after three days.

What can I do?
Clean your baby's eyes twice a day with a cotton ball dipped in warm boiled water. Wipe outward from the inner corner of her eye, and use a fresh cotton ball for cleaning each eye. Gently rub the inner portion of the eye three times a day, which is said to speed up the opening of the tear ducts. Conjunctivitis can be contagious so don't share his washcloth or towel with other family members.

What the doctor might do
If the doctor thinks your baby has conjunctivitis, he may prescribe an antibiotic eye ointment.

CHILLING

Why are babies at risk?
A baby's large surface area makes it difficult for him to internally correct extremes of temperature. If he gets cold, his body temperature will drop and he may become dangerously chilled quickly. Premature babies are particularly vulnerable to this.

What can I do?

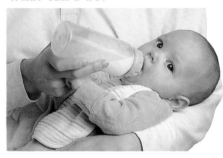

Warm your baby up by picking him up and holding him close to you. It may also help to feed him. Once he has become chilled, it doesn't help just to pile on extra clothes or blankets.

■   SYMPTOMS   ■

First signs
▲ Crying and restless behavior
▲ cold hands and feet.

As the baby gets colder
▲ Quiet, listless behavior
▲ cool skin on the chest and stomach
▲ pink, flushed face, hands, and feet.

How can I prevent chilling?
Keep the room your baby sleeps in at about 75–79°F (23.8–26.1°C). When you undress and bathe him, the room should be even warmer. Keep your baby away from cold surfaces, such as windows, especially when he is undressed. Be sensible about taking him out in cold weather —wrap him up well and don't stay out for too long.

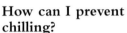

Put on a hat
under the hood to keep his head warm

In cold weather, dress your baby in a one piece outdoor suit, or wrap a blanket over his other clothes and use mittens and bootees.

OVERHEATING

Why are babies at risk?
As young babies are very sensitive to extremes of temperature (see Chilling, above), they can become overheated just as easily as they become chilled.

What can I do?

1 Take your baby to a cooler place and remove a layer of clothing.

2 Take your baby's temperature (see page 187) and, if it is raised, try to reduce it by sponging her with lukewarm water (see page 188).

3 When she seems comfortable, dress your baby in light clothes.

■   SYMPTOMS   ■

▲ Restless behavior
▲ hot, sweaty skin
▲ raised temperature.

■   CALL THE DOCTOR   ■

Call your doctor now if your baby has a temperature over 100.4°F (38°C).

How can I prevent overheating?
Dress your baby according to the weather—on very hot days, she can sleep in just a diaper and a shirt, but always remember the danger of chilling (see above). Never leave her to sleep directly in the sun, because her skin will burn easily. Provide shade and check her often as the sun moves around.

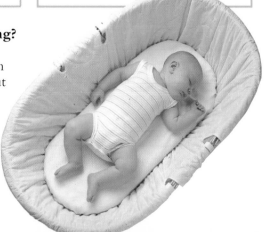

VOMITING

Why do babies vomit?

All babies spit up a small amount of milk during or just after feeding. This is perfectly normal and does not mean that your baby is ill, but until you are used to it, you may think that she is vomiting. If your baby truly has indigestion or nausea, she will vomit most of her feeding. Frequent vomiting, especially if your baby also has diarrhea, may be caused by gastroenteritis (see page 214). This is very serious because it can cause dehydration (see page 214).

FORCEFUL VOMITING

Sometimes a baby throws up with great force, so that the vomit shoots across the room. If your baby does this at two successive feedings, **consult your doctor as soon as possible.**

The most likely reason is that she has thrown up part of her feeding with a large burp of gas behind it. However, if it happens after every feeding, especially if your baby seems hungry all the time, she may have a condition called pyloric stenosis, in which the outlet from the stomach becomes blocked. This conditions runs in families, occurs more frequently in boys, and usually develops when the baby is about two to eight weeks old. If your baby has this, she will need an operation.

What can I do?

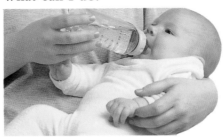

Bottle-fed (formula-fed) baby: If your baby is not becoming dehydrated, continue normal feeding. One sign of dehydration to watch for is a reduction in your baby's urine output. (About four well-soaked diapers in a 24-hour period is usually considered a good output.) The recommended treatment for mild to moderate dehydration is to supplement or replace formula feeding with a commercial oral rehydration solution (ORS—ask your pharmacist to recommend a brand). Especially when dehydration is mild, formula-feeding does not have to be stopped completely. Feed your baby small amounts of ORS frequently, either by bottle, medicine dropper, or small spoon—about 5cc as often as every 1 to 2 minutes. Once dehydration is corrected, resume normal formula-feeding.

Get medical advice if your baby's condition has not improved within 24 hours.

Breast-fed baby: Continue feeding normally if your baby is not dehydrated (see above). To treat mild to moderate dehydration, supplement or replace breast-feeding with an oral rehydration solution given at a rate of about 5cc as often as every 1 to 2 minutes. If your baby refuses the bottle, use a medicine dropper or a small spoon. Resume normal breast-feeding once your baby is rehydrated. If you stop nursing during ORS treatment, make sure to pump breast milk in order to keep up your supply.

What the doctor might do

The doctor may prescribe an oral hydrating solution, but if your baby is severely dehydrated, she may have to be given fluid intravenously in a hospital.

■ EMERGENCY SIGNS ■

Call for emergency help immediately if your baby:
▲ has a dry diaper for more than six hours
▲ vomits all feedings in a four-to six-hour period, despite treatment
▲ brings up green, bilious vomit
▲ has a dry mouth
▲ has sunken eyes
▲ has a sunken fontanelle.

■ CALL THE DOCTOR ■

Call your doctor now if:
▲ your baby vomits and shows any other signs of illness
▲ your baby vomits all of two successive feedings.

DIARRHEA

What is it?

Until babies start eating solid food, they may have fairly runny bowel movements a few times a day. If your baby's BMs are very watery, greenish, and frequent, he has diarrhea. This is serious in a young baby, since it may dehydrate him quickly.

What can I do?

Make sure that your baby has plenty to drink so that he doesn't become dehydrated. Follow the advice above under Vomiting: What can I do? Make sure your baby is wetting his diapers and staying alert.

■ CALL THE DOCTOR ■

Call for emergency help immediately if your baby has any of the signs listed for vomiting. Call the doctor now if your baby has had diarrhea for six hours.

DIAGNOSIS GUIDE

If your child seems sick, try to identify her symptoms in the guide below. If she has more than one symptom, look up the one which seems to be most severe. This gives you a possible diagnosis and refers you to a section covering the complaint that your child might be suffering from. As well as giving a more detailed list of symptoms for the complaint, the section contains a brief explanation of the nature of the illness, with information about how you can help your child, and advice on whether you need to call a doctor. Bear in mind that the guide below is not intended to give an accurate diagnosis—only a doctor can do that—and that your child may not develop all the symptoms listed for an illness. If your baby is under three months old, look also at the guide on pages 174–75, which covers special health risks for young babies.

Fever
A raised temperature, or fever, may mean that your child has an infection, so look for other signs of illness. However, sometimes healthy children run a slight fever during energetic play or in very hot weather, so check your child's temperature again after she has rested for half an hour. If it is still over 100.4°F (38°C), she may have an infection.

Changed behavior
If your child is less energetic than usual, more irritable, whiny, or simply unhappy, she may be sick.

Unusual paleness
If your child looks white-faced or pale she may be sick.

Hot, flushed face
This may be a sign of a fever.

Loss of appetite
Although a child's appetite varies, a sudden loss of appetite may be a sign of illness. If your baby is under six months old and has refused two successive feedings, or has not demanded to be fed for more than eight hours, **call your doctor immediately**. If your child stops eating for more than 24 hours, look for other signs of illness (see page 183).

Eyes looking in different directions, *see Squint (page 203)*

Red, sore, or sticky eyes or eyelids, *see Eye problems (pages 202–3); if combined with a* **rash and fever**, *see Measles (page 198)*

Itchy eyes, *especially if accompanied by* **runny nose** *or* **sneezing**, *see Colds and flu (pages 194–95). Could also be hay fever, particularly if it occurs in summer—consult your doctor*

Aversion to bright light, *especially if accompanied by* **fever, headache, and stiff neck,** *see Meningitis and encephalitis (page 225)*

Runny or blocked nose, **sneezing,** *see Colds and flu (pages 194–95)*

Sore mouth, *see page 206*

Momentary lapses of attention, *see Absence attacks (page 225)*

Loss of consciousness, *see Fainting (page 225); if combined with* **stiffness and twitching movements,** *see Convulsions (page 225)*

Itchy head or tiny white grains in the hair, *see Lice and nits (page 224)*

Earache, partial deafness, discharge from ears, itchy ears, *see Ear problems (pages 204–5)*

Puffy face, swollen glands, *at the angle of the jawbone and on the sides of the neck, see Mumps (page 200);* swollen glands *accompanied by* **sore throat,** *see Tonsillitis (page 207) and German measles (page 197)*

Stiff neck, *if accompanied by* **fever and headache,** *see Meningitis and encephalitis (page 225)*

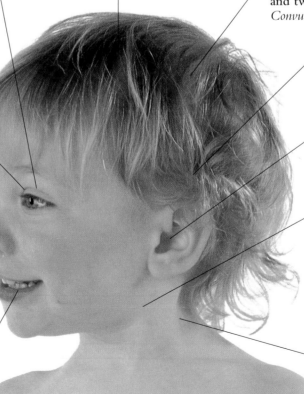

Red lump, perhaps with pus-filled center, *anywhere on the body, see Spots and boils (page 218)*

Red, raw skin, *see Chapped skin (page 221)*

Sore throat, *see Throat infections (page 207); if accompanied by* fever and general illness, *see Colds and flu (pages 194–95); if also accompanied by a* rash, *see German measles (page 197); if accompanied by* puffy face, *see Mumps (page 200)*

Spots or rash *anywhere on the body, if accompanied by* sore throat *or* fever*, see Infectious illnesses (pages 197–99); if without other symptoms, see Skin disorders (pages 218–23) and Insect stings (page 244)*

Stomach pain, *see page 212; if accompanied by nausea, vomiting, or diarrhea, see Gastroenteritis (page 214)*

Abnormal-looking feces, *see page 215*

Diarrhea, *see page 215*

Constipation, *see page 213*

Intense itching around the anus, *see Pinworms (page 224)*

Pain when urinating, odd-colored urine, frequent urination, *see Urinary tract infections (page 216)*

Vomiting with great force *in babies, see Forceful vomiting (page 179)*

Vomiting or nausea, *see page 214*

Sores around the mouth, *see Cold sores (page 222) and Impetigo (page 223)*

Faint red rash over the face or in skin creases, *see Heat rash (page 219)*

Cough, *see Coughs and chest infections (pages 208–11) and Whooping cough (page 201); if accompanied by a* rash, *see Measles (page 198)*

Breathing difficulty, wheezing, rapid breathing, *see Chest infections (pages 208–11)*

Areas of very itchy, dry, red, scaly skin *anywhere on the body, see Eczema (page 220)*

Red, tender skin *anywhere on the body, see Sunburn (page 221) or Burns and scalds (page 237)*

Dry, painless lump *anywhere on the body, see Warts (page 222)*

Soreness, itching, or redness around the vagina, vaginal discharge, *see Genital problems in girls (page 217)*

Intense itching around the vagina, *see Pinworms (page 224)*

Sore tip of penis, *see Genital problems in boys (page 217)*

Painless bulge in the groin or scrotum, *see Genital problems in boys (page 217)*

White or brown lump on sole of foot, *see Warts (page 222)*

FIRST SIGNS OF ILLNESS

Even if your child has no definite symptoms, often you can tell he is getting sick by his whiny, clingy behavior. Children may become pale, lose their appetite, and drive their parents crazy with irritable temper tantrums. With a teething baby, there's always a tendency to dismiss the change in behavior to new teeth on the way. That can be dangerous, though, so don't do it. Take symptoms seriously, because no studies have yet confirmed the connection between illness and teething. Try to isolate the origin of all symptoms by using the guide here. Follow the directions for diagnosing and, above all, stay calm. Sick children can be very frustrating, testing even the most patient parents. If your child is under a year, watch especially carefully, because babies can become very ill very quickly.

Feeling sick
Your child may become more clingy, and demand extra attention when she is sick.

SHOULD I CALL THE DOCTOR?

If you think you know what is wrong, read the relevant section about complaints on pages 194–225 to determine whether you need to call the doctor. As a general rule, the younger the child, the more quickly he should be seen by a doctor. When you phone your doctor, describe your child's symptoms and remind him of your child's age.

Don't ever hesitate to call your pediatrician, even if you are not absolutely certain that something is wrong. Some have regular morning calling hours.

Degree of urgency
Whenever you are instructed to call the doctor, you will be told how quickly your child needs medical help.

■ **Call for emergency help immediately:** this is a life-threatening emergency. Call 911 or an ambulance, or go to the nearest hospital emergency room.

■ **Call your doctor now:** your child needs medical help now, so contact your doctor immediately, even if it is the middle of the night. If you can't reach him, call 911 for immediate emergency help.

■ **Consult your doctor as soon as possible:** your child needs to be seen by a doctor within the next 24 hours.

■ **Consult your doctor:** your child should be seen by a doctor within the next few days.

SYMPTOMS

Common early symptoms of illness in children are:
▲ raised temperature—38°C (100.4°F) or more
▲ crying and irritability
▲ vomiting or diarrhea
▲ refusal to eat or drink
▲ sore or red throat, or a cough
▲ runny nose
▲ rash
▲ swollen glands in the neck or behind the jaw.

EMERGENCY SIGNS

Call for emergency help immediately if your child:
▲ is breathing very noisily, rapidly, or with difficulty
▲ has a convulsion
▲ loses consciousness after a fall
▲ is in severe, persistent pain
▲ has a fever and is unusually irritable or drowsy
▲ has a rash of flat dark red or purplish blood spots (a petechial rash—a sign of bleeding under the skin).

CHECKING FOR SYMPTOMS

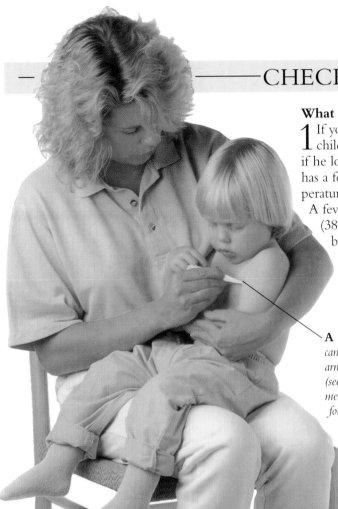

What can I do?

1 If you think your child is feeling sick, or if he looks as though he has a fever, take his temperature (see page 187). A fever of 100.4°F (38°C) or above can be a symptom of illness.

A child's temperature *can be taken under the armpit or in the rectum (see page 187). The oral method should be used only for children over four years of age who can cooperate in the procedure.*

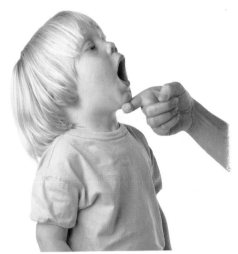

2 Check your child's throat to see if it's inflamed or infected, but don't try to examine the throat of a baby under a year old. Ask your child to face a bright light and open his mouth. If he is old enough to understand, tell him to say "Aah" to open the back of his throat. If his throat looks red or you can see creamy spots, he has a sore throat (see Throat Infections, page 207).

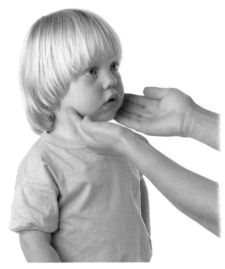

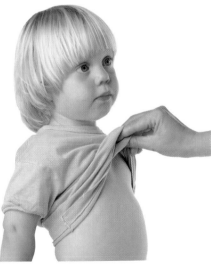

3 Feel gently along your child's jaw-bone and down either side of the back of his neck. Tiny lumps under the skin, or any swollen or tender areas, indicate swollen glands, a common sign of illness. Your doctor can show you how to locate your child's glands.

4 Check your child for a rash, particularly on his chest and behind his ears—the most common areas for one to start. If he has a rash and a fever, he may have one of the common childhood infectious illnesses (see pages 197–99).

QUESTION & ANSWER

"Is my child in pain?"

If your baby is in pain, his crying may sound different from normal. When a baby or small child cries or complains of pain, it can be difficult to discover where the pain is, let alone how bad it is.

Serious pain will affect your child's behavior, so watch him to find out how severe his pain is. Does it make him cry or stop him from sleeping, eating, or playing? Does his face look drawn or has his color changed? Would you know he was in pain if he didn't tell you? If not, his pain isn't severe.

Call your physician and describe your child's symptoms before offering pain medication.

THE DOCTOR'S EXAMINATION

Even though you may have a great relationship with your pediatrician, that initial visit to his office with your sick child can be troubling. His examination may differ from an ordinary checkup and you'll be asked to describe the symptoms in detail. It may help to make notes about your child's illness before you leave home.

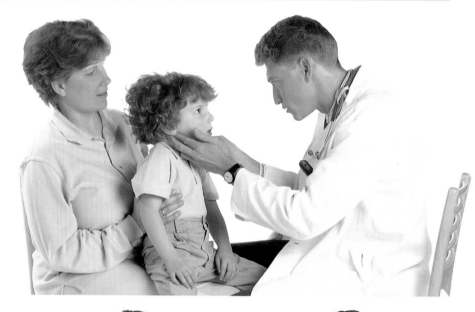

1 The doctor will feel the glands that lie along your child's jawbone, down the back of his neck, and in his armpits and groin. These may become swollen during an infectious illness.

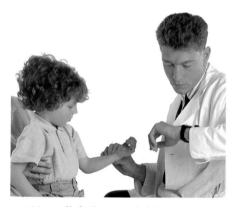

2 He will feel your child's pulse or use a stethoscope to check if his heart is beating faster than usual. This is often a sign of a fever. The doctor may also take your child's temperature.

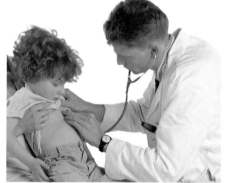

3 By listening to your child's chest and back with a stethoscope, and asking your child to breathe deeply, the doctor will check the condition of his heart and lungs.

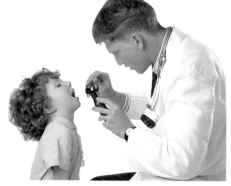

4 If your child has a sore or inflamed throat, the doctor will examine his throat using a small light, pressing his tongue down with a tongue depressor.

5 The doctor may ask your child to lie down on the examining couch so that he can gently feel his abdomen. He's checking for swelling or tenderness in any internal organs.

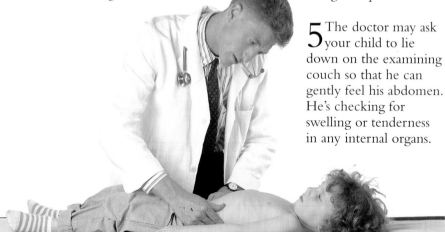

QUESTIONS TO ASK THE DOCTOR

Don't hesitate to question your doctor about anything. If it worries you, then ask:
- how long your child may be sick, and what to expect
- whether he is infectious, and needs to be isolated particularly from small babies and pregnant women
- how you can make your child more comfortable while he is sick.

GOING INTO THE HOSPITAL

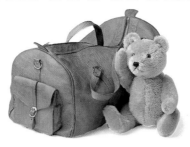

Going into the hospital is stressful for anyone. For a child who is too young to understand why he is there or, indeed, whether he will ever come out, it can be terrifying, especially if it also means that he is separated from his parents. While it helps to explain to your child what is happening, you can't do much to prepare him if he is under two—all he really needs at this age is your presence.

If your child is over two, using a favorite toy to explain why he is going to the hospital can help. Tell him, for instance, that even Teddy bears go to the hospital to get better, not as a punishment. Assure him that you will stay with him or visit often, and do what you promise. Keep explanations simple but truthful; your child will be upset or angry if you tell him something won't hurt, and then it does.

VISITING YOUR CHILD
Hospital personnel know how important it is for a parent to be with a child to comfort and reassure him, and should make it easy for you to visit him at any time. Some even provide accommodations so that you can stay with your child—find out about this before his admission. He won't find the hospital so frightening if you continue to care for him as you would at home, so ask the nurses whether you can still dress, bathe, and feed him as normal.

If you can't stay in the hospital with your child, visit him as often as you can, and arrange to bring brothers and sisters to see him if possible. Visiting policies have become more lenient in recent years. Make a special effort to be with him around the clock for the first day or two, and to be there when he has any unpleasant procedures such as injections, or having his stitches removed.

WHAT TO PACK
Your child may need the following things while she is in the hospital. Call the admissions office to ask for specific guidelines, for instance, on diapers. Label everything clearly.

Bathrobe

Bib and feeding equipment

Three pairs of pajamas or three nightgowns

Slippers

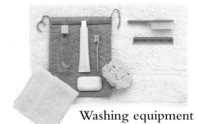

Washing equipment

Favorite toys

Consider packing soap, washcloth, toothbrush and toothpaste, brush, comb, and a favorite bath towel.

HAVING AN OPERATION
If your child is old enough to understand, explain what will happen on the day of his operation. Ask the doctor how the anesthesia will be administered (it may be injected or inhaled through a mask), and find out whether you will be allowed to stay with your child while he is given the anesthesia. Try to be with him when he wakes up after surgery since he may be frightened.

1 Warn your child that he may not be allowed to eat or drink anything on the day of his operation.

2 Tell your child that he will be dressed up for the operation in a hospital gown, and will wear a bracelet with his name on it.

3 While he is still in his room, your child will be given an injection to make him sleepy.

4 Warn your child that he may feel sick when he wakes up.

5 Your child will be wheeled in his bed to the operating room, where the anesthesia is administered. He should fall asleep quickly.

6 If your child has stitches, discourage him from scratching them. If they must be removed, it will hurt only momentarily.

THE CHILD WITH A FEVER

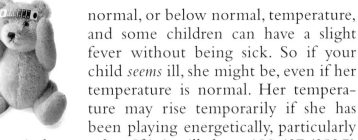

In children, normal body temperature is between 96.8° and 99.5° (36° and 37.5°C), depending on the time of day. Body temperature is usually lowest in the middle of the night and highest in the afternoon. A temperature above 100.4°F (38°C) may be a sign of illness. A child's temperature can shoot up alarmingly quickly when she is sick, but a slightly raised temperature is not a reliable guide to your child's health. Babies and children can be ill with a normal, or below normal, temperature, and some children can have a slight fever without being sick. So if your child *seems* ill, she might be, even if her temperature is normal. Her temperature may rise temporarily if she has been playing energetically, particularly in hot weather. If it is still above 100.4°F (38°C) after she has rested for about half an hour, she may be ill, so check for other signs of illness (see pages 182–83).

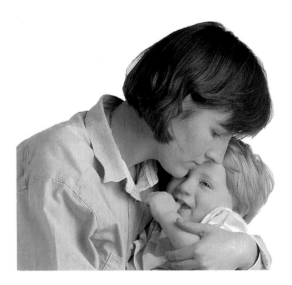

SIGNS OF A FEVER

Your child may have a fever if:
▲ she complains of feeling sick
▲ she looks pale and feels cold and shivery
▲ she looks flushed and her forehead feels hot.

CALL THE DOCTOR

Call the doctor now if your child:
▲ has a fever over 103°F (39.4°C)—over 101°F (38.3°C) if she is under a year old—and you can't bring it down
▲ has a fever for 24 hours.

CHOOSING A THERMOMETER

The best thermometer for taking the temperature of a baby or young child is the fast and easy-to-use digital thermometer, available inexpensively at supermarkets and pharmacies. Digital thermometers emit a beep or a series of beeps when the temperature is ready to be read.

Once the mainstay of home medicine cabinets, the mercury-in-glass thermometer is no longer recommended because it can break easily and expose a child to toxic mercury.

The tympanic, or ear, thermometer gives a fast, digital temperature reading, but it is not as accurate as a regular digital thermometer and is not recommended for young infants.

Heat sensitive panels on a temperature indicator strip glow in sequence and stop when they reach your child's temperature. Indicator strips are probably the easiest way to take a child's temperture, but they are also the least accurate.

Lens filter *protects lens from damage and dirt*

Window *with temperature reading*

98.6°F

Digital thermometer

Window *with temperature reading*

Tympanic thermometer

Panels *marked with a temperature*

Temperature reading

°F	95	96.8	98.6	100.4	102.2	104
°C	35	36	37	38	39	40

Temperature indicator strip

TAKING YOUR CHILD'S TEMPERATURE

When your child is sick, take her temperature at least twice a day, morning and evening. The rectal method gives the most accurate reading, but if you're uncomfortable taking your baby's rectal temperature, taking an axillary (armpit) temperature is your next best choice. Armpit temperature is 1°F (0.6°C) lower than true temperature, but is easier to take than rectal temperature. Use the oral method only if your child is old enough to hold a thermometer correctly in her mouth. A digital thermometer is the best choice for home use. Avoid mercury-in-glass thermometers since they can break and expose your baby to toxic mercury. Temperature indicator strips and tympanic thermometers are easy ways to take a young child's temperature, but give less accurate readings than standard thermometers.

TAKING RECTAL TEMPERATURE

1 Lubricate the tip of a digital thermometer and turn on the switch. Remove your baby's diaper, place him stomach down on your lap or on a changing table, and spread his buttocks. Gently insert the thermometer bulb no more than 1 inch into the rectum, and try to keep him from squirming. Soothe your baby while you hold the thermometer in place until it starts beeping or otherwise indicates that the temperature is ready to be read.

2 Remove the thermometer and read and record the number in the window. Fever is a rectal temperature over 100.4°F (38°C) Clean the thermometer according to manufacturer's directions (usually with warm, soapy water or rubbing alcohol).

TAKING ARMPIT TEMPERATURE

1 Turn on the switch of a digital thermometer. Sit your child on your lap, lift her arm and tuck the bulb end of the thermometer into her armpit.(Make sure the bulb touches skin, not clothing.)

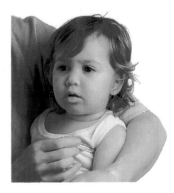

2 Bring your child's arm down and fold it over her chest. Leave the thermometer in place until it starts beeping or otherwise indicates that temperature is ready to be read.

3 Remove the thermometer and read and record the number in the thermometer window. Anything over 99°F (37.2°C) is a fever. (Armpit temperature is lower than rectal.) Switch the thermometer off, then clean according to manufacturer's directions.

TAKING ORAL TEMPERATURE

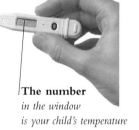

1 Switch the thermometer on and ask your child to open her mouth. Place the thermometer under her tongue and ask her to close her mouth. Hold the thermometer in place until it starts beeping or otherwise signals that the temperature is ready to be read.

2 Remove the thermometer and read and record the number in the thermometer's window. Anything over 99.5°F (37.5°C) is a fever. Switch the thermometer off, then clean it according to manufacturer's directions.

The number *in the window is your child's temperature*

USING AN INDICATOR STRIP

Hold the strip on your child's forehead for about 15 seconds. The highest panel that glows indicates your child's temperature. Anything over 99.5°F (37.5°C) is a fever.

USING A TYMPANIC (EAR) THERMOMETER

Make sure a clean lens filter is in place. For children under four years, select the rectal indicator then switch the thermometer on. Gently pull the ear back and, with a slight back and forth motion, insert the thermometer until the ear canal is sealed off. Press the button on top of the thermometer for one second, then remove the thermometer and read your child's temperature. Before storing, change the lens filter.

WARNING

- Don't take your baby's temperature right after he's had a bath or has been bundled tightly for a while, since this can affect the reading.
- Never leave your baby unattended while taking his temperature.

BRINGING DOWN A FEVER

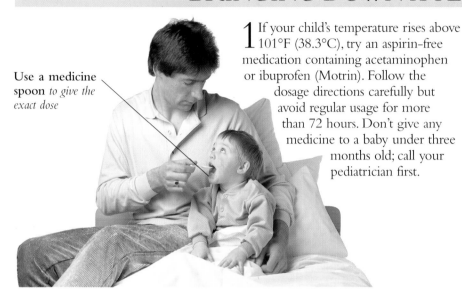

Use a medicine spoon *to give the exact dose*

1 If your child's temperature rises above 101°F (38.3°C), try an aspirin-free medication containing acetaminophen or ibuprofen (Motrin). Follow the dosage directions carefully but avoid regular usage for more than 72 hours. Don't give any medicine to a baby under three months old; call your pediatrician first.

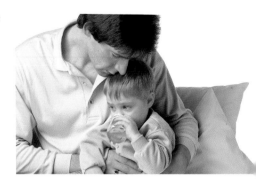

2 Encourage your child to drink plenty of fluids. Cover him with a warm cotton sheet to discourage shivering, which produces heat, and keep his room cool.

ADDITIONAL MEASURES

If your child's temperature rises above 103°F (39.4°C) and medication fails to bring it down, try a tepid bath and then sponging with lukewarm water. If your baby is under three months, try sponging first to reduce fever.

1 Take off your child's blankets and remove her pajama top. Put towels under her so that the bed does not get damp, then fill a bowl with lukewarm water and wring out a sponge in it.

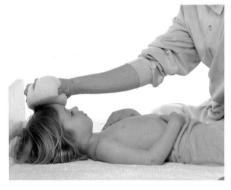

2 Gently wipe your child's face, neck, and arms. Remove her pajama bottoms and sponge her legs. Let her skin dry naturally. Continue for about half an hour, then take her temperature. If it is still above 103°F (39.4°C), **call your doctor now.**

FEBRILE CONVULSIONS

A rapid and sudden rise in temperature can cause convulsions in some children. They'll lose consciousness and go rigid for a few seconds, then twitch uncontrollably.

What can I do?

Put your child on the floor and stay with her, but do not try to restrain her. Call your doctor as soon as the convulsion stops.

How can I prevent febrile convulsions?

Prevention can be difficult as there may be no warning. If a tendency to have febrile convulsions runs in your family, follow the cooling methods shown above, and try not to let her temperature rise above 102.2°F (39°C). Your doctor may instruct you to give her children's medicine with acetaminophen or ibuprofen at the first signs of illness, to prevent a fever.

DELIRIOUS CHILDREN

Some children become delirious when they have a high fever. A delirious child is very agitated, and may hallucinate and seem very frightened. This state is alarming, but it isn't dangerous. Stay with her to comfort and calm her. When her temperature drops, she will probably fall asleep and be back to normal when she wakes up after a good rest.

ALL ABOUT MEDICINES

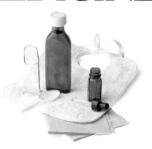

Most minor illnesses get better on their own, with or without treatment. Even if you have to consult your doctor, he may not prescribe a medicine. However, if one is necessary, the doctor will tell you how often, and for how long, your child should take it. It is important to follow the directions carefully. Always shake the bottle before pouring out liquid medicine, and measure doses exactly. You can buy child-sized medicine spoons, droppers, and tubes for giving medication to babies at most drugstores. Never mix medicine into your baby's food or bottle or a child's drink, since he may not finish it, or somebody else may, unwittingly, drink it themselves. If your baby or child struggles when you give him medicine or put drops into his nose,

ears, or eyes, ask another adult to hold him still while you administer it. You can prevent a baby from wiggling by swaddling or wrapping him firmly in a receiving blanket. If the doctor prescribes antibiotics, your child must take the full course, even if he seems better before the course is finished; otherwise the infection may recur. However, antibiotics aren't effective against all illnesses: infectious diseases are caused by either viruses or bacteria, and antibiotics destroy bacteria, but don't affect viruses. There is no real cure for viral illnesses such as colds, measles, mumps, and chicken pox. They simply have to run their course. Other diseases, such as chest and urinary tract infections, may be caused by bacteria and can be treated with antibiotics.

GIVING MEDICINE TO BABIES

When you give medicine to your baby, put a bib on him in case of a spill, and keep some tissues handy. Sterilize all the equipment in boiling water before giving medicine to a baby under six months. If your baby cannot sit up yet, hold him as if you were going to feed him. If he can sit up, hold him on your lap and tuck one of his arms behind your back. Keep your hand firmly on his other arm to prevent him from struggling.

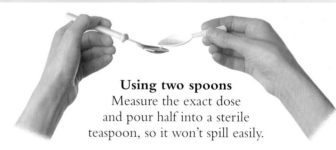

Using two spoons
Measure the exact dose and pour half into a sterile teaspoon, so it won't spill easily.

| **MEDICINE SPOON** | **MEDICINE DROPPER** | **MEDICINE TUBE** | **FINGERTIP** |

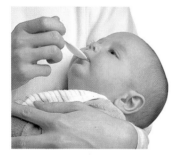

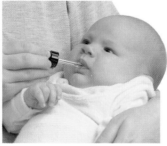

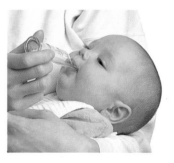

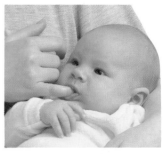

Measure your baby's dose and pour half into another spoon (see above). Keep both spoons nearby, then pick up your baby. Hold him so that he can't wiggle, then pick up one spoon and rest it on his lower lip. Let him suck the medicine off, then repeat with the rest of the dose.

Measure the dose in a medicine spoon, then squeeze the end of the dropper and suck some of it up into the tube. Put the dropper into your baby's mouth and squirt in the medicine. Repeat until your baby has taken an accurate dose. Don't use a glass dropper if your baby has teeth.

Measure the correct dose and pour it into the medicine tube, then pick up your baby and rest the mouthpiece of the tube on his lower lip. Tilt the tube slightly so that the medicine runs into your baby's mouth, but don't tilt it too much, or the medicine will run out too quickly.

When all else fails, try letting her suck medicine off your finger. Measure the dose in a medicine spoon, then pick up your baby, keeping the spoon nearby. Dip your finger into it and let her suck the medicine off. It may take time, but continue until she has taken the whole dose.

GIVING MEDICINES TO CHILDREN

Most medicines for children are sweetened or pleasantly flavored, but if your child dislikes the taste, these tips may help to make it more acceptable.

■ Have a favorite drink poured and ready to take away the taste of the medicine.

■ Try bribery—a small treat or reward may help.

■ Tell your child to hold her nose so that she can't taste the medicine, but never do this forcibly for her.

■ If your child is old enough to understand, explain why she has to take the medicine—if she knows that it will make her feel better, she may be more inclined to take it.

■ If you really find it impossible to get the medicine into your child, ask your doctor if he can prescribe it with a different flavor or in a different form.

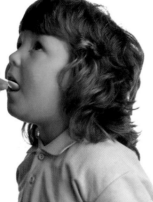

A taste tip
If your child dislikes the taste of the medicine, pour it onto the back of her tongue—it won't taste so strong, because her taste buds are at the front.

■ **MEDICINE AND SAFETY** ■

Make sure that your child can't help herself to any medicines in your home.

▲ Keep all medications out of her reach, preferably in a locked cabinet.

▲ Buy medicines with childproof lids or packaging.

▲ Don't disguise medicine by letting your child think she is having a normal soft drink.

Medicine and tooth decay
Clean your child's teeth after giving her medicine, because many medicines for children contain sugar. If your child must take medicine for any prolonged period of time, ask your doctor whether a sugar-free alternative is available.

■ **WARNING** ■

Never give aspirin to your child when she is sick. Use any child's medication with acetaminophen. A few children given aspirin for viral illnesses, such as the flu or chicken pox, develop a rare, but serious illness called Reye's syndrome. If your child suddenly vomits and develops a high fever while recovering from an illness, **call for emergency help immediately.**

NOSE DROPS

CHILDREN

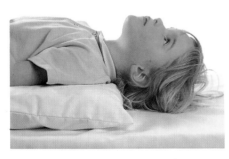

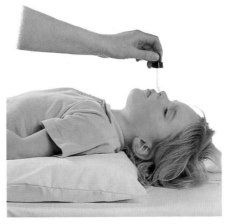

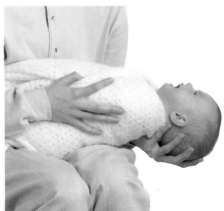

1 Place a small pillow or cushion on a bed and help your child to lie on her back with the pillow beneath her shoulders and her head dropped back. If your child is likely to wriggle as you give her the drops, ask another adult to help you by holding her head.

2 Put the tip of the dropper just above your child's nostril and squeeze out the prescribed number of drops. If the dropper touches her nose, wash it before using it again. Keep your child prone and still for about a minute.

BABIES
Swaddle your baby in a blanket, then lay her on her back across your knees, so that her head falls back over your left thigh. Put your left hand beneath her head to support it, then administer the drops as instructed for a child.

EAR DROPS

CHILDREN

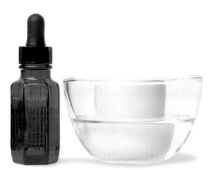

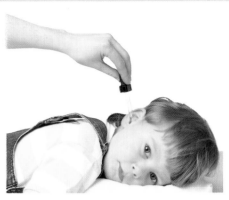

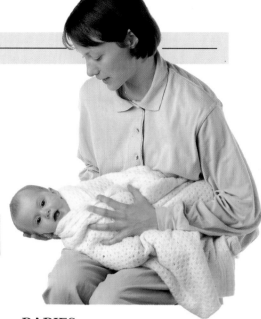

1 Most children find ear drops too cold as they go into their ears, so ask your doctor whether you can warm up the medication (some spoil when they are warmed). Place a few drops in a little cup and place that in warm, not hot, water for a few minutes. Check the temperature on the inside of your wrist: it should not be too hot.

2 Ask your child to lie on his side, with the affected ear facing up, then place the dropper close to his ear and squeeze the prescribed number of drops into the ear canal. Keep your child prone for about a minute and place a cotton ball very lightly in his ear to prevent excess liquid from running out.

BABIES
Swaddle your baby and lay her on her side across your lap with the affected ear facing up. Support her head with one hand, then administer the ear drops as instructed for a child.

EYE DROPS

CHILDREN

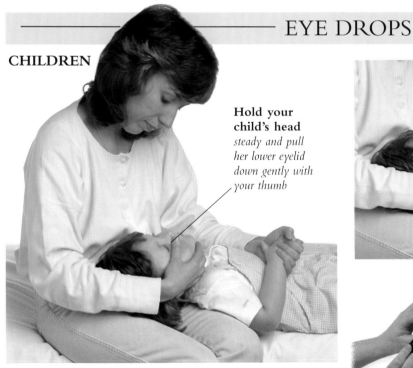

Hold your child's head *steady and pull her lower eyelid down gently with your thumb*

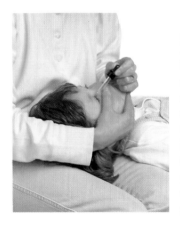

2 Hold the dropper over the gap between the lower lip and the eye, angling it so that it is out of your child's sight. If necessary, ask someone to hold her head steady. Squeeze out the prescribed number of drops, being careful not to touch the eye or the lid. Even if your child cries, enough of the medicine is likely to stay in her eye.

BABIES
Choose a time when your baby is relaxed, then swaddle her and lay her on a firm surface or across your knee. Administer the drops as for a child.

EYE OINTMENT
If your child is prescribed eye ointment, squeeze a tiny amount into the inner corner of her eye.

1 Bathe your child's affected eye with absorbent cotton dipped in warm boiled water, then ask your child to lie on her back across your knee or with her head in your lap. Put one arm around your child's head with your palm against her cheek, then tilt her head so that the affected eye is slightly lower than the other. Draw her lower eyelid gently down with your thumb.

CARING FOR A SICK CHILD

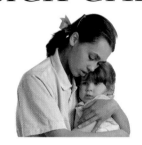

While your child is feeling sick, she will probably demand a great deal of attention, and may be irritable or easily bored. Most children become more babyish when they are sick, and both babies and children need a lot of extra cuddling and reassurance. Try to be very patient and avoid letting your child know you are anxious. Keep your baby with you during the day—let her sleep in her carriage or infant seat, so that you can check on her frequently. Let your child lie down in the living room, or somewhere near you. At night, sleep in the same room as your child if she is very sick. If possible, try to alternate with your partner, so that you have some nights of uninterrupted sleep. Many children vomit when they are ill, so keep a bowl nearby. Vomiting isn't always serious and can be brought on by emotional upset or excitement. However, frequent vomiting can be a sign of a serious condition, and may lead to dehydration. See page 214 for advice about calling your pediatrician and preventing dehydration.

EATING AND DRINKING

Your child will probably have a smaller appetite than usual while she is ill. Because she is not running around as much, she will use less energy, so don't worry if she doesn't want to eat much for a few days—it won't do her any harm. Allow her to choose favorite foods, and offer small helpings. Let her eat as much or as little as she wants: when she is feeling better, her appetite will return. Babies may demand to be fed more frequently than usual, but take very little each time. Be patient if your baby behaves like this—she needs the comfort and reassurance of feeling close to you as she sucks.

Drinking is much more important than eating when your child is ill. To make sure that she doesn't become dehydrated, give her plenty to drink—about 3 pints ($1\frac{1}{2}$ liters) a day. Track her urinations, too—there should be about three to four every 24 hours. A reduction in urine output is a sign of dehydration.

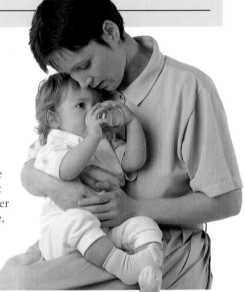

Giving your child a drink
Let your child choose her favorite drink—it doesn't matter whether this is soda, fruit juice, milk, or water.

ENCOURAGING YOUR CHILD TO DRINK
If it's difficult to get your child to drink enough, make her choices more appetizing by trying some of these ideas.

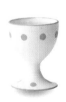

Small container
Offer frequent small drinks from a doll's cup or an egg cup, rather than forcing large amounts.

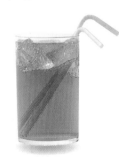

Straws
Make drinks look more appetizing and fun by letting your child use a straw.

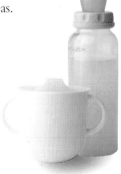

Training cup
If weaning has been difficult, a training cup or bottle should be used only as a last resort.

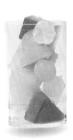

Ice cubes
For a child over a year, freeze diluted fruit juice into cubes, then let her suck the cubes.

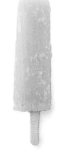

Ice popsicle
Your child may prefer an ice pop—the "drink on a stick." Try to avoid ones with artificial coloring.

NAUSEA AND VOMITING

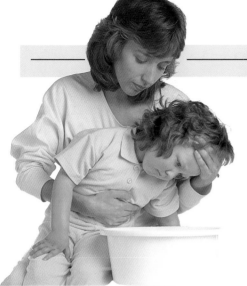
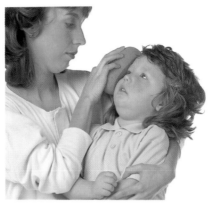
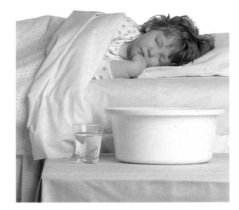

1 Hold your baby or child while she is vomiting to reassure her. Put a big plastic container nearby for her to be sick into. Support her head with one hand on her forehead, and put your other hand over her stomach, just below her rib cage.

2 After she has finished vomiting, reassure your child, then sponge her face and wipe around her mouth. Give her a few sips of water, let her rinse her mouth out, or help her to clean her teeth, to take away the unpleasant taste.

3 Let your child rest quietly after vomiting; she may want to lie down and sleep for a while. Wash the container and put it near her, in case she vomits again. If your child vomits frequently, she may have gastro-enteritis (see page 214).

COMFORT AND ENTERTAINMENT

STAYING IN BED

There is no need to insist that your child stays in bed. If he is feeling very ill, he'll probably want to remain there. If he wants to get up, make sure he keeps warm and that the room he is playing in isn't drafty. However, your child may want to lie down and go to sleep during the day, even if it isn't his usual naptime. If he doesn't want to be alone, let him snuggle with a pillow and a blanket on the sofa in the living room, or make up a bed for him wherever you are. Your child still wants to feel like part of the family even though he's sick.

Playing in bed

If your child feels like staying in bed, but wants to sit up, prop him up with pillows. Make a tray-table by resting a large tray or board on piles of books.

ENTERTAINING YOUR CHILD

Try to keep your child occupied, so that he doesn't get bored, but remember that he will act younger than his age while he is ill. He won't be able to concentrate for very long, and won't want to do anything too demanding. Bring out an old favorite toy he hasn't played with in a while. If you give him small presents to keep him entertained, don't be tempted to buy toys that are advanced for his age. Babies will enjoy a new mobile or a rattle that makes a new sound. Quiet activities such as interlocking building bricks, felt pictures, simple jigsaws, crayons or felt tip pens, a kaleidoscope or Play-Doh are ideal for sick toddlers and children. Protect the bedding with a towel if your child wants to play with something messy while he is in bed.

COLDS AND FLU

All children get occasional colds and bouts of flu. As soon as your child comes into contact with other children, he may get one cold after another—some children under six have up to ten a year. Don't worry. As a child grows older, he develops resistance to many of the viruses that cause colds and flu.

Wiping your child's nose
When a child has a non-stop runny nose, it's nearly impossible to prevent the tender skin beneath the nostrils from becoming sore. Use extra-soft tissues, dab gently, and coat the area with a barrier ointment, such as petroleum jelly, when he is asleep.

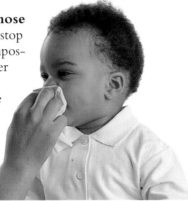

EMERGENCY SIGNS
Call for emergency help immediately if your child develops a rash of flat, dark red or purplish blood spots. Doctors refer to this as a petechial rash.

CALL THE DOCTOR
If your child has been feeling absolutely miserable, and especially if he is not yet one year old, consult your doctor as soon as possible if he has:
▲ a temperature over 102.2°F (39°C)
▲ wheezy, fast, or labored breathing
▲ earache
▲ a throat so sore that swallowing is painful
▲ a severe cough
▲ no improvement after three days.

COLDS

What are they?
Perhaps the most common of all illnesses, a cold is a viral infection that irritates the nose and throat, so children don't catch a cold simply by being cold, by going out without wearing a coat, or by getting their feet wet. While it is not a severe illness, a cold should be taken more seriously in babies and children than in adults, because of the risk of a chest or ear infection developing. Coughs often accompany a cold because, instead of blowing the nose, children tend to sniff mucus down into the throat, which irritates it.

SYMPTOMS
▲ Runny or blocked nose and sneezing
▲ slightly raised temperature
▲ sore throat
▲ cough.

What the doctor might do
If your baby has trouble sucking because her nose is blocked, your doctor may prescribe nose drops to be given just before a feeding.

Nose drops and decongestants
Use these only if your doctor has prescribed them, and never use them for more than three days. Sterile saline nose drops used with gentle suctioning may assist in removal of mucus and help your baby's breathing.

What can I do?
1 Take your child's temperature (see page 187), and give her aspirin-free children's medication to bring it down if necessary. Make sure that she has plenty to drink, but don't force her to eat if she's not hungry. A drink before bedtime may help to keep her nose clear at night.

SINUSITIS
The sinuses are air-filled cavities in the bones of the face. The lining of the nose extends into them, so they can easily become infected after a cold. This infection, sinusitis, causes a stuffed nose or a persistently runny one, and facial pain. The sinuses prone to infection don't develop until age three or four, so for younger children, sinusitis isn't a problem.

FLU

What is it ?

Flu (also known as influenza) is a very infectious illness caused by hundreds of related viruses. It tends to occur in epidemics every two or three years, when a new strain of the virus appears to which people have not yet developed immunity. If your child has caught the flu, he will develop symptoms a day or two later, and will probably be unwell for about three or four days. He may feel ill enough to want to stay in bed and could feel weak for several days after his temperature goes down. A few children develop a chest infection such as bronchitis or pneumonia (see pages 210–11) after having the flu.

SYMPTOMS

▲ Raised temperature
▲ headache
▲ aching all over the body
▲ shivery feeling
▲ runny nose
▲ cough
▲ sore throat.

What can I do?

Take your child's temperature (see page 187) and give him aspirin-free medicine with acetaminophen to reduce his fever if necessary. Make sure he has plenty to drink. Offer your baby cooled water.

QUESTION & ANSWER

"Should I have my child vaccinated against flu?"
If your child has a medical condition making him at risk for complications, a vaccination may be a good idea, so discuss it with your doctor. It will protect him from the flu for about a year. However, since new strains of the virus develop every two or three years, the vaccine (which can only be made from existing forms of the virus) does not give lifelong protection.

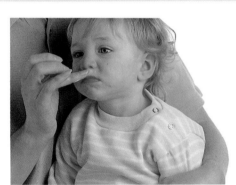

2 Smear a barrier ointment, such as petroleum jelly, under your child's nose and around her nostrils, if the area has become red and sore from a constantly runny nose or frequent wiping.

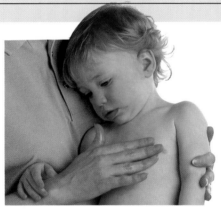

3 If your baby has a cold, she will be able to breathe more easily if you raise the head of the crib mattress slightly. Put a small pillow or a folded towel underneath it, then lay your baby in her crib so that her head and chest are slightly raised.

4 Keep your child's room warm, but make sure that the air isn't too dry. Breathing very dry air can be uncomfortable. Ask your doctor about a humidifier, or hang a wet towel near the heater in your child's room, to add moisture to the air.

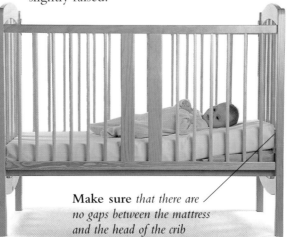

Make sure *that there are no gaps between the mattress and the head of the crib*

HAVING YOUR CHILD IMMUNIZED

At the two-month pediatric checkup, your baby will probably receive her first in a series of immunizations designed to protect her from severe infectious diseases. A vaccine is a small harmless dose of the germ or an inactivated toxin that causes the disease. This dose is too weak to cause dangerous problems in your baby but it will make her body produce special cells called antibodies that will immunize her from the disease in the future. Unfortunately, some babies become fussy or run slight fevers after certain immunizations like the DTP (diphtheria, tetanus, and pertussis) shot.

Why should my baby be immunized?

Some parents decide against immunization because they are worried about possible risks or because they think that a disease is so rare that it is unnecessary. Unfortunately, if the number of children being immunized against a particular disease drops dramatically, epidemics are much more likely to occur. Immunization not only protects your child but also helps to eradicate the disease altogether.

What are the risks?

Immunization is safe, although it may make your baby mildly sick for a short time. However, if your baby has had a nervous system problem, a convulsion, or has a close relative with epilepsy, she may have an increased risk of a serious reaction to the whooping cough (pertussis) vaccine, so tell your doctor. With the newer pertussis vaccines, the risk of complications is even smaller. Do not take her to be immunized if she has a cold, is sick, or has recently had antibiotics.

What are the aftereffects?

Immunization may include a slight fever, so watch her temperature for 24 hours; if it rises, give her the recommended dose of acetaminophen.

Your baby may develop a small, hard lump at the injection site. This will disappear in a few weeks. The measles vaccine may give her a rash and a fever up to ten days later, and the mumps vaccine might make her face swell slightly three weeks later. If her crying sounds unusual, her temperature rises above 100.4°F (38°C), or she develops any other symptoms, **call your doctor immediately.**

Where is it given?

The doctor may inject her in the top of her arm, in her bottom, or in her thigh. Hold your baby firmly while she has the injection.

YOUR CHILD'S IMMUNIZATION PROGRAM ■ Denotes each vaccination ---> Arrows denote a range of acceptable ages for a vaccination											
Vaccine Age	Birth	1 month	2 months	4 months	6 months	12 months	15 months	18 months	4-6 years	11-12 years	13-18 years
Hepatitis B	Hep B-1 ------- / Hep B-2 -------	--->	--->		Hep B-3 -------		-------	--->			
Diphtheria, Tetanus, Pertussis			■	■	■		■ ----	--->	■		
Haemophilus influenzae b			■	■	■	■ ----	--->				
Polio			■	■	■ ----			--->	■		
Measles, Mumps, Rubella						■ ----	--->		■		
Varicella						■ ----		--->			
Pneumococcal			■	■	■	■ ----	--->				

When are the shots given?

Childhood immunization means protection against eleven major diseases: hepatitis B, diphtheria, tetanus, whooping cough (pertussis), hemophilus (Hib) infections, polio, measles, mumps, rubella (German measles), chicken pox, and pneumococcal disease. All these diseases are preventable, so check the table and ask your pediatrician if your child is up to date on the following vaccines:
Hepatitis B All infants should receive the first dose shortly after birth. If the mother is hepatitis B surface antigen (HBsAg) negative, the first dose may be given by age 2 months, but no later. Dose 2 should be given at least one month after the first; dose 3, at least two months after the second, but not before age 6 months. The same intervals apply even if the series is begun later than recommended.
Diphtheria, tetanus, pertussis (DTP) Given at 2, 4, and 6 months, from 15 to 18 months, and prior to school

entry at 4 to 6 years. A tetanus-diptheria (Td) booster is recommended at 11 to 12 years (if at least 5 years have elapsed since the last dose) and every 10 years thereafter.
Haemophilus influenzae type b (Hib) Given at 2, 4, and 6 months and from 12 to 15 months. Depending on the type of vaccine used, the 6 months dose may be omitted.
Polio Vaccinations should be given at 2 and 4 months and then, depending on the type of vaccine, some time between 6 and 18 months, with a booster at 4 to 6 years.
Measles, mumps, and rubella (MMR) The first dose should be given at 12 to 15 months; the second, at 4 to 6 years. Children who miss the second dose should complete the schedule by ages 11 to 12.
Varicella Should be given between 12 and 18 months to children who have not yet had chicken pox. Children who've not been vaccinated or had the disease by age 13 years should receive 2 doses at least 4 weeks apart.

Pneumococcal Four doses of pneumococcal conjugate vaccine (PCV) are recommended at 2, 4, and 6 months and from 12 to 15 months.
Vaccines for high-risk groups
Your pediatrician may recommend additional vaccines if your child is at high risk of contracting certain diseases. These include **pneumococcal polysaccharide vaccine,** or PPV (given at age 2 or older), **hepatitis A** (given at age 2 years or older in 2 doses at least 6 months apart); **influenza** (given annually from 6 months on; also recommended, if possible, for healthy children age 6 to 23 months). A **tuberculosis** risk assessment and, if needed, a TB test are recommended at age 12 months.

If you don't have a pediatrician or family physician, your local public health authority should have vaccine supplies and may give shots free.

INFECTIOUS ILLNESSES

Because most children are immunized, many of the ailments in this section are uncommon. If your child catches an infectious disease, he will most likely develop a lifelong immunity to it. Most infectious diseases are caused by viruses, so medicines can't cure them (see page 189).

Fifth Disease It is marked by bright red raised patches on both cheeks, then a pink, lacy, slightly raised rash on the rest of the body. Fifth disease normally lasts five to ten days during which time your child will feel generally well. It is contagious until the rash appears, so isolation is difficult.

Roseola More common in children under three, roseola starts with a sudden fever of over 101°F (38°C) that continues for up to 4 days. As the fever subsides, a pink rash, which lasts for up to 48 hours, develops on the body. Treat the fever (see below) and keep her cool.

WARNING

If your child has a raised temperature while he is ill with one of these diseases, **DO NOT** give him aspirin to bring the fever down, since it can cause a serious disease called Reye's syndrome (see page 190). Give him an aspirin-free medication with acetaminophen.

EMERGENCY SIGNS

Call for emergency help immediately if your child has an infectious disease and develops any of these signs:
▲ unusual and increasing drowsiness
▲ headache or stiff neck
▲ convulsions
▲ rash of flat, dark red or purplish blood spots.

GERMAN MEASLES (RUBELLA)

What is it?
German measles is a very mild illness, so your child may feel perfectly well and may not want to stay in bed. She will develop symptoms two to three weeks after she has been infected.

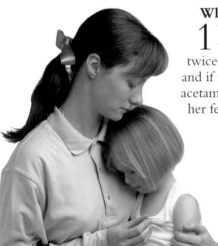

What can I do?
1 Take your child's temperature at least twice a day (see page 187), and if necessary give her acetaminophen to reduce her fever.

2 Make sure that your child has plenty to drink, especially if she has a fever.

SYMPTOMS

Days 1 and 2
▲ Symptoms of a mild cold
▲ slightly sore throat
▲ swollen glands behind the ears, on the sides of the neck, and on the nape of the neck.

Day 2 or 3
▲ Blotchy rash of flat, pink spots appearing first on the face, then spreading down the body
▲ slightly raised temperature.

Day 4 or 5
▲ Fading rash and general improvement.

Day 6
▲ Your child is back to normal.

Day 9 or 10
▲ Your child is no longer infectious.

CALL THE DOCTOR

Call for emergency help immediately if your child develops any of the emergency signs above. Consult your doctor as soon as possible if you think your child has German measles, but check with him before taking your child to his office, to avoid the possibility of her coming into contact with a pregnant woman.

What the doctor might do
Your doctor will confirm that your child has German measles, but there is no treatment for it.

German measles and pregnancy
While your child is infectious, prevent her from coming into contact with pregnant women. Although German measles is a mild disease, it can cause defects in a fetus if a pregnant woman catches it.

MEASLES (RUBEOLA)

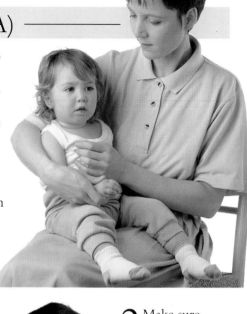

What is it?

Measles is a very infectious illness that causes a rash, fever, and cough. Symptoms appear one or two weeks after your child has been infected.

Children usually feel uncomfortably ill with measles, and your child will probably want to stay in bed while her temperature is high. A few children develop complications such as earache.

What can I do?

1 Check your child's temperature (see page 187) at least twice a day, and every five to six hours when her fever is high on days four and five. Stay with her if she is feeling very miserable while her temperature is high.

SYMPTOMS

Days 1 and 2
▲ Runny nose
▲ dry cough
▲ red, sore, watering eyes
▲ temperature that gets steadily higher.

Day 3
▲ Slight fall in temperature
▲ continuing cough
▲ tiny white spots, like grains of salt, in the mouth.

Days 4 and 5
▲ Rising temperature—it may reach 104°F (40°C)
▲ dull red rash of slightly raised spots, appears first on the forehead and behind the ears, gradually spreading to the rest of the face and trunk.

Days 6 and 7
▲ Fading rash and disappearance of other symptoms.

Day 9
▲ Your child is no longer infectious.

---

2 Make sure your child is comfortable. Try to bring down her temperature with an aspirin-free medicine containing acetaminophen and by giving a tepid bath or sponging (see also page 188).

3 Make sure that your child has plenty to drink, especially when her temperature is high.

CALL THE DOCTOR

Call for emergency help immediately if your child develops any of the signs listed on page 197. Consult your doctor as soon as possible if you think your child has measles. Call him again if:
▲ your child is no better three days after the rash develops
▲ your child's temperature rises suddenly
▲ your child's condition worsens after she seemed to be getting better
▲ your child has an earache
▲ your child's breathing becomes noisy or difficult.

4 If your child's eyes are sore, bathe them with cotton balls dipped in cool water. Although bright light won't damage her eyes, keep her room dark if this makes her more comfortable.

What the doctor might do

There is no medical treatment for measles, but your doctor will confirm the diagnosis and may want to check your child and have you watch her closely until she has recovered. He will treat any complications as they develop.

CHICKEN POX (VARICELLA)

What is it?

This very infectious illness produces a rash of itchy spots. Your child may not feel very ill, but if she has a lot of spots, she may itch all over. Symptoms appear two to three weeks after your child has been infected, but the virus is infectious 24–48 hours before the rash appears.

Chicken pox is caused by the same virus that causes shingles in adults. Keep your child away from the elderly or seriously ill while she is infectious.

The varicella vaccine (see page 196) effectively prevents illness in the majority of cases. However, it is possible to get a milder form of the disease even after immunization.

SYMPTOMS

Days 1 to 6

▲ Groups of small, red, very itchy spots with fluid-filled centers, appearing in batches, first on the scalp and behind the ears, then on the trunk, and later elsewhere on the body

▲ fluid within the spots becomes white and cloudy
▲ slight temperature.

Days 5 to 9

▲ The spots burst, leaving small craters
▲ scabs form over the spots and drop off a few days later

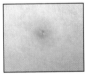

▲ about 24 hours after the last blister has crusted over, the virus is no longer contagious.

Day 10

▲ Your child is back to normal.

CALL THE DOCTOR

Call for emergency help immediately if your child develops any of the emergency signs listed on page 197. Consult your doctor as soon as possible if you think your child has chicken pox, and call him again if your child has any of these symptoms:

▲ very severe itching
▲ redness or swelling around any spots, or pus oozing from the spots—this means they have become infected by bacteria.

What can I do?

1 Take your child's temperature (see page 187), and, if raised, give her the recommended dose of ibuprofen or a children's medicine containing acetaminophen to bring it down, and plenty to drink.

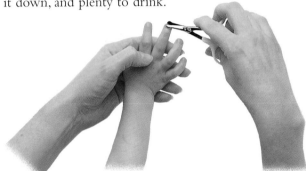

2 Try to discourage your child from scratching the spots, because they can become infected and may cause scarring when they heal. Cut your child's fingernails short and keep them clean so that the spots are less likely to become infected if she does scratch them.

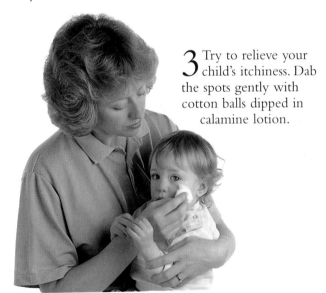

3 Try to relieve your child's itchiness. Dab the spots gently with cotton balls dipped in calamine lotion.

4 Give your child regular warm baths, each with a handful of baking soda dissolved in the water to help reduce the itching.

5 If your child is very itchy, she will probably find loose cotton clothes the most comfortable

What the doctor might do.

Your doctor will confirm the diagnosis and may prescribe an antihistamine cream or medicine to relieve your child's itching if it is very severe. If any of the spots have become infected, he may prescribe an antibiotic.

MUMPS

What is it?

Mumps is an infection that causes swollen glands. It specifically affects the glands in front of the ears, making your child's cheeks look puffy. Your child will develop symptoms two to four weeks after he has been infected.

Occasionally mumps causes inflammation of the testicles or ovaries, but this is very rare before puberty. Headache and vomiting may also occur.

■ SYMPTOMS ■

Day 1
▲ Pain when chewing, or facial pain that your child can't locate
▲ raised temperature.

Day 2
▲ Swelling and tenderness on one side of the face

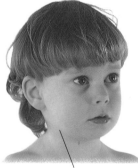

Area of swelling

▲ pain when opening the mouth
▲ fever
▲ sore throat, and pain when swallowing
▲ dry mouth.

Day 3
▲ Increased facial swelling, usually on both sides.

Days 4 to 6
▲ Gradual reduction of swelling and improvement in other symptoms.

Day 13
▲ Your child is no longer infectious.

What can I do?

1 Very gently feel your child's glands (see page 183) if he complains of facial pain, or if his face looks swollen.

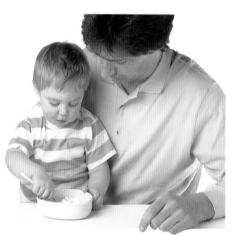

4 If it hurts your child to swallow, give him liquid or semi-liquid foods such as ice cream and soup.

■ CALL THE DOCTOR ■

Call for emergency help if your child shows any of the emergency signs on page 197. Consult your doctor as soon as possible if you think your child has the mumps, and call him again if he develops stomach pain or a red testicle.

2 Check his temperature (see page 187) and give him children's medication with acetaminophen to reduce his temperature if it is raised.

3 Encourage your child to drink liquids, but avoid acidic fruit juices. Let him drink through a straw if it hurts him to open his mouth. Be patient when feeding your baby, since he may find sucking painful.

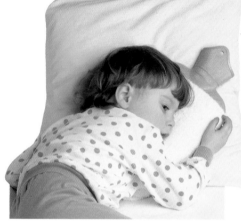

5 Fill a hot water bottle with warm water and wrap it in a towel, then let your child rest his cheek against it to soothe the swelling. Don't give a hot water bottle to a baby who may be too young to push it away if it is too hot: heat a soft cloth and hold it gently against his face instead.

What the doctor might do

There is no cure for the mumps, but your doctor can offer suggestions for making your child as comfortable as possible.

WHOOPING COUGH (PERTUSSIS)

What is it?
One of the most serious childhood diseases, whooping cough is a severe and persistent cough. Caused by a bacteria, it is highly infectious, so keep your child away from unimmunized babies and children. Even a child who has been immunized can get a mild form of the illness. A few children with whooping cough also develop a secondary infection, such as bronchitis or pneumonia (see pages 210–11).

SYMPTOMS

Week 1
▲ Symptoms of a normal cough and cold
▲ slight temperature.

Week 2
▲ Worsening cough, with frequent coughing fits lasting up to a minute, after which your child has to fight for breath
▲ if your child is over 18 months, he may make a "whooping" sound on inspiration after a coughing fit
▲ vomiting after a coughing fit.

Weeks 3 to 10
▲ Cough improves, but may worsen if your child gets a cold
▲ your child is unlikely to be infectious after the third week.

What can I do?
1 Stay with your child during coughing fits, since he may be very distressed. Sit him on your lap and hold him leaning slightly forward. Keep a bowl or plastic container nearby so that he can spit out any phlegm he coughs up, and in case he vomits afterward. Clean the bowl thoroughly with boiling water, to make sure that the infection doesn't spread.

2 If your child often coughs and vomits after meals, offer him small meals at frequent intervals, if possible just after a coughing fit.

3 Keep your child entertained—he will have fewer coughing fits if his attention is distracted, but don't let him get too excited or overtired since this may bring on a coughing fit.

EMERGENCY SIGNS
Call for emergency help immediately if your child turns blue during a coughing fit.

CALL THE DOCTOR
Consult your doctor as soon as possible if you suspect that your child has whooping cough.

4 Sleep in the same room as your child, so that you can be with him if he has a coughing fit at night.

5 Don't let anyone smoke near your child, and don't give him any cough medicines, unless prescribed.

What the doctor might do
The doctor might prescribe a cough suppressant and an antibiotic. Although the antibiotic won't cure your child's cough, it may reduce its severity and make your child less infectious. This is particularly important if you have a baby who is at risk of catching whooping cough from an older sibling who already has the disease. However, the antibiotic is only really effective if it is given right at the beginning of the infection.

CARING FOR A BABY
Whooping cough is dangerous in babies as they may not be able to draw breath properly after coughing. Your baby will need careful nursing and may be admitted to the hospital. She may find sucking difficult if she vomits frequently, so abandon your regular feeding schedule, and feed her as soon as she has calmed down after coughing or vomiting.

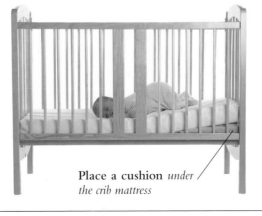

Place a cushion under the crib mattress

Coughing fits
When your baby has a coughing fit, lay her in her crib on her stomach with the foot of her crib mattress slightly raised, or face down across your lap. Stay with her until she has stopped coughing and is breathing normally again. Cuddle her to comfort her after a bout of coughing or vomiting.

EYE PROBLEMS

Although most eye disorders clear up quickly when they are treated, all problems affecting the eye should be taken seriously. Eye infections spread easily to other people, so give your child her own washcloth and towel, and change them frequently. Dry her eyes with tissues, using a clean one for each eye. Keep your child's hands clean and try to stop her from rubbing her eyes. These steps will help prevent an infection, and stop one from spreading.

> ### ■ EMERGENCY SIGNS ■
> Call for emergency help immediately if your child has an injury that has damaged her eye, or if you think that she is not seeing clearly after an injury.

BLEPHARITIS

What is it?
Blepharitis is an inflammation of the edges of the eyelids, which usually affects both eyes. Children with dandruff often have blepharitis.

> ### ■ SYMPTOMS ■
> ▲ Red and scaly eyelids.
>

What can I do?
1 Dissolve a teaspoon of baking soda or salt in a glass of warm boiled water and use this to bathe your child's eyelids. Wash your hands before and afterward, and use a fresh cotton ball for each eye. Do this twice a day, making a fresh solution each time.

2 If your child has dandruff, wash her hair with an antidandruff shampoo. Use an anticradle cap shampoo for a baby.

> ### ■ CALL THE DOCTOR ■
> Consult your doctor as soon as possible if:
> ▲ your child's eyes are sticky
> ▲ there is no improvement after about a week of home treatment.

What the doctor might do
The doctor might prescribe a cream to soothe your child's eyelids, or an antibiotic ointment.

CONJUNCTIVITIS

What is it?
Also known as "pink eye," because the white of the eye may turn pink, conjunctivitis is an inflammation of the lining of the eye and the eyelids. It can be caused by a virus or by bacteria. It is milder when caused by a virus. If your child's eyelids are gummed together with pus when she wakes up, she probably has bacterial, rather than viral, conjunctivitis. If your baby develops any of the symptoms in the box (right) in the first day or two of life, see Sticky eye, page 177.

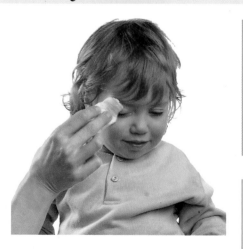

> ### ■ SYMPTOMS ■
> ▲ Bloodshot eye
> ▲ gritty, sore eye
> ▲ discharge of pus
> ▲ eyelids gummed together after sleep.
>

What can I do?
1 Try to find out whether your child's symptoms are caused by something other than conjunctivitis. She might have a corneal abrasion, an allergy such as hay fever, or she may have a speck of dust or an eyelash in her eye. If she has an allergy, her eyes may be itchy and watering as well as red and sore.

2 If you think she has conjunctivitis, dissolve a teaspoon of salt in a glass of warm boiled water, and dip a cotton ball in this. Bathe both of her eyes, using fresh cotton balls for each one. Start with the infected one, and wipe from the outside corner to the inside. Wash your hands before and after this procedure.

> ### ■ CALL THE DOCTOR ■
> Consult your doctor as soon as possible if you think your child has conjunctivitis or if her eyes are bloodshot and sore.

What the doctor might do
The doctor may prescribe antibiotic drops or ointment for a bacterial infection. Viral conjunctivitis needs no treatment, but may last a few weeks.

STYE

What is it?

A stye is a painful, pus-filled swelling on the upper or lower eyelid, caused by infection at the base of an eyelash. Some styes simply dry up, but most come to a head and burst within a week, relieving the pain. Styes are not serious and you can treat them at home.

SYMPTOMS

▲ Red, painful swelling on the eyelid
▲ pus-filled center appearing in the swelling.

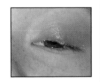

CALL THE DOCTOR

Consult your doctor as soon as possible if:
▲ the stye does not improve after a week
▲ your child's whole eyelid is swollen
▲ the skin all around your child's eye turns red
▲ your child also has blepharitis.

What can I do?

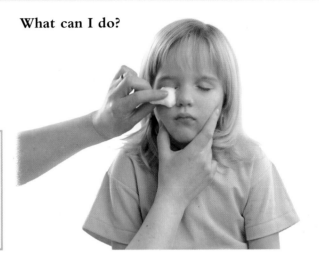

1 Dip a cotton ball in hot water, squeeze it, and press it gently onto your child's stye for two or three minutes, to help bring the stye to a head more quickly. Repeat this three times a day until the stye bursts.

2 When the stye bursts, the pain is relieved. Wash the pus away very gently using a fresh cotton ball dipped in warm boiled water for each wipe.

SQUINT

What is it?

Normally, both eyes look in the same direction at the same time, but in a child with a squint, one eye focuses on an object, while the other does not follow it properly.

A newborn baby's eyes do not always work together correctly, so intermittent squinting is common. This is nothing to worry about—your baby is simply learning to use his eyes. But if your baby's eyes don't move together after he is about three months old, he may have a squint.

Squinting may be constant, but in some children it comes and goes. However, children do not grow out of a squint, so it is essential to have it treated. The younger the child, the more successful the treatment.

SYMPTOMS

▲ Eyes looking in different directions.

CALL THE DOCTOR

Consult your doctor if you think your child has a squint.

How can I check for a squint?

When your baby is about three months old, hold a toy 8in (20cm) from his face and move it slowly from side to side. Check that his eyes work together to follow the moving object.

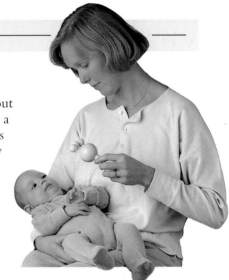

What the doctor might do

The doctor will check your child's vision and may give him a patch to wear over his stronger eye for several hours each day. This forces him to use his weak eye. A toddler may need to wear glasses. If your child is under two, this treatment will probably cure his squint in a few months. If your child has a severe squint caused by muscle weakness, he may need to have surgery to correct the problem.

EAR PROBLEMS

Most ear problems in small children come from an infection of the outer or middle ear, or because the tube connecting the ear and throat becomes blocked. Ear infections should be taken seriously, but they are dangerous only if they are not treated promptly: there is a risk that pus may build up behind the eardrum, and eventually burst it, or that infection might spread into a bone behind the ear (mastoiditis).

Anatomy of the ear
The ear consists of three parts. From the outer ear (the only visible part) a slightly curved canal leads to the eardrum. The middle ear lies just behind the eardrum and is a cavity housing three small bones that transmit sound vibrations. The inner ear contains the delicate structures that allow you to hear and to balance yourself.

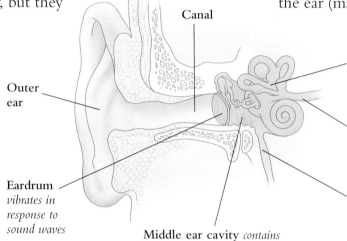

Canal

Outer ear

Eardrum *vibrates in response to sound waves*

Inner ear *contains the mechanisms for hearing and balance*

Auditory nerve *takes sound signals to the brain*

Eustachian tube *leads to the back of the throat. It is much shorter in children than in adults, so infection can spread easily*

Middle ear cavity *contains three tiny bones that transmit sound signals to the inner ear*

——— OUTER EAR INFECTION (OTITIS EXTERNA) ———

What is it?
The skin lining the outer ear canal becomes inflamed when your child has an outer ear infection. This may happen if he swims in water a lot, or because he has poked or scratched his ear and it has become infected. Children with eczema are especially prone to such infections if they get water in their ears.

SYMPTOMS
▲ Pain in the ear that is worse when the child touches his ear or lies on it
▲ redness in the ear canal
▲ discharge from the ear
▲ itchiness inside the ear.

CALL THE DOCTOR
Consult your doctor as soon as possible if you think your child has an outer ear infection.

What can I do?
1 Give your child the recommended dose of a children's medication containing acetaminophen.

2 Make sure that water doesn't get into the affected ear at bathtime, and just sponge his hair clean. Don't let your child go swimming until the infection clears up.

What the doctor might do
Your doctor will probably prescribe antibiotic or anti-inflammatory ear drops to treat the infection.

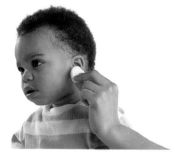

WAX IN THE EAR
Wax sometimes accumulates in the ear, giving a feeling of fullness or partial deafness. If your child has a lot of ear wax, very gently wipe away any visible wax with a cotton ball, but don't poke anything into the ear. If this doesn't help, consult your doctor.

To administer ear drops, ask your child to lie still on his side while you squeeze drops into the affected ear. It may be difficult, but try to keep him in this position for about a minute afterward.

MIDDLE EAR INFECTION (OTITIS MEDIA)

What is it?
If your child has a middle ear infection, the cavity behind his eardrum becomes inflamed, usually because an infection has spread from his throat. The tube that runs from the throat to the ear is very short and narrow in a child, allowing infection to spread extremely easily. Generally, only one ear is infected. Viruses cause most episodes, although bacteria may be responsible. Otitis media may reoccur in children who are less than 2 years of age.

What can I do?
1 Try to relieve your child's earache. Fill a hot water bottle with warm, not hot, water and wrap it in a towel, then let him rest his ear against it. Don't give a hot water bottle to a baby who is too young to push it away if it too hot. Heat a soft cloth and hold it against his ear instead.

2 If your child's ear is very painful, give him the recommended dose of children's aspirin-free pain medication.

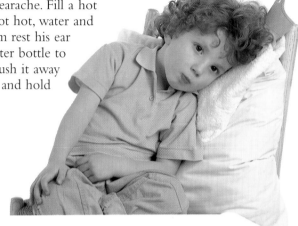

3 If you notice a discharge, don't clear it away or probe into his ear—just put a clean handkerchief over his ear. Encourage him to rest his head on the affected side, so that any discharge can drain away.

■ SYMPTOMS ■
▲ Very painful ear, which may stop your child from sleeping
▲ crying and rubbing or tugging at the ear, if your child can't talk yet or easily explain that his ear aches
▲ crying, loss of appetite, and general signs of illness in young babies, especially following a cold
▲ fever
▲ partial deafness.

■ CALL THE DOCTOR ■
Consult your doctor as soon as possible if your child's ear is infected or has a discharge.

What the doctor might do
The doctor may prescribe an antibiotic to clear the infection. If fluid builds up behind the eardrum, an antibiotic may also be prescribed to help clear it up. If this is not effective, your child may need the minor surgery described below.

OTITIS MEDIA WITH EFFUSION

What is it?
Common in infants and preschoolers, this condition is a build-up of fluid in the middle ear without the symptoms of a middle-ear infection (see above).

SYMPTOMS
• Discomfort or behavior changes
• Persistent cases may result in partial hearing loss.

■ CALL THE DOCTOR ■
Consult your doctor as soon as possible if you think your child has an ear infection or shows signs of a hearing loss.

What the doctor might do
Your doctor may prescribe antibiotics, but most cases of middle ear fluid clear up without treatment in about three months. A child who has had fluid in both middle ears for three months should have a hearing test. Persistent cases accompanied by hearing loss may require a simple operation. Under anesthesia, a tiny tube is inserted in the eardrum. The tube is not uncomfortable and will not affect your child's hearing, but he can't go swimming while it's in place. After several months, the tube will fall out, the hole will heal, and his hearing will be back to normal.

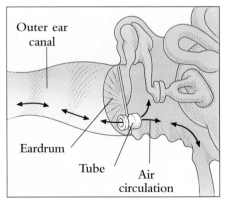

The tube is implanted in the eardrum to equalize air pressure on either side of the eardrum and to allow the ear to dry out.

MOUTH INFECTIONS

When a baby or young child has a mouth infection, two of life's simple yet satisfying pleasures—sucking and eating—become very painful. Thrush is the most common mouth affliction in babies, while older children may be prone to cold sores (see page 222).

Helping the child with a sore mouth

If your child's mouth is sore, try to make eating and drinking as painless as you can. Allow warm meals to cool before giving them to your child, since hot food generally hurts more than cold, and offer her plenty of very cold drinks. If she is reluctant to eat or drink, try some of the suggestions given here.

Let your child drink through a straw or

use a training cup, since this may be less painful than drinking straight from a glass.

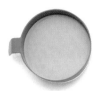

Soup This is nourishing, easy to eat, and can be served cold. Mix or chop solid food into very small bites.

Cold drinks Serve drinks very cold; avoid fruit juice, since it is very acidic.

Ice cream Your child may find cold food such as ice cream easy to eat.

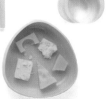

Water

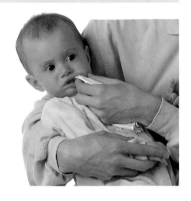

Cheese Encourage your child to finish meals with cheese and a drink of water to help keep her teeth clean without brushing.

THRUSH

What is it?

Thrush is an infection caused by candida, a type of yeast that lives in the mouth and intestines. The yeast normally does not cause an infection, but sometimes it multiplies wildly, producing a sore, irritating rash. Occasionally, it spreads through the intestines and causes a rash around the anus. It is not a serious infection and, although it does not ordinarily respond to home remedies, it usually clears up quickly under a doctor's care.

What can I do?

1 Wipe the patches in your child's mouth very gently with a clean handkerchief. If they don't come off easily, she probably has thrush. Don't rub them hard, because if you scrape them off there will be sore, bleeding patches beneath.

2 Give your child food that is easy to eat (see above). If you are bottle-feeding, buy a special soft nipple and clean it carefully, then sterilize it after each feeding.

3 If you are breast-feeding, continue to nurse normally, but take extra care with nipple hygiene to prevent your nipples from becoming infected. Wash them in water only, not soap, after each feeding, and don't wear breast pads. If they are sore or develop white spots, consult your doctor.

What the doctor might do

Your doctor will usually prescribe a medicine to be dropped into your baby's mouth just before a feeding, or for a child over two, lozenges to suck. If you are breast-feeding, the doctor may check your nipples for signs of infection.

SYMPTOMS

▲ Reluctance to eat due to a sore mouth
▲ creamy yellow, slightly raised patches on the inside of the cheeks, tongue, or the roof of the mouth, which do not come away easily if you try to wipe them off
▲ in babies, a rash around the anus that looks like diaper rash.

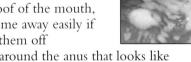

CALL THE DOCTOR

Consult your doctor as soon as possible if you think your baby or child has thrush.

THROAT INFECTIONS

S ore throats are common in children of all ages, and often accompany a cold or the flu. Most of the time they are caused by viruses and clear up quickly. Call your doctor because it's important to rule out more severe throat ailments, which might require a prescription medication or signal a bacterial infection of the tonsils.

■ CALL THE DOCTOR ■

Consult your doctor as soon as possible if your child:
▲ has a throat so sore that swallowing is painful
▲ seems generally sick with a fever or rash
▲ has infected tonsils.

SORE THROAT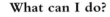

What is it?
A sore throat may be caused by infection with *Streptococcus pyogenes* (causing a strep throat) or by a virus. It may be part of a cold or flu (see pages 194–95), or indicate German measles or mumps (see pages 197 and 200). Children are prone to earache when they have a throat infection (see pages 204–5).

■ SYMPTOMS ■
▲ Reluctance to eat, because it hurts to swallow
▲ red, raw-looking throat
▲ earache (see pages 204–5)
▲ slightly raised temperature
▲ swollen glands
▲ stomach ache in young children.

What can I do?
1 Ask your child to face a bright light and open his mouth. Examine the back of his throat carefully (see page 183). If it is sore, it will look red and raw and you may be able to see creamy spots.

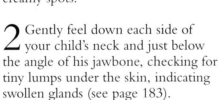

2 Gently feel down each side of your child's neck and just below the angle of his jawbone, checking for tiny lumps under the skin, indicating swollen glands (see page 183).

3 Give your child plenty of cold drinks, and mash solid foods if it hurts him to swallow. Very cold food such as ice cream is less painful to eat than warm food.

4 Take your child's temperature (see page 187), and if it is above normal, give him pain medication containing acetaminophen to bring his fever down.

What the doctor might do
Most mild sore throats need no treatment, but if the doctor suspects that the infection is caused by bacteria, he may prescribe an antibiotic.

TONSILLITIS

■ SYMPTOMS ■
▲ Very sore throat
▲ red and enlarged tonsils, possibly covered with creamy spots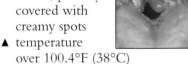
▲ temperature over 100.4°F (38°C)
▲ swollen glands on the neck.

What is it?
Tonsillitis is an inflammation of the tonsils, causing a very sore throat and other symptoms of illness. The tonsils are glands at the back of the throat, one on either side, which trap infection and prevent it from spreading.

What can I do?
1 Examine your child's tonsils and feel his glands (see page 183). If infected, his tonsils will be large and red, and may have creamy spots.
2 Take his temperature (see page 187) and give him an aspirin-free pain medication containing acetaminophen to bring it down.

3 Encourage your child to have plenty to drink, especially if he has a fever. Offer him cold drinks and liquid or semi-liquid foods.

What the doctor might do
Your doctor will examine your child's throat, and may take a throat culture or other test by wiping a sterile swab across it. He may prescribe an antibiotic to clear up the infection quickly.

If your child has recurring bouts of severe tonsillitis, your doctor may recommend that he has his tonsils removed. This operation is rarely performed on a child under four years of age.

COUGHS AND CHEST INFECTIONS

Coughs in small children are often a symptom of a cold or the flu (see pages 194–95), which produces a dry, ticklish cough. A cough may also signal a chest infection (see pages 209–11) or be an early sign of the measles (see page 198). A severe, persistent cough might be whooping cough (see page 201) or asthma (see pages 210–11).

Your child may get a chest infection after a cold or the flu if the infection spreads down toward his lungs. He may find breathing difficult, and might cough up some mucus. However, slightly wheezy breathing is normal for a small child with a cold or the flu, because his airways are very narrow and become even narrower if they are swollen when he is ill. Occasionally, a chest infection develops as a complication of the measles or whooping cough.

Respiratory Syncytial Virus (RSV) can cause bronchiolitis (infection of the small airways of the lung) as well as more serious lung infections. It may begin with cold symptoms, such as a runny nose, mild fever, and cough; if your child begins wheezing and has difficulty breathing, call the doctor. There is no vaccine, but the best way to prevent RSV is good handwashing as it is transmitted by rubbing the eyes. Wash your hands before handling your baby and try to keep him away from other sick children during the winter months.

| | EMERGENCY SIGNS | |

Call for emergency help immediately if your child:
▲ has a bluish tinge around his face, mouth, and tongue
▲ is breathing very rapidly
▲ is breathing so noisily that it can be heard across the room
▲ seems to be fighting for breath
▲ deteriorates suddenly when he has a cold or the flu
▲ is abnormally drowsy
▲ is unable to speak or make sounds as usual.

FREQUENT CHEST INFECTIONS

Babies under a year old and children with a long-term chest disorder such as asthma (see page 210) are prone to chest infections. If you smoke, your children are much more likely to develop chest infections than the children of nonsmoking parents.

Breathing

As your child breathes in, air is sucked down his windpipe and bronchi (the airways) into his lungs, where oxygen is absorbed into his bloodstream. His blood then carries the oxygen around his body.

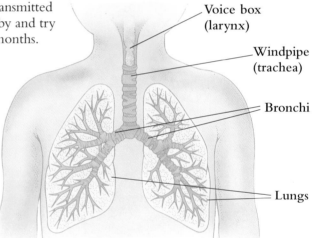

Voice box (larynx)

Windpipe (trachea)

Bronchi

Lungs

CROUP

What is it?
Croup is an inflammation of the larynx or voice box, which makes it swell, so that your child finds it difficult to breathe. Attacks of croup tend to occur at night, and usually last about two hours.

| | SYMPTOMS | |

▲ Breathing difficulty
▲ loud, crowing sound as breath is drawn in
▲ barking cough.

What can I do?
1 Keep calm, and reassure your child. He may be very frightened, but if he panics, it will be even harder for him to breathe.

2 Take your child into the bathroom and create a steamy atmosphere by turning on the hot water full blast. Moist air will help him to breathe more easily. Meanwhile put a cold-mist humidifier in his room to moisten the air there, too.

3 Prop your child up on pillows, or sit him on your lap—he will then be able to breathe more easily.

| | CALL THE DOCTOR | |

Call your doctor now if your child has difficulty breathing, or if you think he has croup.

What the doctor might do
The doctor will reassure you and tell you what to do if your child's croup recurs. He might prescribe an antibiotic, and, in case of another attack, may also give some medication to ease your child's breathing. If your child seems very ill, the doctor might recommend going to the hospital.

COUGH

What is it?

A cough can be either a reaction to irritation in the throat or windpipe, or the result of a chest infection. A dry, ticklish cough is rarely serious. It probably means that your child's throat or windpipe is irritated, which may be a by-product of a cold, because mucus dribbles down the throat and irritates it. Her throat might also be irritated by smoke, if she is with adults who smoke. An ear infection can also cause a dry cough.

If your child's cough sounds moist, particularly if she spits up mucus, she probably has a chest infection. While most coughs like this are not serious, they can be a symptom of pneumonia (see page 210).

■ CALL THE DOCTOR ■

Call your doctor now if, over a period of about half an hour, your child is breathing faster than usual, or if his breathing is labored or very noisy. Consult your doctor as soon as possible if:
▲ your baby is under six months old and has a cough
▲ your child's cough prevents him from sleeping
▲ the cough does not improve in three days
▲ your child has a recurrent cough.

What the doctor might do

The doctor will listen to your child's breathing. If he has a dry cough, the doctor may prescribe a cough suppressant medication to soothe his throat. If the cough is deep, the doctor may carry out some diagnostic tests. He may prescribe antibiotics and perhaps a cough medication to make the mucus easier to cough up.

What can I do?

1 If your child has a sudden attack of coughing, make sure she hasn't inhaled a small object such as a piece of candy or a button. If she has, try to remove it (see Choking, page 234), but don't put your fingers down her throat to pull it out.

2 If your child has a deep cough, try to help her clear the mucus from her chest when she is coughing. Lay her on her stomach across your lap, then pat her back rhythmically but not too hard.

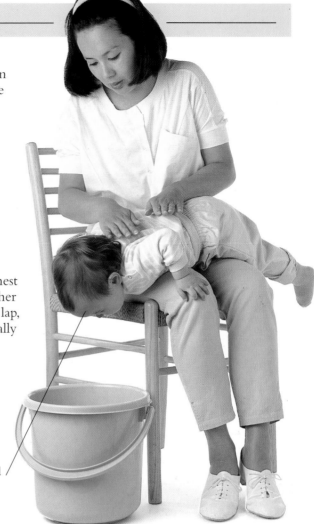

Keep your child's head *slightly tipped down*

3 Have a bucket or bowl nearby and encourage her to spit out any mucus that she has coughed up. Productive coughing is nature's way of clearing airways that are clogged by mucus.

4 If your child has a dry cough, give her a warm drink at bedtime. For a child over 18 months, make a soothing drink by dissolving a teaspoon of honey in a glass of warm water and adding a few drops of fresh lemon juice.

5 Prop your child up with extra pillows at night to help prevent mucus from dribbling down his throat. For a baby, put a pillow under the head of the mattress.

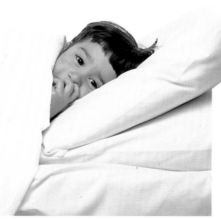

6 If your child's cough is worse in a smoky atmosphere, don't let anyone smoke near him and keep him away from smoky areas.

7 Don't give a cough medication unless your doctor prescribes one.

BRONCHIOLITIS

What is it?
Bronchiolitis is a viral infection of the lungs that causes inflammation and swelling of the bronchioles, the smallest airways in the lungs. The condition occurs in children under 2 years of age (average age: 6 months). Symptoms—similar to those of asthma (see below)—typically become worse for 2 or 3 days, then begin to improve. The most worrisome complication is difficulty breathing.

■ SYMPTOMS ■
- ▲ Wheezing
- ▲ rapid or tight breathing
- ▲ coughing
- ▲ fever and runny nose preceding breathing problems and cough

What can I do?
1 Take your child's temperature (see page 187) and if it is raised, give him aspirin-free medication with acetaminophen, and plenty to drink. Warm liquids also help to relax the airways and loosen secretions.

2 To relieve wheezing and clear your child's lungs during a coughing fit, lay him across your lap on his stomach and pat his back (see page 209).

3 To ease breathing, put a pillow under the head of your baby's mattress. Prop up an older child in bed with extra pillows (see page 209).

4 Use a cool-mist vaporizer to humidify the air in his room.

■ CALL THE DOCTOR ■
Call your doctor immediately if:
- ▲ your child's breathing becomes difficult or faster than 60 breaths per minute
- ▲ his wheezing becomes severe
- ▲ he shows any of the emergency signs on page 208

Consult your doctor if you think your child has bronchiolitis and again if his fever lasts more than 2 days or his coughing more than 2 weeks.

What the doctor might do
In some cases, a doctor may prescribe an asthma-type medication to relieve symptoms. A child with severe breathing difficulty may require hospitalization.

ASTHMA

What is it?
Asthma is a recurrent narrowing of the tiny airways leading to the lungs. During an asthma attack, breathing, especially exhaling, is difficult. Asthma may be caused by an allergy. If other members of your family have asthma, eczema, or hay fever, your baby is susceptible too. Mild asthma is common, and your child may outgrow it.

■ SYMPTOMS ■
- ▲ Coughing, particularly at night or after exercise
- ▲ slight wheeziness and breathlessness, especially during a cold
- ▲ attacks of severe breathlessness, when breathing is shallow and difficult
- ▲ feeling of suffocation during an asthma attack
- ▲ pale, sweaty skin during an attack
- ▲ bluish tinge around the lips during a severe attack.

What can I do?
1 Keep calm and reassure your child. If he has had previous attacks, give him whatever medication the doctor has prescribed. If this has no effect, call for emergency help.

2 Sit your child on your lap and help him to lean slightly forward—this makes it easier for him to breath. Don't hold him tightly; let him settle into the most comfortable position.

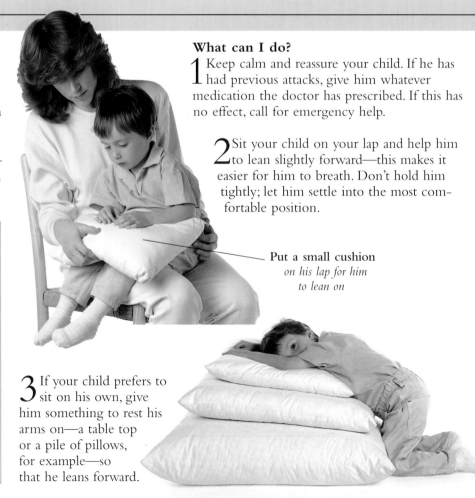

Put a small cushion *on his lap for him to lean on*

3 If your child prefers to sit on his own, give him something to rest his arms on—a table top or a pile of pillows, for example—so that he leans forward.

PNEUMONIA

What is it?

Pneumonia is an inflammation of the lungs, which causes breathing difficulty. In young children it is nearly always due to the spread of an infection such as a cold or the flu, and is usually caused by a virus, not bacteria. Occasionally pneumonia is the result of a tiny amount of food being inhaled into the lungs and causing a small patch of inflammation and infection to occur.

Pneumonia is a serious disease, but most healthy babies—even those under a year old—recover completely in about a week.

■ SYMPTOMS ■

▲ Deterioration in a sick child
▲ raised temperature
▲ dry cough
▲ rapid breathing
▲ difficult or noisy breathing.

What can I do?

1 Prop your child up with extra pillows in bed, so that he can breathe more easily. For a baby, put a pillow under the head of the mattress.

2 Take your child's temperature (see page 187) and, if it is raised, try to reduce it by giving an aspirin-free medication with acetaminophen or by sponging him (see page 188).

■ CALL THE DOCTOR ■

Call for emergency help immediately if your child develops any of the emergency signs on page 208. Call your doctor now if you think your child has pneumonia.

3 Make sure that your child has plenty to drink, especially if his temperature is raised. Offer your baby cool water.

What the doctor might do

The doctor will advise you how to nurse your child, and, if the infection is bacterial, he may prescribe an antibiotic. If your child is very ill, he might need to be treated in a hospital.

PREVENTING ASTHMA ATTACKS

Try to find out what causes your child's asthma attacks by keeping a record of when they occur. Vigorous exercise and overexcitement can bring on an attack. Some other common triggers are shown here.

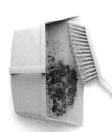

Dust
Reduce dust in your house by vacuuming and damp-mopping, rather than sweeping and dusting. Cover your child's mattress with a plastic sheet.

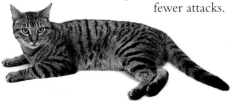

Animal fur If you have a pet, let it stay somewhere else for a while, and note whether your child has fewer attacks.

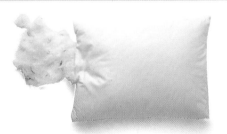

Feather-filled cushions or pillows
Change these for ones with synthetic filling.

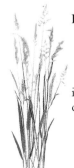

Pollen, especially from grass and trees
Discourage your child from playing in tall grass, and keep him inside when the pollen count is high.

Cigarette smoke
Don't let people smoke near your child.

■ EMERGENCY SIGNS ■

Call for emergency help immediately if your child:
▲ has a bluish tinge on his tongue or around his lips
▲ is severely breathless
▲ does not start to breathe more easily 10 minutes after taking his medication
▲ becomes abnormally drowsy.

■ CALL THE DOCTOR ■

Call your doctor now if this is your child's first asthma attack. Consult your doctor as soon as possible if you think your child may have asthma.

What the doctor might do

The doctor may prescribe a drug to be given at the beginning of an attack, or before any activity that causes one. During a severe attack, he may send your child to the hospital.

STOMACH PAIN

Pain between the bottom of the ribs and the groin, or "stomach pain," can be a symptom of many disorders, including gastroenteritis (see page 214) and urinary tract infections (see page 216). It may also be caused by vomiting, and can accompany illnesses such as tonsillitis and the measles. Your child may complain of a stomach ache if he feels generally sick, knows he is about to be sick, or if he has a pain somewhere else, but can't easily describe its exact location.

DEALING WITH A STOMACH ACHE

What causes stomach pain?

Many children have recurrent bouts of stomach pain when something makes them feel anxious or insecure. Provided that your child's pain is not severe and lasts for only an hour or two, you needn't worry; try to find out what is bothering him, and reassure him.

However, if your child is in severe pain for a few hours, you should take it seriously. He might have appendicitis—inflammation of the appendix, a small blind-ended tube attached to the intestines—though this is extremely rare in children who are under the age of three.

Waves of severe stomach pain at intervals of about 15 to 20 minutes in a baby or toddler may mean that his bowel has become blocked.

What can I do?

1 Take your child's temperature. If it is slightly raised, he may have appendicitis, especially if the stomach pain is severe or seems to be located around his navel. Don't give him medication to ease it, or anything to reduce his temperature.

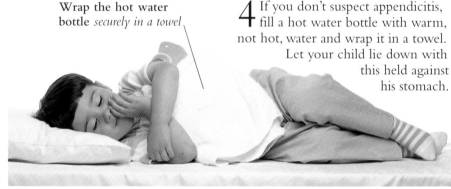

Wrap the hot water bottle *securely in a towel*

2 If you think your child may have appendicitis, don't give him anything to eat or drink. Otherwise give him some water if he is thirsty, but don't let him eat anything.

3 Comfort your child by giving him cuddles and extra attention.

4 If you don't suspect appendicitis, fill a hot water bottle with warm, not hot, water and wrap it in a towel. Let your child lie down with this held against his stomach.

■ EMERGENCY SIGNS ■

Call for emergency help immediately if your baby or child:
▲ screams with pain at intervals of about 15 to 20 minutes, and goes pale when he screams
▲ has a dark red bowel movement that resembles red currant jelly
▲ has severe stomach pain for longer than three hours
▲ has severe stomach pain combined with a fever.

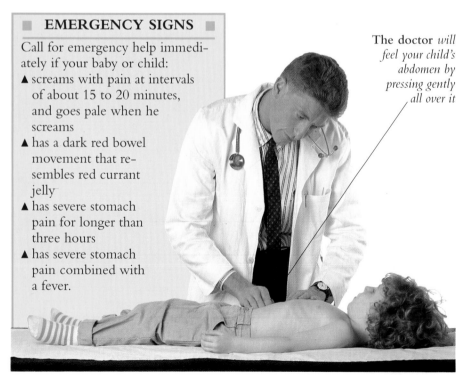

The doctor will feel your child's abdomen by pressing gently all over it

■ CALL THE DOCTOR ■

Call your doctor now if your child:
▲ develops any other symptoms
▲ has stomach pain for longer than three hours.
Consult your doctor if your child frequently has stomach pain.

What the doctor might do

The doctor will examine your child to try to find out the cause of his stomach pain. The treatment will depend on his diagnosis, but most of the time, stomach pain disappears on its own. If the doctor suspects appendicitis or a blocked bowel, he will arrange for your child to go to the hospital for emergency surgery.

CONSTIPATION, VOMITING, AND DIARRHEA

A minor change in diet can cause temporary constipation or diarrhea. Vomiting or diarrhea may accompany almost any illness, and can also be caused by excitement or anxiety. If your child vomits or has mild diarrhea, check for other signs of illness (see paged 182–3). Frequent vomiting or severe diarrhea can quickly make a baby or young child dehydrated. This is a serious condition and must be treated promptly (see page 214), before the body loses too much fluid

CONSTIPATION

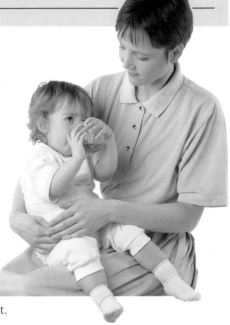

What is it?
If your child has constipation, she has bowel movements less frequently than usual, and they are harder than normal. Children's toilet habits vary greatly: some children have a bowel movement twice a day, others go only once every two or three days. Whatever your child's pattern, it is quite normal—don't tamper with it. Babies often become slightly constipated when they learn to sit up or crawl, and before they can walk.

■ CALL THE DOCTOR ■
Consult your doctor as soon as possible if your child:
▲ cries or complains of pain when moving her bowels
▲ has streaks of blood in her bowel movement, on her diaper, or underpants
▲ has constipation for more than three days.

What can I do?
1 A temporary bout of constipation won't do your child any harm. Don't give her a laxative, since this will upset the normal action of her bowels and don't add sugar to her bottle.

2 Give your child plenty to drink, especially if the weather is hot, to soften her stool. Fruit juice helps to ease her constipation,

3 Don't hurry your child when she is on the toilet, but don't let her stay there for too long. If she's constipated, dab petroleum jelly on her bottom before sitting her on the toilet. This will help ease her bowel movement.

4 Dairy foods can be constipating. Limit milk, cheese, and yogurt to two or three servings a day.

5 Try to include more fiber in your child's diet (see below). This provides the bulk that helps the bowel to grip and move its contents along.

What the doctor might do
The doctor may prescribe a mild laxative and give you some advice on your child's diet. If your child had streaks of blood in her stool, she could have a small tear in the lining of her anus, so the doctor may lubricate the area very gently.

GOOD SOURCES OF FIBER
Some examples of foods rich in fiber are shown here. Fresh foods are always best. Wash vegetables and fruit thoroughly, remove pips and strings, and peel for a child under one year. Purée the food for a baby under eight months (see pages 110–11).

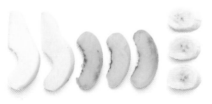

Fresh fruit Give your child slices of peeled pear, peach, banana, and other fruit.

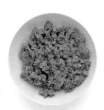

Wholegrain bread　　**Wholegrain breakfast cereal**

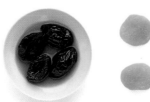

Dried fruit Prunes and apricots are ideal for young children.

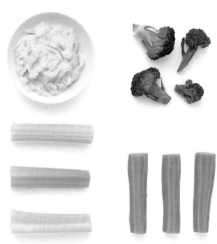

Fresh vegetables Mashed potatoes and lightly cooked broccoli are high in fiber (so are peas and beans). Celery and carrots can be served raw.

VOMITING

What is it?
When your child vomits, she may throw up most of the contents of her stomach. Babies under about six months old often regurgitate a small amount of their feedings. This is perfectly normal, so don't worry.

■ CALL THE DOCTOR ■

Call your doctor if your child:
▲ vomits and seems abnormally drowsy
▲ throws up green-yellow vomit
▲ has vomited repeatedly for more than six hours
▲ shows any signs of dehydration.

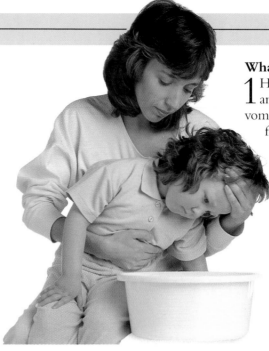

What can I do?
1 Hold your child over a bowl and comfort her while she is vomiting (see page 193). Wipe her face afterward and give her some sips of water.

2 Make sure that your child has plenty to drink: she needs more than the usual amount of fluid to make up for her losses (see Dehydration). If your baby won't take a bottle, try using a teaspoon or a medicine dropper (see page 189) to feed it to her.

What the doctor might do
The doctor will examine your child to find out what is making her vomit, and will then treat her according to the diagnosis.

If she shows signs of dehydration, the doctor may prescribe an oral rehydration solution for her to drink. If she is very dehydrated, the doctor might arrange for her to be admitted to the hospital, where she can be given fluid intravenously.

IDENTIFYING AND TREATING DEHYDRATION

Your child may be dehydrated if she shows one or more of these symptoms:
▲ dry mouth and lips
▲ dark, concentrated urine
▲ no urine passed for six hours
▲ sunken eyes
▲ sunken fontanelle
▲ abnormal drowsiness or lethargy.

One way to detect dehydration is to track your child's urinations. There should be about three or four every 24 hours. Reduced urine output is a sign of dehydration. If your child is dehydrated or in danger of becoming so, call your doctor. Oral rehydration products are available at your drugstore to replace lost salts and sugar.

GASTROENTERITIS

What is it?
Gastroenteritis is an inflammation in the stomach and intestines that can be caused by a virus infection or contaminated food. It is serious in babies, since they can dehydrate quickly, but it is rare in breast-fed babies. A mild attack in a child over two is generally not a cause for alarm.

■ SYMPTOMS ■
▲ Vomiting and nausea
▲ diarrhea
▲ stomach cramps
▲ loss of appetite
▲ fever.

What can I do?
1 Make sure that your child drinks about 2 to 3 pints (1 to 1½ liters) a day. An oral rehydration solution, as described above, should be given.

2 Don't give your child anything to eat until he stops vomiting, then introduce bland foods. Give your baby the usual formula in small frequent feedings (see page 179).

3 If your child has a fever, give him an aspirin-free medication with acetaminophen to reduce it.

4 Let your child wear a diaper again if he has outgrown them.

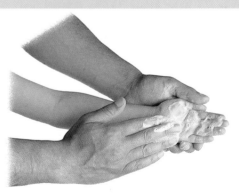

5 Make sure that your child washes his hands after going to the bathroom and before eating. Wash your own hands after changing his diaper and before preparing his food.

DIARRHEA

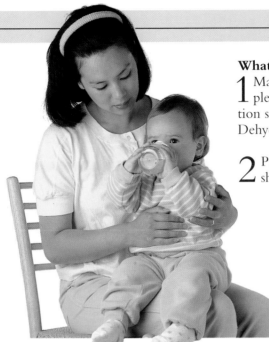

What is it?
If your child has diarrhea, her bowel movements will be watery and more frequent than normal. This may be the result of eating contaminated food or food that is too rich or oily. It may also be caused by a viral infection.

■ CALL THE DOCTOR ■
Call your doctor now if your child:
▲ has had diarrhea for more than six hours
▲ has blood in her stool
▲ shows any signs of dehydration (see page 214).

What can I do?
1 Make sure that your child has plenty to drink. An oral rehydration solution (ORS—see Dehydration, page 214) is ideal.

2 Put your child in a diaper again if she has outgrown them.

3 Pay careful attention to hygiene: wash your hands after changing your baby's diaper and before preparing her food, and make sure that your child always washes her hands after using the toilet and before eating.

What the doctor might do
The doctor will examine your child to find out the cause of her diarrhea, and will treat her according to the diagnosis. If your child has become dehydrated, the doctor will prescribe an oral rehydration solution for her to drink. If she is very dehydrated, he might arrange for her to be admitted to the hospital, where she can be given the extra liquid she needs intravenously.

TREATMENT OF DIARRHEA
The standard treatment for diarrhea used to be to replace all food and drink (including breast milk) with an oral rehydration solution (ORS) available at your pharmacy. This is no longer the case. A baby or child with diarrhea should continue to be fed his regular diet, whether it's breast milk or formula (see page 179) or solid foods. Give him plenty to drink (but avoid undiluted fruit juice and sweetened beverages). If he is dehydrated or in danger of becoming so (see page 214), supplement his diet with oral rehydration solution. Recommended foods for babies who take solids include bananas, rice cereals, apple sauce, and toast.

■ CALL THE DOCTOR ■
Call your doctor now if your child:
▲ is under two and may have gastroenteritis
▲ is over two and has had symptoms of gastroenteritis for more than two days.

What the doctor might do
The doctor will probably treat your child for dehydration and may advise you to give him only liquids for a few days. He may ask for a sample of your child's stool.

QUESTION & ANSWER

"What steps can I take to prevent gastroenteritis?"
Clean all your baby's feeding equipment thoroughly for as long as he drinks formula or milk from a bottle (see pages 100–01). Put prepared bottles in the refrigerator—never store them warm in an insulated container, since bacteria thrive in warm conditions.

Pay careful attention to hygiene when preparing food. Don't store cooked food in the refrigerator for longer than two days, and make sure it is heated thoroughly when you serve it, because heat kills the bacteria that could cause gastroenteritis.

If you are traveling with a baby or a small child in a foreign country, ask your doctor about any precautions you should take, particularly with water, fruit, and salads.

Prevention can be difficult since often diarrhea and vomiting occur as a result of a viral infection.

BLADDER, KIDNEY, AND GENITAL PROBLEMS

Most urinary tract infections are caused by bacteria entering the urethra (see diagram below) and spreading up into the bladder. They are reasonably common in young children, and are usually not serious. Some children are born with minor abnormalities of the urinary tract, which make them prone to such infections. Minor infections of the genitals are also quite common, and in babies and young children they are often part of the symptoms of diaper rash (see page 176).

The urinary tract
Your child has two kidneys which filter his blood. The clean blood returns to his bloodstream, while the waste product (the urine) drains into his bladder, where it collects until he is ready to urinate.

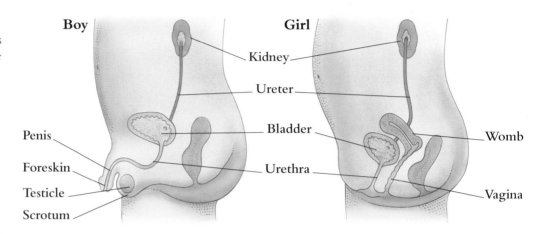

Boy — Girl
Kidney
Ureter
Penis
Bladder
Womb
Foreskin
Urethra
Testicle
Scrotum
Vagina

— URINARY TRACT INFECTIONS —

What are they?
Any part of the urinary tract—the kidneys, the bladder, and the connecting tubes—can become infected with bacteria. Infections are more common in girls, because the tube from the bladder (the urethra) is shorter in a girl than in a boy, and its opening is nearer to the anus, so germs can spread to it more easily.

What can I do?
1 If your child seems sick, check to see whether her urine looks pink or cloudy. Note whether she is urinating more frequently than usual and whether it seems to hurt when she goes to the bathroom. If your child is still in diapers, you probably won't be able to tell if urination is frequent or painful, but you will probably notice a change in odor.

2 Make sure that your child has plenty to drink, to keep her kidneys flushed.

3 If your child has a fever, give her a dose of aspirin-free children's medication with acetaminophen to reduce it.

SYMPTOMS
▲ Urinating more often than usual
▲ pain when urinating
  ▲ pink, red, or cloudy urine
  ▲ change in odor of the urine
  ▲ fever
  ▲ listlessness
    ▲ loss of appetite
    ▲ abdominal pain.

CALL THE DOCTOR
Consult your doctor as soon as possible if you think your child has a urinary tract infection.

What the doctor might do
The doctor will examine your child and may ask you to take a sample of her urine (ask your doctor how you should collect this). He may prescribe an antibiotic.

216

GENITAL PROBLEMS IN GIRLS

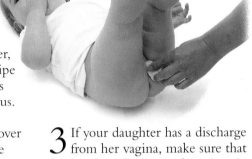

What can go wrong?
A little girl's vagina can become sore due to diaper rash (see page 176), an infection such as thrush (see page 206), pinworms (see page 224) or irritation caused by bubble bath. If your daughter has a blood-stained or smelly discharge from her vagina, she may have pushed something into it. Newborn girls often produce a white or blood-stained discharge for a week or two after birth. After this age until just before puberty, a discharge is abnormal.

What can I do?
1 If your daughter's bottom is sore or red, don't use soap when you wash it—just use water, and dry it thoroughly. Always wipe from front to back, so that germs can't spread forward from her anus.

2 Don't put waterproof pants over your daughter's diapers, since they prevent air from circulating to her bottom. Dress an older child in 100% pure cotton underpants.

3 If your daughter has a discharge from her vagina, make sure that she hasn't pushed something into it. If she has, **consult your doctor as soon as possible**.

What the doctor might do
The doctor will examine your daughter and may take a sample of the discharge. If she has something lodged in her vagina, he will remove it gently. If she has an infection, he may prescribe antibiotics to be taken by mouth, or a cream to be applied to the affected area, depending on the cause of her symptoms.

■ **SYMPTOMS** ■

▲ Soreness or itching in or around the vagina
▲ redness around the vagina
▲ discharge from the vagina.

■ **CALL THE DOCTOR** ■

Consult your doctor as soon as possible if your daughter:
▲ has a discharge from her vagina
▲ still has symptoms after two days of home treatment
▲ has pushed something into her vagina.

GENITAL PROBLEMS IN BOYS

What can go wrong?
In an uncircumcised boy, the foreskin, which covers the tip of the penis, can become inflamed or infected (balanitis), often as part of diaper rash (see page 176).

If a swelling develops in your son's groin or scrotum, he may have a hernia (intestines bulging through a weak area in the abdomen).

What can I do?
If your son's foreskin is inflamed, wash it without using soap and dry it thoroughly at each diaper change, or at least once a day. Change to a mild laundry soap and rinse his diapers or underpants thoroughly.

How can I prevent inflammation?
Don't try to pull your son's foreskin back—it won't retract until he is at least four. If you try to force it, you may make his foreskin inflamed.

■ **SYMPTOMS** ■

Inflamed foreskin
▲ Red, swollen foreskin
▲ discharge of pus from the penis.

Hernia
▲ Soft, painless bulge in the groin or scrotum, which may disappear when your child lies down and get bigger when he coughs, sneezes, or cries.

What the doctor might do
If your son's foreskin is inflamed, the doctor may prescribe an antibiotic cream. If he has a hernia, he may need no treatment, but if he is under six months old, or if the lump feels hard or does not disappear when he lies down, your doctor may recommend surgery to repair the hernia in his groin or scrotum.

■ **CALL THE DOCTOR** ■

Consult your doctor as soon as possible if:
▲ your son's foreskin looks red or swollen, or if there is any discharge
▲ your son's hernia becomes painful, or changes in any other way.
Consult your doctor if you think your son may have a hernia.

CIRCUMCISION
This is a surgical procedure to remove the foreskin. If you want your son circumcised, discuss it with your doctor. Once considered routine for newborn boys, it is now done electively or for religious, cultural, or specific medical reasons.

SKIN PROBLEMS

Minor skin problems are common in childhood. Most clear up quickly, but some are very contagious, and must be treated promptly. If your child has a rash combined with other signs of illness, he may have an infectious illness (see pages 197–99). For other problems, see the guide below.

QUICK DIAGNOSIS GUIDE

One or more red spots, or a rash, see Spots and boils, Hives, Heat rash (below and opposite), Insect stings (page 244) or, if dry and scaly, see Eczema (page 220).
Raw, cracked areas, usually on or around the lips, or on the cheeks and hands, see Chapped skin (page 221).
Small blisters or crusty patches on or around the mouth, see Cold sores and Impetigo (pages 222–23).
Hard lump of skin, usually on the hands or feet, see Warts (page 222).
Itchy head, see Lice and nits (page 224).
Intense itching around the anus, see Pinworms (page 224).

DEALING WITH ITCHING

Many skin problems cause itching, and since scratching can make the skin infected, it is important to relieve your child's itchiness.
■ Dress him in cotton clothes, since cotton is less irritating to the skin than other fabrics.
■ Gently dab the area with cotton balls soaked in calamine lotion, to soothe inflamed or irritated skin.
■ Dissolve a handful of baking soda in your child's bathwater and let him have a good soak.
■ Put cotton socks on his hands when he is in bed.

SPOTS AND BOILS

What are they?

A spot is a small red swelling, usually on the face. A boil is an infection in the skin that causes a large, painful lump, which then festers to produce a head of pus in the middle. Boils are most likely to occur on the face or on pressure points such as the buttocks, but they can appear anywhere on the body.

Don't worry if your child gets occasional spots, but recurrent boils may be a sign of illness.

SYMPTOMS

Spot
▲ Small, red, painless lump.

Boil
▲ Painful, red lump that gradually gets larger
▲ white or yellow center of pus appearing after a day or two.

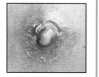

CALL THE DOCTOR

Consult your doctor as soon as possible if:
▲ your child has a spot that looks inflamed
▲ your child has a boil in an awkward or painful place
▲ the center of pus does not appear three days after the boil first developed
▲ red streaks spread out from the boil.
  Consult your doctor if your child often gets boils.

What can I do?

1 If your child gets occasional spots, simply ignore them. They will clear up in a few days without treatment. If she tends to drool, and the spots appear around her mouth, smear a barrier ointment over the area.

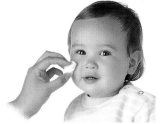

2 If your child has a boil, or a spot that looks inflamed, gently clean it, and the skin around it, with a cotton ball dipped in antiseptic.

3 Cover it with an adhesive bandage. If it is rubbed by clothing, or is in a painful place such as the buttocks, cushion it with a large adhesive bandage or sterile gauze pad and surgical tape.

4 The boil will come to a head and burst of its own accord in a few days. Don't squeeze it—this may spread the infection. After it has burst, clean it gently with a cotton ball dipped in antiseptic, and keep it covered with a bandage or gauze pad until it has healed.

What the doctor might do

The doctor may lance the boil and drain away the pus, to reduce the pain and swelling, and might prescribe a cream. If your child has a lot of boils, the doctor may prescribe a course of antibiotics.

HIVES

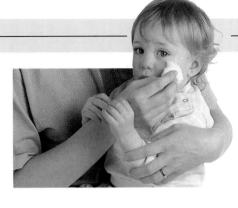

What are they?
Hives (also known as urticaria) are itchy red patches on the skin. They usually fade after a few hours, but can recur. They may be caused by a prickly plant, such as a nettle, harsh sunshine, an allergy to a food or drug, or a viral or bacterial infection.

▲ welts varying in length from $\frac{1}{16}-\frac{1}{2}$in (1mm–1cm)
▲ larger welts joining together.

What can I do?
1 Dab your child's rash with cotton balls dipped in calamine lotion.

2 If the rash is caused by an allergy, try to find out what your child is allergic to, so that you can help her avoid it in the future. Such a rash usually develops a few hours after contact with an allergen, so try to remember whether, for example, she has recently eaten a new food.

■ CALL THE DOCTOR ■
Call your doctor now if your child's face or neck is swollen, or if she is wheezing.
Consult your doctor as soon as possible if:
▲ the rash does not disappear within four hours
▲ your child has frequent attacks of hives.

What the doctor might do
The doctor may prescribe an antihistamine cream or medication for your child. He might also test her to find the cause of the allergy. If her face or neck is swollen, she might need to be given an injection to reduce the swelling.

HEAT RASH

What is it?
Heat rash is a faint rash caused by overheating. It is more common in babies than in children, and usually appears on the face or in skin creases, where sweat can gather. It is not a serious disorder, and you can treat it yourself at home.

■ SYMPTOMS ■

▲ Pink rash on the face or in skin creases.

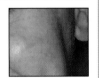

■ CALL THE DOCTOR ■
Consult your doctor as soon as possible if the rash has not faded 12 hours after your child cools down.

What can I do?
1 Take off any heavy bedding and remove a layer of your baby's clothing. Let him sleep dressed in just a T-shirt and diaper.

2 Give him a bath in luke-warm water. Pat his skin dry gently, leaving it slightly damp so that he cools down as his skin dries. When he is dry, apply a little baby powder to absorb new sweat.

3 Take your baby's temperature; if it is raised, give him an aspirin-free children's medication with acetaminophen or sponge bath him (see page 188).

How can I prevent heat rash?
Dress your baby in light clothes when the weather is hot, with cotton next to his skin rather than wool or a manmade fiber. Make sure he's well protected from the sun.

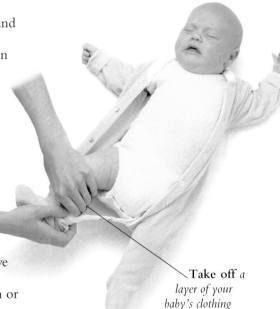

Take off *a layer of your baby's clothing*

What the doctor might do
The doctor will check that the rash is just a heat rash. If it is, your baby needs no medical treatment. If the rash has another cause, the doctor will treat that.

ECZEMA

What is it?

Eczema is a skin reaction resulting in areas of itchy, red, scaly skin. It most commonly affects the face and skin creases, such as the inside of the elbows and the back of the knees, but it can be more widespread.

It usually first appears between the ages of three months and two years, then improves as the child grows older. About half of all children with eczema grow out of it by age six, and nearly all of them grow out of it by puberty. Your child is more likely to develop eczema if other people in the family suffer from allergies such as eczema, asthma, and hay fever.

What can I do?

1 Try to prevent the skin from becoming too dry. When you bathe your child, use a mild nondrying soap such as Dove. Clean the affected areas by wiping them with emollients to prevent drying of the skin, rather than washing with soap. Don't bathe your child excessively.

Use cotton balls to apply the emollient

SYMPTOMS

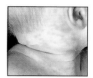

▲ Itchy, read, scaly dry patches, usually on the face or in skin creases
▲ clear fluid oozing from the affected areas.

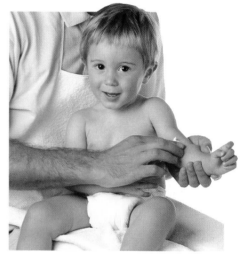

2 After a bath, apply an unscented ointment to your child's skin, since it may be very dry. Avoid products with water or alcohol as the first ingredient.

3 Dress your child in cotton, rather than wool. In cold weather, put cotton clothing under warmer layers.

4 Try to stop your child from scratching the affected areas—put cotton socks on his hands at night and keep his fingernails short.

5 Try to discover a possible cause of the eczema. It may result from an allergy to a food (especially dairy products and wheat), animal fur, woolen clothes, and laundry detergents, but anxiety can also trigger it.

6 When your child's eczema is bad, keep him away from anyone with chicken pox or cold sores because of a greater infection risk.

CALL THE DOCTOR

Consult your doctor if you think your child has eczema. Call your doctor as soon as possible if:
▲ your child's eczema is very widespread or very itchy
▲ fluid is oozing from the eczema.

What the doctor might do

The doctor may prescribe a cream, and if the area is infected, an antibiotic. Most importantly, he'll try to determine the exact allergen and advise you on how to eliminate it from your child's daily environment, if at all possible.

SUNBURN

What is it?
Sunburn is sore or reddened skin caused by exposure to the sun. Babies and young children, especially those with fair hair and blue eyes, have very sensitive skin, so they are particularly vulnerable to it.

SYMPTOMS
▲ Red, sore areas of skin
▲ blisters appearing on badly affected areas
▲ flaking or peeling of skin a day or two later.

What can I do?
1 Take your child out of the sun as soon as her skin begins to look red—symptoms will most likely worsen in a few hours. Encourage her to drink as she may become dehydrated.

2 Cool any reddened areas of skin with cold water, then apply a soothing after-sun lotion or dab on some calamine lotion.

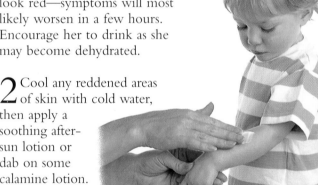

PREVENTING SUNBURN
Under six months of age, a baby's skin is too sensitive for sunscreen. Until she's six months old, keep your baby out of the sun whenever possible or dress her in protective clothes and a hat. Beginning at six months, protect your child with sunscreen whenever she's in the sun. Apply a waterproof UVA and UVB sunscreen with an SFP (sun protection factor) of 30 or higher about 30 minutes before she goes out, and then reapply every hour or two. Dress her in a T-shirt and a sun hat. Make her keep the T-shirt on when she is swimming or playing near water. If her skin is red the next day, keep her out of the sun.

CALL THE DOCTOR
Consult your doctor as soon as possible if:
▲ your child has a fever and seems sick
▲ blisters appear over a large area

What the doctor might do
The doctor may prescribe a soothing and healing cream.

CHAPPED SKIN

What is it?
Chaps are small cracks in the skin that occur when the skin becomes dry after being exposed to cold or hot, dry air. Chapping is not serious, but it can be painful.

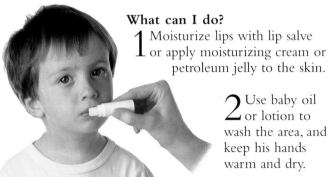

What can I do?
1 Moisturize lips with lip salve or apply moisturizing cream or petroleum jelly to the skin.

2 Use baby oil or lotion to wash the area, and keep his hands warm and dry.

3 If the cracks bleed, put a bandage or gauze pad over them.

SYMPTOMS
▲ Tiny cracks in the skin, usually on or around the lips or on the cheeks or hands
▲ bleeding if the cracks are deep.

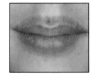

CALL THE DOCTOR
Consult the doctor as soon as possible if:
▲ the cracks do not heal after three days
▲ the cracks become red, sore, or pus-filled.

What the doctor might do
If the chapped area has become infected, the doctor may prescribe an antibiotic. Otherwise there is no treatment.

COLD SORES

What are they?

Cold sores are small blisters, usually on or around the lips but they sometimes develop inside the mouth or elsewhere on the face.

They are caused by a virus which, once it has infected a child, lies dormant in the skin and tends to flare up occasionally, so if your child has had a cold sore, he is liable to get others in the future. Strong sunlight can trigger a recurrence, and so can a minor illness, such as a cold (which is why they are called cold sores).

What can I do?

1 At the first sign of a cold sore, hold an ice cube wrapped in cloth against the affected area for 10 minutes. This may prevent the blister from developing.

Wrap an ice cube *in a cloth and hold it against your child's lip*

2 If your child develops a blister, apply a cream such as petroleum jelly.

3 Keep his hands clean, and stop him from touching the sore, which could spread infection.

4 Since cold sores are very contagious, don't let your child kiss other people, and if he tends to put toys into his mouth, don't let him share them with other children until the sore has gone.

SYMPTOMS

▲ Raised, red area that tingles or itches, usually around the mouth
▲ small, painful yellow blisters forming about a day later
▲ blisters crusting over after a day or two
▲ fever and general illness during the first attack.

5 If your child has ever had a cold sore, protect his lips from strong sunlight with a sunscreen, because sunlight can trigger a recurrence.

CALL THE DOCTOR

Consult your doctor as soon as possible if:
▲ your child has a cold sore for the first time
▲ your child's cold sore starts to ooze or spread
▲ your child has a cold sore near his eyes.

What the doctor might do

The doctor will probably prescribe a cream to be spread over the affected area several times a day, which will help the blister to heal.

WARTS

What are they?

A wart is a lump of hard, dry skin; a plantar wart (verruca) is a wart on the sole of the foot. Warts are caused by a virus that invades the skin, and most children get them occasionally.

Warts are not painful, and disappear spontaneously, usually after a few months, so treatment is not necessary. Plantar warts tend to be painful because of the pressure put on them whenever your child walks or wears shoes, so they should be treated promptly.

SYMPTOMS

Wart
▲ Hard lump of dry skin.

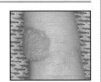

Plantar wart (verruca)
▲ Hard, painful area on the sole of the foot, perhaps with a tiny black center.

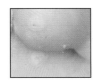

What can I do?

1 If your child has a wart, simply ignore it, unless it is on his genitals or near his anus; in that case call your doctor. It will disappear on its own after a few months, though some last for a year or more.

IMPETIGO

What is it?

Impetigo is a bacterial skin infection that may develop when a rash such as eczema, or a cold sore becomes infected, though healthy skin can sometimes become infected with impetigo. It usually affects the skin around the mouth and nose, but it can occur anywhere on the body. Impetigo isn't a serious disorder in children, but in a young baby it can spread over a large area and make him seriously ill. It is very contagious, so it is important to have it treated promptly.

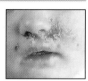

SYMPTOMS

▲ Rash of small red spots
▲ blisters forming over the spots
▲ the spots burst, then form large brownish-yellow scabs
▲ fever and general malaise in a young baby.

What can I do?

1 Keep your child's washcloth and towel separate from those of the rest of the family, and wash them frequently, so the infection doesn't spread.

2 Try to keep your child from touching the affected area—don't let him suck his thumb or pick his nose, because this could spread the infection.

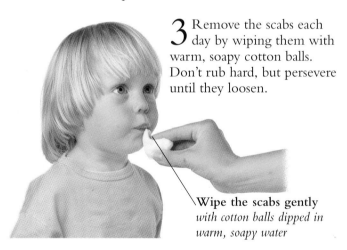

3 Remove the scabs each day by wiping them with warm, soapy cotton balls. Don't rub hard, but persevere until they loosen.

Wipe the scabs gently *with cotton balls dipped in warm, soapy water*

4 Pat the area dry with a tissue or paper towel and throw it away immediately, so that the infection can't spread. After drying, apply an antibiotic ointment.

5 Keep your child away from other children, especially young babies, until he is better.

CALL THE DOCTOR

Call your doctor now if your baby is under three months old and suddenly develops widespread impetigo. Consult your doctor as soon as possible if you think your child has impetigo.

What the doctor might do

The doctor may prescribe oral antibiotics or a cream and tell you to wipe the scabs away (see left). If the infection is still there after five days, consult your doctor again.

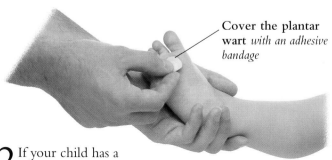

Cover the plantar wart *with an adhesive bandage*

2 If your child has a plantar wart, keep it covered with an adhesive bandage and don't let him go barefoot until it has cleared up. It may disappear spontaneously. Keep his towel and washcloth separate.

CALL THE DOCTOR

Consult your doctor if:
▲ your child's warts multiply
▲ your child has a wart on his genitals or anus
▲ your child has a plantar wart, or verruca.

What the doctor might do

Your doctor may prescribe a lotion to be applied regularly to the wart until it gradually disappears. Alternatively, he may refer your child to a podiatrist or dermatologist to have it burnt or frozen off under local anesthesia.

LICE AND NITS

What are they?
Lice are tiny insects that infest the hair, and make the child's head itchy. Their minute white eggs (nits) cling to the hair roots. Lice spread very easily from one head to another, so treat the whole family if your child picks up lice, and tell your friends to check their children's heads.

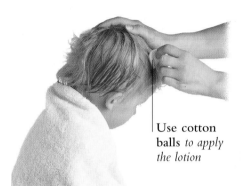

Use cotton balls *to apply the lotion*

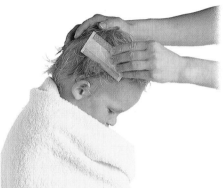

■ SYMPTOMS ■

▲ Itchy head
▲ tiny white grains firmly attached to the hairs near the roots
▲ red bite marks on the scalp.

What can I do?
1 Ask your pharmacist for a lotion or shampoo to kill the lice and nits. Apply it all over your child's head, and leave it on his hair for as long as the instructions specify.

3 Clean your child's brush and comb by covering them with the lotion or shampoo for 15 minutes, then soaking them in rubbing alcohol for 15 minutes before rinsing them.

2 Wash and rinse the hair, then comb it thoroughly with a special fine comb to release the dead lice and nits. You may need to repeat this treatment. Wash all bed linen and hats and vacuum the furniture.

4 If your child goes to a toddler group, nursery school, or child care center, inform the staff that he has lice, and keep him at home until they have been completely eradicated.

PINWORMS

What are they?
Pinworms are tiny, white thread-like worms, about $\frac{1}{2}$ in (1cm) long. They can enter the body in contaminated food, and then live in the bowels, coming out at night to lay eggs around the anus, and causing intense itchiness. They are common in children, and are harmless, though the itching may be extremely uncomfortable. In little girls, the worms may crawl forward to the vagina.

■ SYMPTOMS ■

▲ Intense itching around the anus, which is usually worse at night
▲ intense itching around the vagina
▲ tiny white worms in the stool.

What can I do?
1 Try to prevent your child from scratching, because she might inflame the skin around her anus.

2 Keep her fingernails short so that, if she scratches, she doesn't pick up any eggs under her nails, which could reinfect her or other people.

3 Make sure that the whole family washes their hands thoroughly after going to the bathroom and before eating. Use a nail brush to clean the nails properly.

■ CALL THE DOCTOR ■

Consult your doctor as soon as possible if you think your child has pinworms.

4 If your child no longer wears diapers, make sure she wears pajamas, or cotton underpants under a nightgown. Change her pants and pajama bottoms every day and sterilize them in boiling water to kill any worms or eggs on them. Change her sheets every day and wash and rinse them thoroughly in very hot water.

5 When she feels itchy, lay her across your lap and look for tiny white worms near her anus. Remove any you see with a damp wad of toilet paper and flush them away.

What might the doctor do?
The doctor will probably prescribe a medication for the whole family, which will kill the worms. He may also prescribe a cream for your child to soothe any inflammation around the anus or vagina.

FAINTING, DIZZINESS, AND CONVULSIONS

Even children under three occasionally feel faint or dizzy. Ordinarily this simply means they need food or to be calmed down after a period of intense excitement or anxiety. A convulsion, however, is worrisome and should send you straight to the telephone for a professional opinion.

FAINTING AND DIZZINESS

What is it?
Fainting is a brief loss of consciousness that is usually preceded by your child feeling lightheaded and looking pale. It may follow a bout of dizziness.

CALL THE DOCTOR

Call your doctor now if your child loses consciousness.

---

1 If your child faints, lay him down with his legs higher than his head. Loosen any tight clothing.

2 As he begins to recover, put him into the recovery position (see page 233). If you are outside under hot sun, find a cooler spot. Let him rest for a few minutes. Once he's fully conscious and recovered, offer him something sweet to drink, such as orange juice.

A CONVULSION

What is it?
A convulsion, seizure, or fit is caused by a departure from normality in the electrical activity of the brain. When it accompanies a high fever, it's called a febrile convulsion (see page 188); a tendency to have convulsions when there is no fever is known as epilepsy.

What can I do?
1 Put your child on his side on the floor. Try to make sure he doesn't injure himself, but don't restrain him or put anything in his mouth.

2 After it's over, put your child into the recovery position (see page 233). Don't wake him, but check his breathing. Reduce any fever.

CALL THE DOCTOR

Call your doctor now if your child has a convulsion.

SYMPTOMS

Convulsions (also known as major seizures or grand mal convulsions)
▲ Sudden unconsciousness
▲ eyes rolling back into the head
▲ clenched teeth
▲ shaking spasms in the muscles
▲ wetting the pants, or loss of bowel control
▲ sleeping, or gradual return to consciousness, when the twitching movements stop.

Absence attacks (also known as petit mal convulsions)
▲ Sudden lack of movement
▲ dazed expression
▲ complete recovery in a few seconds.

MENINGITIS

What is it?
Meningitis is an inflammation of the tissues that cover the brain. It is a very serious disease, and must be treated promptly. Inflammation of the brain itself (encephalitis) causes similar symptoms.

CALL THE DOCTOR

Call your doctor now if you think your child may have meningitis or encephalitis.

SYMPTOMS

▲ Fever
▲ listlessness and drowsiness, or sudden irritability
▲ change for the worse in a child who has recently had an infectious illness such as measles or mumps
▲ vomiting
▲ loss of appetite
▲ headache or, in babies, slightly bulging fontanelle
▲ reluctance to bend the neck forward
▲ convulsions.

ELECTRICITY

Electric shocks from any power source can be very serious, so minimize the chances of your child receiving a shock:

- Turn off electrical appliances when you are not using them.
- Never leave a socket switched on with nothing plugged into it.
- Cover unused sockets with childproof socket covers, or mask them with heavy insulating tape.
- Check electrical cords regularly, and repair any with exposed wires.
- Don't let your child play with electrically powered toys until he is at least four.

LIVING ROOM

When you buy upholstered furniture, ask the salesperson about the fabric content. You don't want it to give off toxic fumes if you have a fire. Always use a fireplace screen. Don't let your child touch the back of your television.

Don't leave cigarettes, matches, alcohol, sewing equipment, or coins lying around. Keep indoor plants out of his reach, as some are poisonous.

If you have low glass panels in doors or windows, use toughened, laminated, or wire-net glass, apply a transparent safety film, or put colored stickers on them, so that your child can see where the glass is. Avoid glass-topped tables.

HALL AND STAIRS

Put safety gates at the top and bottom of the stairs before your child can crawl or climb. Make sure that the hall, stairs, and landings are well lit, and that your banisters aren't so wide apart that your child could fall through. Don't leave toys, piles of laundry, or anything else on steps. Make sure that the door knobs and locks are out of his reach or not easily opened. Install smoke detectors.

Repair loose tiles or tears in rugs or flooring, and, if your floors are polished, put a nonslip backing on any rugs. On polished floors, don't let your child wear socks without shoes, and if you let him go barefoot, make sure there are no splinters.

IN THE YARD

Keep an eye on your child when he is playing in the yard, and if you put your baby to sleep outside, have a mosquito net handy to slip over the carriage. Never let your child play in or near a wading pool without an adult supervising him, and empty the pool after use. If you are near a stream or a pond, fence your yard securely. Keep all your walks in good condition—remove weeds regularly so that they don't become slippery in wet weather, and repair walks if they are uneven. Don't let your child play in an area of your yard where you have recently used pesticide, weedkiller, or fertilizer, as these can be poisonous.

CARS

Your child should always travel in a car seat that is officially approved for his age and weight (see page 157). Use the locks on car doors and don't let your child lean out of the window or put his hand out while the car is moving. Never leave your child alone in the car, even if it is only for a moment.

Check where your child is before closing the car door. When you are backing out of a driveway always take note of where your child is. Don't take any chances when he is just behind the car, you won't see him in the rearview mirror.

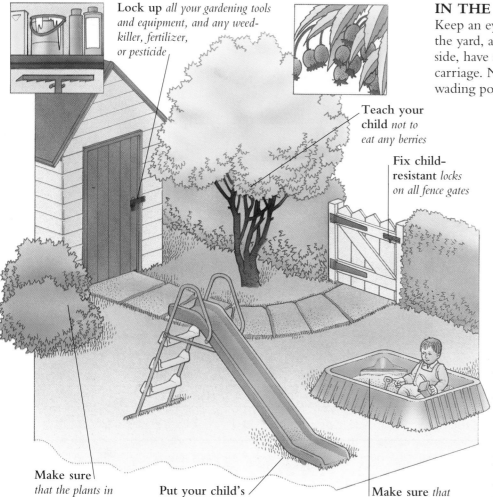

Lock up *all your gardening tools and equipment, and any weed-killer, fertilizer, or pesticide*

Teach your child *not to eat any berries*

Fix child-resistant *locks on all fence gates*

Make sure *that the plants in your garden aren't poisonous, and pull up mushrooms or fungi as soon as they appear*

Put your child's *play equipment on grass or sand, not on a hard surface*

Make sure *that the sand in your child's sandbox is too shallow for him to bury himself and teach him not to throw sand. Cover the sandbox when he is not playing in it*

FIRST AID

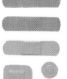

If your child is injured, always treat the most serious injury first. If he is unconscious, check his breathing, and resuscitate him if necessary (see pages 230–32), before giving first aid for any other injury. If he is breathing, first treat anything that might prevent him from breathing properly, such as choking, suffocation, or drowning (see pages 234–35), then control any heavy bleeding (see page 238). If your child is badly injured or in shock, he will need urgent medical treatment, but you should give first aid before calling for medical help. The instructions in this chapter explain how to cope with various injuries and tell you when help is necessary. If you need to get your child to the hospital quickly, it may be faster to take him there yourself, rather than to call for an ambulance, but check this page for occasions when you must call an ambulance.

GETTING YOUR CHILD TO A HOSPITAL
Call for an ambulance, or ask someone else to phone if:
- you think your child might have a spinal injury
- you think he'll need special treatment on the way to the hospital
- you have no suitable transportation of your own.

If you take your child to a hospital yourself, have someone else drive while you sit with your child and continue to give first aid.

If your child is unconscious, don't leave him alone for more than a minute or so while you call for help. If he is not breathing, resuscitate him before phoning for an ambulance. Don't stop until he is breathing again, but shout to other people between breaths if necessary.

WARNING
If there is a chance that your child has injured his neck or spine—for example, after a bad fall—don't move him unless it is absolutely essential. Leave him in whatever position you found him while you check to see if he is breathing. If you need to perform artificial respiration, get someone to help you if possible. Turn your child on his back very gently without twisting his spine—try to hold his head, shoulders, and hips so that his body turns as a single unit.

FIRST AID KIT
Keep a supply of first aid equipment in a clean, dry container, and replace anything you use as soon as possible. Take some antiseptic wipes with you on outings, to clean cuts and scrapes.

Surgical tape This is useful for sticking on bandages, and drawing together the edges of large cuts.

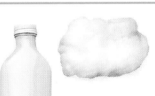

Cotton

Calamine lotion Soothes sunburn, insect bites, and any stings.

Eye bath

Nonadherent, absorbent, sterile gauze bandages These peel off a wound easily.

One elastic bandage

Triangular bandage This can be used to make a sling or secure a dressing.

Scissors

Tweezers

Safety pins

Gauze bandage rolls

Prepared wound dressings These consist of a pad attached to a bandage, and are easy to put on.

Assorted adhesive bandages Use these for dressing minor cuts and scrapes.

LIFESAVING TECHNIQUES

FAMILIARIZE YOURSELF with these instructions so that you can act quickly in an emergency. Every second counts. If your baby or child seems to be unconscious, follow these procedures before treating any injuries. If he has stopped breathing, it is vital to get air into his lungs quickly, so that he doesn't suffer brain damage. By breathing your own air into his lungs, you can prevent this, and revive your child. If his heart has stopped beating, you can pump it manually to keep his blood circulating round his body. Don't give up—children have revived after several hours of resuscitation.

> ### EMERGENCY
> Call for emergency help if your child becomes unconscious, even if this is only for a few seconds.

CHECKING FOR UNCONSCIOUSNESS
Tap the soles of your child's feet, and call his name. Note whether he responds.
Don't shake him, since this could worsen any injuries he may have.

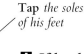

Tap *the soles of his feet*

✚ **If he doesn't respond,** he is unconscious, so check his breathing immediately.

✚ **If he responds,** check for injury and treat any he may have (see pages 234–45).

CHECKING BREATHING

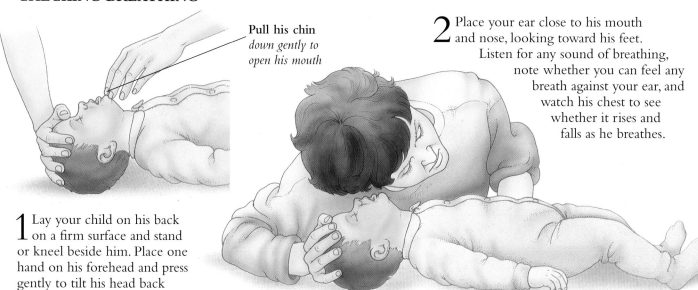

Pull his chin *down gently to open his mouth*

2 Place your ear close to his mouth and nose, looking toward his feet. Listen for any sound of breathing, note whether you can feel any breath against your ear, and watch his chest to see whether it rises and falls as he breathes.

1 Lay your child on his back on a firm surface and stand or kneel beside him. Place one hand on his forehead and press gently to tilt his head back slightly. Open his mouth.

✚ **If there are no signs of breathing,** start artificial respiration immediately (see opposite).

✚ **If your child is breathing,** put him on his side in the recovery position (see page 233) and call for emergency help immediately.

ARTIFICIAL RESPIRATION FOR A BABY

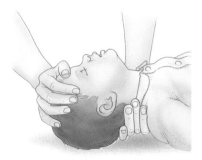

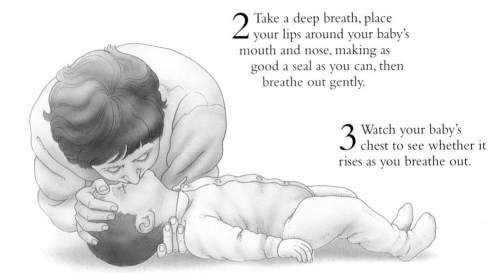

2 Take a deep breath, place your lips around your baby's mouth and nose, making as good a seal as you can, then breathe out gently.

3 Watch your baby's chest to see whether it rises as you breathe out.

1 Slide one hand under your baby's neck, cupping the base of his head, to support him and keep his head tilted back. Leave your other hand on his forehead.

✚ **If his chest doesn't rise,** he probably has something blocking his windpipe. Treat him for choking (see page 234), then continue with artificial respiration if necessary.

✚ **If his chest rises,** remove your mouth from his face and let his chest fall. Give two quick, gentle breaths, then check his heartbeat (see next page).

ARTIFICIAL RESPIRATION FOR A CHILD

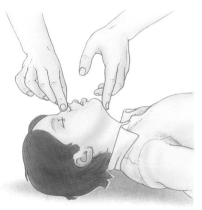

Pinch *his nostrils as you breathe into his mouth*

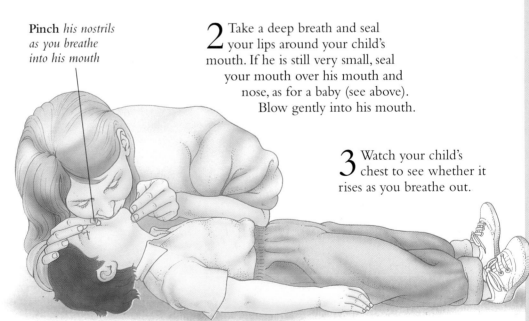

2 Take a deep breath and seal your lips around your child's mouth. If he is still very small, seal your mouth over his mouth and nose, as for a baby (see above). Blow gently into his mouth.

3 Watch your child's chest to see whether it rises as you breathe out.

1 Lift your child's chin to pull his jaw forward. Open his mouth and pinch his nostrils together.

✚ **If his chest doesn't rise,** he probably has something blocking his windpipe. Treat him for choking (see page 234), then continue with artificial respiration if necessary.

✚ **If his chest rises,** remove your mouth from his face and let his chest fall. Give two quick, gentle breaths, then check his heartbeat (see next page).

LIFESAVING TECHNIQUES *continued*

CHECKING PULSE

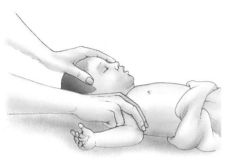

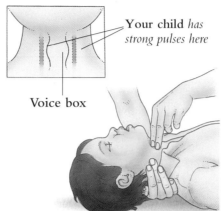

Your child *has strong pulses here*

Voice box

For a baby
Feel the pulse in the baby's armpit by gently pressing on the inside of the arm between shoulder and elbow with index and middle fingers.

For a child over two
Place the pads of two fingers over the voice box at the front of his neck, then slide them into the slight hollow beside this. Feel for five seconds.

For a baby or a child

✚ **If you can't feel a pulse,** his heart may have stopped. Start external chest compression immediately (see below).

✚ **If his heart is beating,** continue breathing gently into his lungs at a rate of about one breath every three seconds, until he starts to breathe on his own, or until emergency help arrives. As soon as he starts to breathe again, turn him on his side in the recovery position (see opposite).

EXTERNAL CHEST COMPRESSION
For a baby

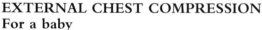

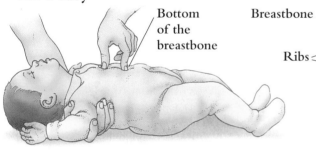

Bottom of the breastbone

Breastbone

Ribs

Press here

You can find *the bottom of the breastbone by feeling where the rib cage forms an inverted V-shape*

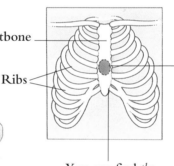

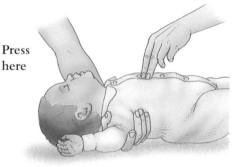

1 Slide one hand under your baby's shoulders and grasp the top of his arm. With your other hand, find the bottom of his breastbone (see right), then measure halfway up to his neck.

2 Place two fingers just below the middle of his breastbone and press down to a depth of about $\frac{1}{2}$–1in (1.5–2.3cm), then release the pressure.

For a child over two

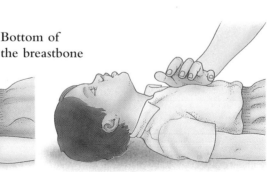

Bottom of the breastbone

1 Find the bottom of your child's breastbone (see diagram above), then measure halfway up to the base of his neck.

2 Place the heel of one hand just below the halfway point and press down to a depth of about 1–1$\frac{1}{2}$in (2.5–3.5cm), then release the pressure.

For a baby or a child

3 Give five compressions at a rate of about two per second, then give a breath into his lungs. Continue with five compressions followed by one breath until his heart starts to beat, or emergency help arrives. Every two or three minutes, check whether he is breathing and whether his heart has started to beat.

4 When his heart starts to beat, stop giving compressions, but continue artificial respiration until he begins to breathe by himself, or help arrives.

THE RECOVERY POSITION

PUT YOUR child into this position if he is unconscious, but breathing. This is the safest position because it prevents his tongue falling back into his throat and obstructing his airway, and avoids the risk of him choking if he vomits.

WARNING

Do not use the recovery position if there is a possibility that your child's neck or spine is damaged, for example, after a bad fall or a car accident.

1 Turn your child's face toward you, keeping his chin pulled forward. Place the arm nearest to you by his side, and tuck his hand under his buttocks, with the palm up. Fold the arm farther from you over his chest, and cross his farther leg over his near leg.

His head *must be turned to one side and tilted well back with the chin jutting forward*

2 Lay a coat or blanket in front of your child, if available. Put one hand by his face to protect it, then grasp his hip with your other hand. Roll him toward you onto the coat or blanket.

3 Make sure that his nose and mouth aren't obstructed, then bend his top arm and leg up to a right angle, so that they support him. Gently pull his lower arm out from under his hip, and leave it by his side.

4 Cover him with a coat or blanket, then call for emergency help. Stay with him until help arrives, and every three minutes check his breathing and his heartbeat (see opposite), if his heart had stopped.

CHOKING

This happens when a small object or piece of food gets lodged in the windpipe, causing a coughing fit. It is important to dislodge the object quickly, so that your child can breathe properly again. Choking is common in very young children, who tend to put everything they get hold of into their mouths. They may find it hard to swallow dry, crumbly foods, so avoid them if possible.

<table>
<tr><td>

EMERGENCY

Call for emergency help immediately if:
▲ your child stops breathing
▲ you cannot remove the blockage
▲ your child continues to choke after you have removed the blockage.
</td></tr>
</table>

HELPING A BABY

1 Hold your baby face down with his head lower than his body and support him along your forearm. Support his head by firmly holding his jaw and rest your forearm on your thigh. Using the heel of your hand, strike your baby between the shoulder blades five times.

2 If he is still choking, place your free arm along his back so that your hand holds his head. One hand should support your baby's head, neck, jaw, and chest while the other supports his back. Turn him over so that he lies draped over your thigh with his head lower than the rest of his body.

3 Do five quick chest thrusts using the same finger position as outlined for chest compressions (see page 232). Repeat back blows and chest compressions alternately until the blockage is removed.

4 If your baby does not start breathing normally when the blockage is removed, carry out artificial respiration immediately (see pages 231–32).

HELPING A CHILD

1 Stay with your child and encourage her to cough up the obstruction. Do not interfere unless her cough becomes weak, or she emits a high-pitched crowing noise when she breathes. Should that happen, tell her that you are going to help her.

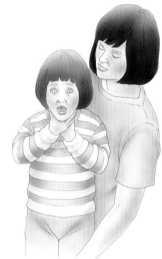

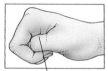

Tuck your thumb *in when you make a fist*

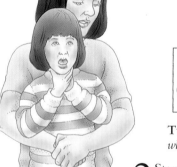

2 Stand behind her, or in the case of a small child, kneel behind her and wrap your arms around her waist. Make a fist and place it, thumb side in, against the child's tummy, above the navel (but well below the breastbone), and using your other hand to exert pressure, quickly press your fist inward and upward into the child's abdomen.

3 Each inward and upward thrust should be a separate, distinct movement. Continue performing thrusts until the obstruction is cleared or the child loses consciousness.

4 If your child does not start breathing normally when the blockage is removed, carry out artificial respiration (see pages 231–32).

SUFFOCATION

Anything lying across your child's face may block her mouth and nose, and prevent her from breathing.

What can I do?

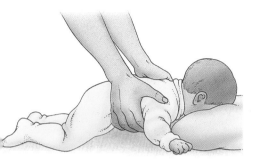

1 Pick your child up or remove whatever is covering her face.

2 Check to see if your child is conscious and breathing (see page 230).

✚ **If she is not breathing,** start artificial respiration immediately (see pages 231–32) and ask someone to call for emergency help.

✚ **If she is breathing but un-conscious,** place her in the recovery position (see page 233), then call for emergency help.

✚ **If she is conscious,** simply comfort and reassure her.

DROWNING

Babies and children can drown in very shallow water. When a young child's face is submerged, his automatic reaction is to take a deep breath to scream, rather than to lift his face up out of the water.

What can I do?
Make sure that your child is conscious and breathing (see page 230). If he is coughing, choking, or vomiting, he is still breathing. If there is any chance that he has injured his neck or back, lift him very gently and be careful not to twist his spine.

✚ **If he is not breathing,** don't waste time trying to drain the water from his lungs. Clear any debris, such as mud or seaweed, from his mouth and start artificial respiration (see pages 231–32) right away— if possible while he is still being carried from the water—and **call for emergency help.** Continue artificial respiration until help arrives or until he starts to breathe again. When he starts to breathe again, put him in the recovery position (see page 233).

Clear any debris *from his mouth with your finger*

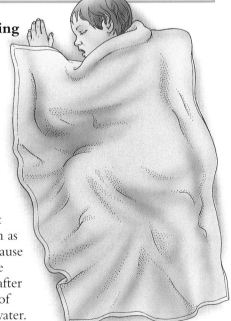

✚ **If he is breathing but unconscious,** place him in the recovery position (see page 233) so that water can drain from his mouth and lungs, and **call for emergency help immediately**. Cover him with a coat or blanket to keep him warm. Get him to a warm room as soon as you can, because he may have become dangerously chilled after even a short period of immersion in cold water.

✚ **If he is conscious,** simply comfort and reassure him, and make sure he keeps warm.

SHOCK

A life-threatening state of collapse, when blood pressure falls dangerously low, shock is a reaction to any severe injury, especially one in which your child has been badly burned or suffered heavy bleeding.

What can I do?

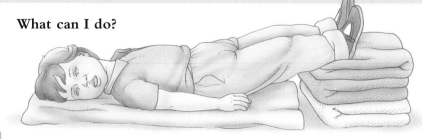

1 Lay your child down on her back, if possible on a coat or blanket. Turn her head to one side, then raise her feet about 8in (20cm) and rest them on something, such as a pile of clothes or a bag.
Don't raise her legs if she has a broken leg or a poisonous bite on her leg.

2 Cover her with a blanket or coat, or cuddle her, to keep her warm.
Don't try to warm her up with a hot water bottle or an electric blanket—this only draws blood away from the vital body organs to the skin.

3 If she complains of thirst, moisten her lips with a damp cloth.
Don't give her anything to eat or drink. There is one exception to this—you can give sips of water to your child if she has been badly burned.

4 If she becomes unconscious, check her breathing (see page 230).

✚ **If she is not breathing,** start artificial respiration (see pages 231–32).

✚ **If she is breathing,** put her into the recovery position (see page 233).

SYMPTOMS

▲ Pale, cold, sweaty skin
▲ blue or grayish tinge inside the lips or under the fingernails
▲ rapid and shallow breathing
▲ restlessness
▲ drowsiness or confusion
▲ unconsciousness.

EMERGENCY

Call for emergency help immediately if your child is in shock.

POISONING

Poisoning is one of the most common emergencies in young children. Keep poisonous substances locked up, and post the number of the nearest Poison Control Center by your telephone. Never hesitate to call.

What can I do?
1 If your child is unconscious, check his breathing (see page 230).

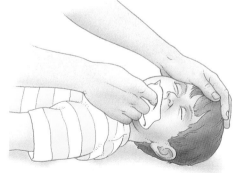

✚ **If he is not breathing,** start artificial respiration immediately (see pages 231–32), but wipe his face first (see above) or place a fine cloth over his mouth and breathe through that, to avoid getting any poison into your own mouth.

✚ **If he is breathing,** put him into the recovery position (see page 233).

EMERGENCY

Call for emergency help immediately if you think your child has swallowed something poisonous.

2 If you see signs of burning around your child's mouth, or think he has swallowed a chemical product, wash his skin and lips with water. If he is conscious and able to breathe and swallow, give him some milk or water to drink.

3 If the doctor recommends that you induce vomiting—**always check first**—use one tablespoon of ipecac syrup for a baby or young child and two for a child over 12 years. Ipecac may not be recommended if the poison is very caustic.

4 If your child vomits, save a sample for medical personnel. If he isn't able to vomit, he may have his stomach emptied at the hospital.

SYMPTOMS

Your child's symptoms will depend on the type of poison he has swallowed. You may notice any of these signs:
▲ stomach pain
▲ vomiting
▲ symptoms of shock (see above)
▲ convulsions
▲ drowsiness
▲ unconsciousness
▲ burns or discoloration around the mouth if your child has swallowed a corrosive poison
▲ poison or empty container nearby.

BURNS AND SCALDS

A small, superficial burn that causes reddening of the skin over an area of about 1in (2–3cm) is a minor burn, and can safely be treated at home. A burn that affects an area greater than this is a major burn, and is dangerous for your child, since fluid is lost from the damaged area and infection can enter it. For sunburn, see page 221.

MINOR BURNS
What can I do?

1 Cool the burn immediately, by holding it under cold, slowly running water until the pain decreases. This will help to prevent blisters from developing.

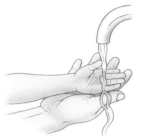

2 If a blister develops, put a pad of clean, non-fluffy material over it and hold it in place with adhesive bandages or surgical tape.
Don't burst the blister—it protects the damaged area underneath while the new skin is growing.
Don't put any cream or lotion on the burn.

BURNING CLOTHES
What can I do?

1 Lay your child on the ground with the burning area up. Avoid touching the burning area with your hands or your own clothes, if possible.

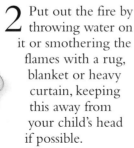

2 Put out the fire by throwing water on it or smothering the flames with a rug, blanket or heavy curtain, keeping this away from your child's head if possible.
Don't throw water over him if he is near an electrical appliance that is turned on.
Don't try to smother the flames with nylon or any other flammable fabric.
Don't let him rush outside—air will only fan the flames.

3 When the flames are out, treat your child for a major burn (see right).

MAJOR BURNS
What can I do?

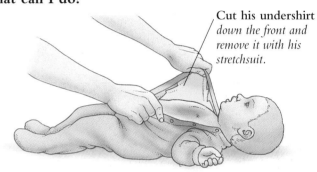

Cut his undershirt *down the front and remove it with his stretchsuit.*

1 Remove any loose clothing that has been soaked in boiling water, fat, or corrosive chemicals, taking care not to let it touch your child's skin anywhere else. Cut his clothes off rather than pull them over his face.
Don't remove dry, burnt clothing, or any clothing that is sticking to the burn.

2 Cool the burn immediately by drenching it with cold water: put your child in a cold bath or soak a sheet or towel in cold water and cover the burn with this.
Don't rub his skin.

✚ **If chemicals have burnt his skin,** wash them off with plenty of cold water, but **don't** let the water run onto unharmed areas.

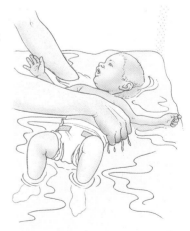

3 Cover the area very loosely with a clean, non-fluffy material. If you don't have a sterile dressing, an ironed handkerchief or pillowcase will do.

4 Check for symptoms of shock, and treat your child for this if necessary (see opposite). If he complains of being thirsty, give him sips of water.

HEAVY BLEEDING

If blood spurts forcefully from a wound, or bleeding continues for more than five minutes, try to stem the flow so that the blood has a chance to clot.

What can I do?

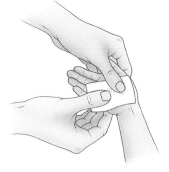

1 Raise the injured part above the level of your child's heart, to reduce the amount of blood flowing through it. Check for embedded objects in the wound; if there are any, treat them as described below.

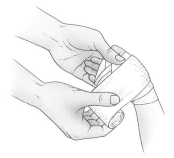

2 Place a pad of clean, non-fluffy material over the wound—a clean handkerchief or dishtowel is ideal—then press hard on it for about 10 minutes. If there is no clean material available, press with your fingers, drawing the edges of the cut firmly together.

3 Leaving the original pad in place, bind a clean pad or dressing firmly over the wound so that the pressure is maintained. If this becomes soaked with blood, don't remove it, just bandage another pad over it, maintaining the pressure all the time.

4 Check for symptoms of shock (see page 236), and treat your child for this if necessary.

EMERGENCY

Get your child professional medical help as soon as you have given first aid if he's been bleeding heavily.

EMBEDDED OBJECTS

Small pieces of dirt in a cut will probably be washed out by bleeding, and larger pieces may wipe easily off the surface of the wound. However, if your child has something embedded in a wound, treat it as shown below.

What can I do?

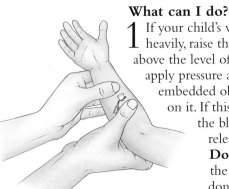

1 If your child's wound is bleeding heavily, raise the injured part above the level of his heart and apply pressure around the embedded object, not directly on it. If this seems to make the bleeding worse, release the pressure. **Don't** try to pull the object out and don't probe or try to clean the wound.

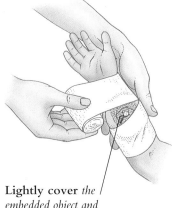

Lightly cover the embedded object and the fabric ring with a piece of gauze

2 Release the pressure for a moment, and roll up a small piece of material, such as a clean handkerchief, into a sausage shape, then twist this into a ring.

3 Place the ring of material round the cut and cover it with gauze, then bandage it in place firmly. **Don't** bandage tightly *over* the embedded object.

EMERGENCY

Get your child professional medical help as soon as you have given first aid if he has an embedded object.

CUTS AND SCRAPES

Cuts and scrapes are common throughout childhood, and you can treat most of them yourself at home. Keep your child's tetanus injections up to date (see page 196), since tetanus can result from dirt entering a wound. Treat an animal bite as a cut, but if your child has a poisonous bite or sting, see page 244.

EMERGENCY

Call your pediatrician and get your child professional medical help as soon as you have given first aid if:
▲ the cut is large or deep
▲ the cut has gaping edges
▲ your child has cut his face badly
▲ the cut or scrape is very dirty
▲ your child has a puncture wound (a deep cut with only a small opening in the skin) caused by something dirty such as a rusty nail or an animal's tooth.
Consult your doctor as soon as possible if the area around the wound later becomes tender and red—it may be infected.

What can I do?

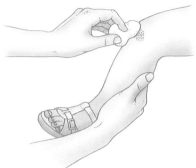

1 Wash your hands first, if possible. Clean the cut by holding it under running water, or wiping gently around it with an antiseptic swab or cotton soaked in warm water. Use a clean ball or piece of cotton for each stroke.
Don't remove anything that is embedded in the cut (see opposite).

✚ **If your child has been bitten by an animal,** wash the wound thoroughly with soap and water.

2 If the cut is still bleeding after five minutes, press a pad such as a clean handkerchief firmly on it for a few minutes.

3 Put an adhesive bandage or dressing over it, to help protect it and keep it clean. **Don't** put any antiseptic ointment on your child's cut.

4 Keep the cut covered with an adhesive bandage or a dressing until it has completely healed. This ensures that the area remains clean, and helps the cut heal more quickly. Change the bandage every day.

NOSEBLEEDS

Nosebleeds can result from a bump on the nose, nose-picking, or excessive nose-blowing. Sometimes there is no apparent reason for them. A few children seem prone to nosebleeds, probably because they have unusually fragile blood vessels in their noses.

CALL THE DOCTOR

Call your doctor now if your child's nose is still bleeding just as badly after half an hour. Consult your doctor if your child has frequent, severe nosebleeds.

What can I do?

1 Help your child to lean forward over a bowl or sink, and pinch her nostrils firmly at the point below the bone for about ten minutes. Try to stop her from sniffing or swallowing the blood—encourage her to spit it out instead.

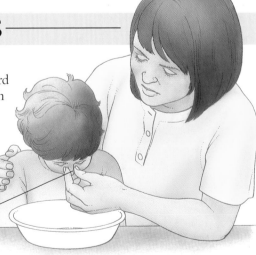

Pinch *your child's nostrils firmly*

2 If her nose is still bleeding, hold a cloth wrung out in very cold water, or an ice pack wrapped in a cloth, over her nose for about two minutes, then pinch her nose again.

3 Don't have your child blow her nose for about four hours after the bleeding has stopped.

HEAD AND FACE INJURY

Bumps on the head are common in young children and may raise a sizeable bruise, but are seldom serious. A cut on the forehead or scalp, however small, is likely to bleed profusely.

If your child has had a severe blow to her head, she may suffer from a concussion, or loss of consciousness. All people must receive medical attention after a concussion. The resulting injuries, such as potential bleeding or bruising to the brain, may not be apparent for several hours. Signs of these injuries are listed below.

■ EMERGENCY ■

Call for emergency help immediately if your child has injured her head and shows any unusual behavior or has any of these symptoms up to 24 hours later:

▲ unconsciousness, however brief
▲ vomiting
▲ noisy breathing or snoring, if your child doesn't normally snore
▲ difficulty in waking, or abnormal drowsiness
▲ discharge of clear or blood-stained fluid from her nose or ear (see point 4 in right column)
▲ unusual crying
▲ severe headache
▲ dislike of bright light.

BROKEN TEETH
If your child has broken a tooth, or one has become dislodged, cover the tooth or broken piece with milk, and take your child and her tooth to your dentist or to the hospital immediately.

What can I do?

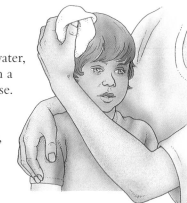

1 If your child's head is bruised, hold a cloth wrung out in very cold water, or an ice pack wrapped in a damp cloth, over the bruise. This may stop it from swelling. Check the skin underneath every minute, and remove the pack if a red patch with a white waxy center develops.

2 If your child's head is bleeding, place a clean cloth over the cut and press on it, just as you would for bleeding anywhere else on the body (see page 238).

3 Watch your child carefully for the next 24 hours, in case she develops any of the emergency signs listed in the box, left. If she bumped her head badly, wake her every three hours. If she won't wake up, **call for emergency help immediately**.

4 If a discharge of clear or blood-stained fluid trickles from your child's nose or ear, put her into the recovery position with a pad of clean material placed under her nose or ear. If the fluid is coming from her ear, lay her on the injured side, so that the fluid can drain away. **Don't** stop it from trickling out.

BRUISES AND SWELLING

A bruise appears when a fall or blow causes bleeding into the tissues beneath the skin, which produces swelling and discoloration. Bruises normally fade gradually, and disappear after about a week.

CRUSHED FINGERS AND TOES
If your child has crushed his fingers in a door or window, or dropped something heavy on his foot, hold the injured area under cold running water for a few minutes. If it is very swollen, or still painful after half an hour, get professional medical help.

What can I do?

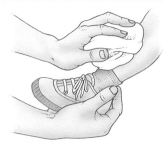

1 Hold a pad wrung out in very cold water, or an ice pack wrapped in a damp cloth, over the bruise for about half an hour. This should help to reduce pain and swelling.

2 If your child seems to be in great pain or if it hurts him to use a bruised limb, especially if the swelling is severe, check for any signs of a sprained joint or a broken bone (see opposite).

SPRAINED JOINTS

When a joint is sprained, the ligaments (tough fibers that support the joint) are damaged. This can cause symptoms very like those of a broken bone: if you are not sure which it is, treat it as a broken bone (see below).

What can I do?

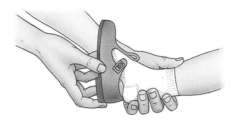

Rest the injured joint on some soft material

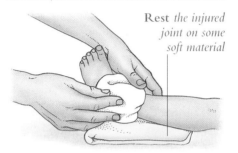

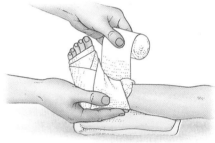

1 Gently take off your child's shoe and sock, or anything else that might constrict swelling around the injured joint.

2 Support the injured joint in the most comfortable position for your child, then hold a cloth wrung out in ice-cold water, or an ice pack wrapped in a damp cloth, on the joint, to reduce swelling and pain.

3 Wrap a thick layer of cotton around the joint, then bandage it firmly, but not so tightly that the beds of his toenails (or fingernails if bandaging a wrist) turn white or pale blue. Keep the joint elevated to reduce swelling.

FRACTURES AND DISLOCATED JOINTS

Broken bones are unusual in babies and young children: their bones have not yet hardened, so they are flexible and tend to bend rather than break. Sometimes there may be a partial break, which mends easily (often called a "greenstick" fracture). A joint is dislocated if one or more bones have slipped out of place.

If you think your child's neck or back might be broken, do not move him or change his position unless he stops breathing (see pages 229–30).

What can I do?

1 Gently take off your child's shoe and sock, or anything else that might constrict swelling around the injured area.
Don't move him unless it is absolutely essential.

2 Support the injured part in the most comfortable position for your child.
For a broken wrist, arm, or collar bone, put padding around the injured area and, if your child will let you, gently fold his arm across his chest, then support it in a sling. Don't try to force his arm into this position.

Tie the bandages on the uninjured side

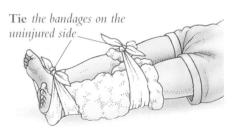

For a broken leg or ankle, lay your child down and put padding around the injured area and between his knees and ankles. Bandage the injured leg to the uninjured one, securing it above and below the injury. Put some padding under the knots.

3 Check for symptoms of shock and treat him for this if necessary (see page 236). If you think he has a broken leg, don't raise his legs.

FOREIGN BODY IN THE EYE

Eyelashes or particles of dust can easily get into the eye. If your child's eye seems irritated but you can't see anything in it, she may have an eye infection (see page 202).

(see page 202)

SYMPTOMS

▲ Pain in the eye
▲ red, watering eye
▲ your child may rub her eye.

CHEMICALS IN THE EYE

If your child splashes chemicals or corrosive fluids in her eyes, wash them out immediately under cold running water for five to ten minutes. Keep her eyelids apart with your fingers. If only one eye is affected, tilt her head so that the injured eye is lower, and the chemical cannot wash over into the uninjured one. Then cover the eye with a pad and take your child to a hospital. If possible, take the chemical bottle with you.

What can I do?

1 Wait a few minutes to see if the natural watering of the eye washes the foreign body away. Try to stop your child from rubbing her eye.

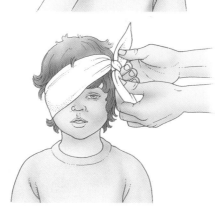

2 If the object is still there, examine your child's eye under a good light. Ask her to look up while you pull her lower eyelid gently down with your thumb.

3 If you can see the object on the white part of your child's eye, try to remove it by sweeping across it very gently with the corner of a clean handkerchief or a piece of damp, twisted cotton.

4 If you can't see anything, hold the eyelashes and draw the upper lid gently outward and down over the lower lid. If the object is under the upper lid, this may dislodge it.

5 If your child's eye still feels gritty or painful, or if the object is not on the white of the eye, or not easily removable, cover the eye with a pad of cotton secured with a bandage and seek professional medical care. Try to stop her from rubbing her eye.
Don't try to remove anything on the central colored part of the eye, or anything that is embedded in the white of the eye.

FOREIGN BODY IN THE EAR

Insects may crawl into your child's ear, and children sometimes push small objects into their ears. Don't let your child play with beads, marbles, or similar small objects until he is old enough to understand that they should not be put into his ears.

What can I do?

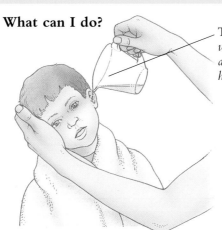

Tip the container *very gently, so just a few drops go into his ear*

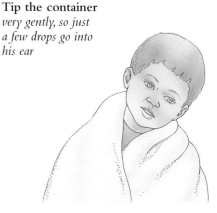

SYMPTOMS

▲ Tickling in the ear
▲ partial deafness
▲ your child may rub or tug at his ear.

1 Put a towel around your child's shoulders, then hold his head on one side, with the affected ear on top, and pour a few drops of lukewarm water into his ear.

2 Tip his head the other way, so that the affected ear is underneath. The water may wash out whatever was in his ear. If this doesn't work, seek professional medical attention for him.

FOREIGN BODY IN THE NOSE

Children sometimes stuff small pieces of food or other objects such as beads up their noses.

■ SYMPTOMS ■

▲ Smelly, blood-stained discharge from the nose.

What can I do?
If your child can blow his nose, help him to blow it, one nostril at a time. If this does not dislodge the object, don't try to remove it yourself—get professional medical help right away.

ELECTRIC SHOCK

A mild electrical shock gives only a brief pins and needles sensation. A severe one can knock your child down, render her unconscious, and stop both breathing and heartbeat. Electric current can also burn.

If your child touches a faulty appliance with wet hands, she will get a worse shock than touching it with dry hands.

■ EMERGENCY ■

Get your child to the hospital as soon as you have given first aid if:
▲ she was unconscious, even if only for a few seconds
▲ she has any electrical burns.

ELECTRICAL BURNS

Electricity can burn where the current enters the body and where it leaves, so your child may have burns where she touched the electrical source and anywhere that was in contact with the ground. Although these burns may look small, they are often very deep.

What can I do?

1 Turn off the electricity, at the source.

✚ **If you can't do this,** stand on an insulating material—such as a rubber mat or a pile of dry newspaper. Separate your child from the electrical source by pushing the cable or your child away, using some dry, non-metal object such as a wooden chair or broom handle.

✚ **If nothing is available,** drag your child away, insulating your hand as much as you can by wrapping it in a dry cloth or newspaper. Grasp your child's clothes, and avoid touching her skin.

Move *the cable rather than your child's arm*

2 Check to see if your child is conscious (see page 230).

✚ **If she is unconscious,** check her breathing: start artificial respiration immediately if necessary (see pages 231–32). If she is breathing, put her in the recovery position (see page 233).

✚ **If she is conscious,** comfort and reassure her. Look for symptoms of shock (see page 236).

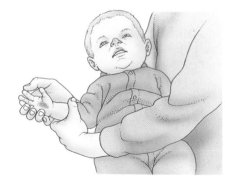

3 Examine her for any burns: check areas that were in contact with the electrical source or the ground (burns will look red or scorched, and may swell up). If you find any, treat them as major burns (see page 237).

INSECT BITES AND STINGS

Most plants, insects, and jellyfish cause only minor stings which, while they may be painful, are not dangerous for your child. However, a few people develop a serious allergic reaction to stings, and therefore need urgent medical treatment.

■ SYMPTOMS ■

▲ Sharp pain
▲ redness
▲ slight swelling
▲ itching.

■ EMERGENCY ■

Get your child to a hospital emergency room as soon as you have given first aid if he:
▲ has difficulty breathing
▲ develops a widespread rash
▲ feels dizzy or faints
▲ develops symptoms of shock (see page 236)
▲ has a sting inside his mouth.

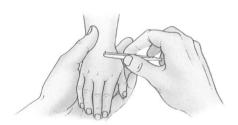

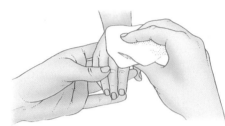

What can I do?

1 If your child has been stung by a bee, see if the stinger has been left in the skin. Scrape it off with a fingernail or credit card, or pull it out with tweezers. If the tiny sac of poison is still intact, try not to squeeze it.

2 Hold a cloth wrung out in ice-cold water over the sting.

If he has been stung in his mouth, give him a cold drink or, if he is over two, let him suck an ice cube. This helps to reduce swelling.

3 Soothe the area around the sting, which will quickly become red, swollen, and itchy, by dabbing it gently with cotton balls dipped in calamine lotion. If itching is trouble-some, ask your pharmacist about an over-the-counter oral antihistamine.

SNAKE AND SPIDER BITES, SCORPION STINGS

Bites from snakes and poisonous spiders, and scorpion stings are always serious for young children. Snake bites carry a risk of tetanus, but your child can be vaccinated against this (see page 196).

Ask your pediatrician for inform-ation about local varieties of snakes, spiders, or scorpions.

■ SYMPTOMS ■

Your child's symptoms will de-pend on what has bitten or stung him; some symptoms may not appear for a few hours:
▲ severe pain
▲ one or two puncture marks
▲ swelling
▲ nausea or vomiting
▲ difficulty breathing
▲ shock (see page 236)
▲ convulsions
▲ drowsiness
▲ unconsciousness.

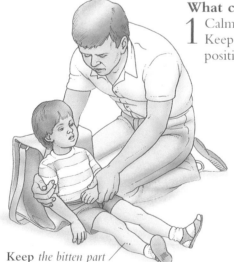

Keep *the bitten part lower than his heart*

■ EMERGENCY ■

Get your child to a hospital as soon as you have given first aid if he has been bitten by a snake or spider, or stung by a scorpion.

What can I do?

1 Calm your child, and help him to sit down. Keep the bitten or stung part still, and position it below the level of his heart.

2 Wash thoroughly around the area, but **don't** suck out any poison.

3 Check for shock, and treat your child for this if necessary (see page 236). If he was bitten or stung on his leg or foot, don't raise his legs.

4 If he becomes unconscious, check his breathing (see page 230).

If he is not breathing, start arti-ficial respiration (see pages 231-32).

If he is breathing, put him into the recovery position (see page 233).

5 Try to identify the snake, spider, or scorpion. If it has been caught, show it to the doctor.

244

SEVERE JELLYFISH STINGS

The type of jellyfish most likely to give you or your child a severe sting is the Portuguese man-of-war. This gelatinous, pale marine creature has tentacles that can be as long as 50 feet and doesn't just live in waters near Portugal. Its sting feels like a hot iron and will make your child very sick.

SYMPTOMS

▲ Burning pain
▲ redness
▲ shortness of breath
▲ fainting.

What can I do?

1 Use wet sand to scrape off any tentacles still stuck to her skin, but avoid touching the tentacles yourself. Make a paste from either meat tenderizer (papain) or baking soda and apply it to the affected area.

2 Put your child into the recovery position (see page 233) and cover her.

EMERGENCY

Get professional medical help as soon as you have given first aid if she has a jellyfish sting.

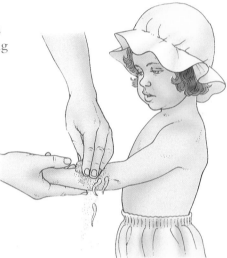

THORNS AND SPLINTERS

Thorns or tiny splinters in a child's hands or feet are quite common. Those on your child's feet may not hurt, but splinters in the tips of his fingers will.

CALL THE DOCTOR

Consult your doctor as soon as possible if:
▲ the area around a splinter becomes red, swollen, or tender up to 48 hours later
▲ you cannot remove a large or painful splinter
▲ your child has a splinter of glass or metal.

What can I do?

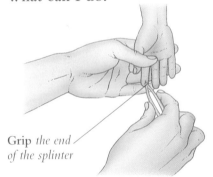

Grip *the end of the splinter*

1 If the end of the splinter is sticking out, sterilize a pair of tweezers in a flame, then pull the splinter straight out gently. Wash the area thoroughly with soap and water.

2 If there is no loose end, but you can see the splinter clearly, it is probably lying just below the surface of the skin. Sterilize a needle in a flame and let it cool, but don't touch the point. Then, starting where the splinter entered, gently tear the skin a little way along the line of the splinter. Carefully lift up the end of the splinter with the needle point and pull it out with tweezers, then wash the area thoroughly with soap and water.

3 If a small splinter has gone straight down into the skin, and is not painful, leave it alone. It will probably work its own way out in time. If your child is in pain, call your pediatrician.

BLISTERS

Blisters form when burns, scalds, or friction damage the skin. The fluid-filled blister protects the new skin forming underneath. It will peel off of its own accord in a few days.

What can I do?

1 Don't burst or prick the blister. Dress your child in clothes that will not rub against it.

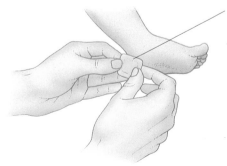

Cover the blister *with an adhesive bandage to prevent your child's shoe from rubbing it*

2 If the blister bursts, leave it uncovered, unless it is likely to be exposed to further friction (for example, if it is on your child's foot). In this case, protect the blister with an adhesive bandage.

GROWTH CHARTS

GIRLS

THE CHARTS BELOW show average growth in children (the solid line), and the range of normal measurements. You can check your baby's progress by weighing and measuring her regularly. The pediatrician will do this, but you too can mark her growth curves on the charts. A healthy rate of growth is indicated by the shape of the average curve.

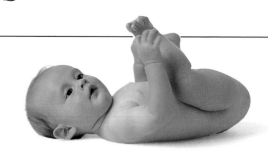

GIRL BABY'S HEAD CIRCUMFERENCE

ins / cms — Age in months

/ average

range of measurements likely in a normal child; 94% of girls fall within this area

HEAD CIRCUMFERENCE
Your pediatrician will measure this for you (see page 81). During the first year of life, head circumference and height are equally essential as yardsticks of healthy growth.

ROUGH GUIDE TO CLOTHES SIZES

Size	Weight
0 to 3 months, infant	up to 13lbs
3 to 6 months	14 to 18lbs
6 to 12 months	19 to 22lbs
12 to 18 months	23 to 25lbs
18 to 24 months	26 to 28lbs

Buy clothing according to the weight marked on it, rather than the age, if you can. After age two, manufacturers often call sizes Toddler, or "T".

GIRL CHILD'S HEIGHT

ins / cms — Age in months

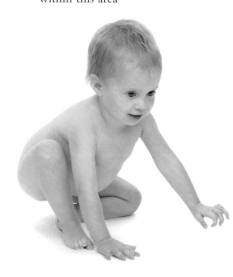

YOUR CHILD'S HEIGHT
About every six months measure your child standing up against the same wall. She should stand close to it, without shoes and with feet together. Use a ruler at right angles to the wall to mark her height lightly in pencil, then measure from mark to floor. Don't worry if she has periods of slow growth interspersed with spurts; but if two consecutive measurements seem very low, ask your doctor about it.

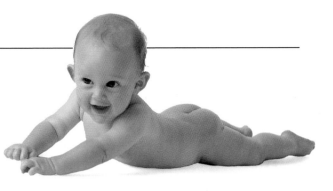

GIRL CHILD'S HEIGHT

Age in months

lbs / kgs

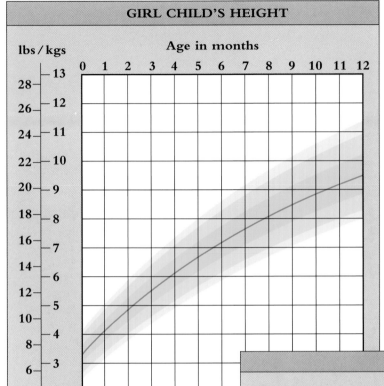

YOUR BABY'S WEIGHT

Your baby's weight is a vital indicator of his general health and well being through the first year. Your pediatrician will weigh him once a month and more often if you are at all worried that he might not be gaining normally.

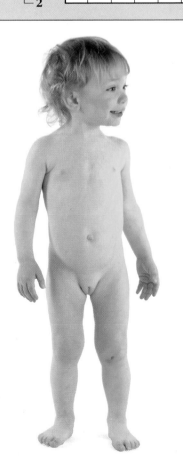

GIRL CHILD'S WEIGHT

Age in months

lbs / kgs

YOUR CHILD'S WEIGHT

After his first birthday, your child won't put weight on steadily, but the periods of slow and rapid growth should balance out. He shouldn't lose weight: even if he looks fat to you, it won't be long before his height catches up to his weight and he slims down. Ask your doctor for advice if your child's weight drops, or if you are worried about him gaining too much too fast.

GROWTH CHARTS

─ BOYS ─

THE CHARTS BELOW show average growth in children (the solid line), and the range of normal measurements. You can check your baby's progress by weighing and measuring him regularly. The pediatrician will do this, but you too can mark his growth curves on the charts. A healthy rate of growth is indicated by the shape of the average curve.

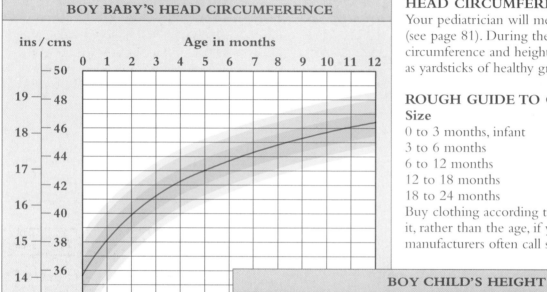

BOY BABY'S HEAD CIRCUMFERENCE

ins / cms   Age in months

HEAD CIRCUMFERENCE

Your pediatrician will measure this for you (see page 81). During the first year of life, head circumference and height are equally essential as yardsticks of healthy growth.

ROUGH GUIDE TO CLOTHES SIZES

Size	Weight
0 to 3 months, infant	up to 13lbs
3 to 6 months	14 to 18lbs
6 to 12 months	19 to 22lbs
12 to 18 months	23 to 25lbs
18 to 24 months	26 to 28lbs

Buy clothing according to the weight marked on it, rather than the age, if you can. After age two, manufacturers often call sizes Toddler, or "T".

/ average

☐ range of measurements likely in a normal child; 94% of boys fall within this area

BOY CHILD'S HEIGHT

ins / cms   Age in months

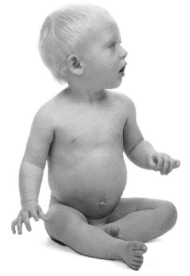

YOUR CHILD'S HEIGHT

About every six months measure your child standing up against the same wall. He should stand close to it, without shoes and with feet together. Use a ruler at right angles to the wall to mark his height lightly in pencil, then measure from mark to floor. Don't worry if he has periods of slow growth interspersed with spurts; but if two consecutive measurements seem very low, ask your doctor about it.

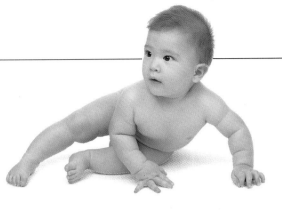

BOY BABY'S WEIGHT

lbs / kgs   **Age in months**

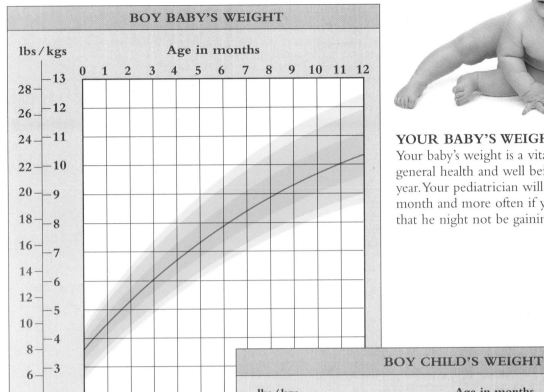

YOUR BABY'S WEIGHT

Your baby's weight is a vital indicator of his general health and well being through the first year. Your pediatrician will weigh him once a month and more often if you are at all worried that he night not be gaining normally.

BOY CHILD'S WEIGHT

lbs / kgs   **Age in months**

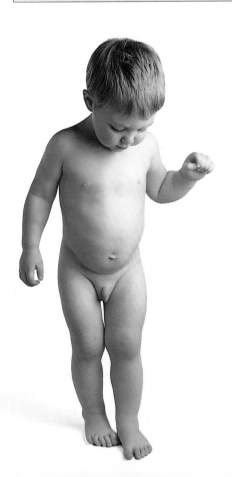

YOUR CHILD'S WEIGHT

After his first birthday, your child won't put weight on steadily, but the periods of slow and rapid growth should balance out. He shouldn't lose weight: even if he looks fat to you, it won't be long before his height catches up to his weight and he slims down. Ask your doctor for advice if your child's weight drops, or if you are worried about him gaining too much too fast.

INDEX

ACKNOWLEDGMENTS

DORLING KINDERSLEY would like to thank **Elizabeth Fenwick**, the author of the English edition, for all the work she put into writing the book; and the following for their design and editorial work on the original edition: Rowena Alsey, Carole Ash, Tina Hill, Tanya Hines, Claire Le Bas, Sarah Pearce, and Daphne Razazan.

Special photography
(numbers indicate pages; t=top, b=below, c=center, l=left, r=right)

Andy Crawford assisted by Gary Ombler: 25, 29t, 53t, 85, 88tr, 106t, 118, 119, 147, 186br, 191tl, 216;

Antonia Deutsch assisted by Pamela Cowan: 2tl, 6: 1st column, 11–13, 17, 19, 21, 27, 29b, 37–42, 43t, 44–49, 56t and br, 57–61, 64, 67, 71–73, 90tr and br, 91tl, tc, and cr, 92bl and br, 94, 95 all except bl, 96, 97;

Dave King: 2cl, 4: 1st column pictures 2–4, 2nd column pictures 1–4; 6: 2nd column t and lower c, 7: 1st column, 2nd column all except bl, 89, 32t, 50–52, 53b, 54 tr and c, 55 all except tr, 74–75, 76–81, 83tr, 88tl, 95bl, 98, 99t, l, and tc, 100bl, 101, 104, 105 all except bl, 101, 104, 105 all except bl 108 all except t and br, 109br, 110–111, 112tl, 114–16, 117t, 2nd row r, 121 all except t and tl, 124bl, 125tr and b, 128–33, 134t, 138–41, 145t, cl, 146t, 149bl and c, 154, 158bl and bc, 159–67, 171–73, 174t and l, 176b, 177tr, cr, and br, 178–96 all except 191tl, 197r, cr, and b, 199tr and br, 200–1, 202br, 203tr and b, 204–5, 206tl, tr, and cr, 207t, 209–15, 217, 218c and 219t and bl, 220cl, cr, and b, 221 tl, tr, and bl, 222tl and cr, 223tl, cr and b, 224c and r, 226t, 229, 246b, 247b, 248–49;

Ray Moller: 6: 2nd column upper cr, 100, 106cl, cr, bl, and br, 107, 136t, cr, and br, 137 all except br, 142bl and br, 143, 146bl, 175c;

Stephen Oliver: 4: 1st column pictures 1 and 5; 10, 15, 54l and b, 55tr, 56bl, 99bc and br, 103, 105bl, 108t and bl, 109l and tr, 120bl and br, 121t and tl, 125tl, 134 all except t, 135, 146br, 148, 149tl, box tr, cl and cr, 153, 155, 156bl and br;

Susanna Price: 1, 2–3 main picture, 6: 2nd column upper cl and b, 7: 2nd column bl, 68–69, 82, 83tl and c, 84, 86–87, bl, and br, 89, 90tl and c, 91tr and bl, 92tl and tr, 93, 112tr, c, and br, 117 2nd row l, 3rd row l and r, 4th row l, c, and r, 120t, 123, 124 all except bl, 125c, 127, 136bl and bc, 137br, 142tl, 144, bc, and br, 150–52, 158t and br, 168, 246t, 247t;

Steve Gorton: 142tr, 145cr, 169;

Steve Shott: 2: 2nd column picture 5; 157–9.

Picture credits
The publishers would like to thank the following for their kind permission to reproduce photographs:
(numbers indicate pages; t=top, b=below, c=center, l=left, r=right)
Sue Ford, Western Ophthalmic Hospital: 175tr, 177bl, 202r; Genesis Film Productions Ltd/Neil Bromhall: Lesley Howling: 43b; 23; Mother and Baby Picture Library/Emap Elan: 16, 18, 20, 22, 24, 26, 28, 30, 31 (posed by model); National Medical Slide Bank: 175br, 198l, 202tl, 206bl, 218l, 219cl, 224l; St. John's Institute of Dermatology: 220tl, 223tr; St. Mary's Hospital: 177tl, 199tl, 199bl; Science Photo Library/Hank Morgan: 70; Ron Sutherland: 67c; Dr. I. Williams: 174br, 175cr, 176t and cr, 197r, 203l, 207b, 219bl, 221br, 222t, bc, and b; ZEFA: 63.

Loan or supply of props
Baby B's, Fulham, London, England; Diana Dolls Fashions Inc., Stoney Creek, Ontario; The Nursery Collection, Watford, England; Porter Nash Medical, London, England; Seward Ltd., London, England;
Special thanks to: Mary Snyder at Snugli, Inc.; Gerry Baby Products Company, Denver, Colorado; Judi's Originals, Scottsdale, Arizona.

Illustrator
Coral Mula: all line artwork except pp. 226–28, 14t; Jim Robins: 226–28; Roy Flooks (colouring) 227, 230–31, 232–33, 234; Nick Hall: 14t.

Consultants
Dorling Kindersley acknowledges the contribution of the following consultants to the original edition.
Professor R. W. Taylor, MD, FRCOG, Head of Departmant of Gynecology, The United Medical Schools of Guy's and St Thomas's Hospitals, London; Professor Jon Scopes, MB, PhD, FRCP, Department of Pediatrics, St Thomas's Hospital, London; Christine Williams, RGN, HV, FWT, Health Visitor and Family Planning Nurse; Janice Leighton, RGN, RM, Community Midwife; Alan McLaughlin, RGN, Department of Clinical Neurology, St Thomas's Hospital, London.